INBORN ERRORS OF SKIN, HAIR AND CONNECTIVE TISSUE

*Previous Symposia of the Society for the
Study of Inborn Errors of Metabolism.
Published by E. and S. Livingstone.*

1. *Neurometabolic Disorders in Childhood. Ed. K. S. Holt and
    J. Milner 1963*
2. *Biochemical Approaches to Mental Handicap in Children. Ed. J. D.
    Allan and K. S. Holt 1964*
3. *Basic Concepts of Inborn Errors and Defects of Steroid Biosynthesis.
    Ed. K. S. Holt and D. N. Raine 1965*
4. *Some Recent Advances in Inborn Errors of Metabolism. Ed. K. S.
    Holt and V. P. Coffey 1966*
5. *Some Inherited Disorders of Brain and Muscle. Ed. J. D. Allan and
    D. N. Raine 1969*
6. *Enzymopenic Anaemias, Lysosomes and other papers. Ed. J. D.
    Allan, K. S. Holt, J. T. Ireland and R. J. Pollitt 1969*
7. *Errors of Phenylalanine Thyroxine and Testosterone Metabolism.
    Ed. W. Hamilton and F. P. Hudson 1970*
8. *Inherited Disorders of Sulphur Metabolism. Ed. N. A. J. Carson and
    D. N. Raine 1971*
9. *Organic Acidurias. Ed. J. Stern and C. Toothill 1972*
10. *Treatment of Inborn Errors of Metabolism. Ed. J. W. T. Seakins,
    R. A. Saunders and C. Toothill 1973*

*The Society exists to promote exchanges of ideas between workers in different
disciplines who are interested in any aspect of inborn metabolic disorders.
Particulars of the Society can be obtained from the Editors of this Symposium.*

INBORN ERRORS OF SKIN, HAIR AND CONNECTIVE TISSUE

MONOGRAPH BASED UPON
*Proceedings of the Eleventh Symposium of
The Society for the Study of Inborn Errors of Metabolism*

EDITED BY
J. B. Holton
and
J. T. Ireland

MTP
Medical & Technical Publishing Co. Ltd.

The editors wish to express the gratitude of all the
members of the Society for the generous grants which
have been received in support of this symposium from
Mr J. Milner of Milner Scientific and Medical Research,
Liverpool.

Published by
MTP, Medical and Technical Publishing Co. Ltd.
PO Box 55, St. Leonards House
St. Leonardgate, Lancaster, Lancs.

ISBN 978-94-011-6617-1   ISBN 978-94-011-6615-7 (eBook)
DOI 10.1007/978-94-011-6615-7

THE GARDEN CITY PRESS LIMITED
LETCHWORTH, HERTFORDSHIRE
SG6 1JS

Preface

Following the pattern of previous years the 11th symposium of the
S.S.I.E.M. held in the beautiful sylvan surroundings of Sussex University, concentrated on a relatively small section of the field of inborn
errors. The subject chosen—Inborn Errors of Skin, Hair and Connective Tissue, was a highly topical one. Intensive research during the
last few years particularly on the structure and disorders of connective
tissue has considerably advanced our knowledge on this subject. We
believe that the range of diseases covered, and the depth in which they
were discussed, made this meeting unique. The proceedings contain
much original material and reference information which should make
them an invaluable addition to the literature on metabolic disorders.

The work involved is multi-disciplinary involving among others
physicists, organic chemists, biochemists, clinical chemists, paediatricians, physicians, geneticists and neurologists. The bringing together
of workers of many disciplines to contribute to the particular subject
under discussion at our Symposia has always been an important
objective of the Society. In this case we were very fortunate in gathering
together experts from all the fields mentioned above. In particular we
were honoured that Professor A. Dorfman of Chicago could accept our
invitation to give the second Milner Lecture. We were also privileged to
have some excellent contributions from the research scientists on whom
we must rely for our ultimate understanding of the diseases, and
rational approach to treatment.

On the medical side, although almost all of the many disorders
described by our medical contributors to this volume are rare, collect-
ively they account for quite a significant proportion of the severe
physical and neurological defects and mental retardation seen by the
paediatricians. Unfortunately, they are almost all untreatable at present
and there was considerable emphasis in the discussions at the Symposium on the possibilities and problems of prenatal diagnosis, which
offer the chance of therapeutic abortion of affected foetuses.

The application of newer techniques such as column chromatography, T.L.C., electrophoresis, cell culture and improved enzymological methods has considerably eased the laboratory problem of diagnosis and classification of these patients. In the last section a number of workers compare their different approaches to this problem.

We are much indebted to all the participants in the Symposium who have made the publication of the proceedings possible, and to Dr. Linda Tyfield, Miss Iris Lynn and the publishers who have given so much help with its preparation.

J. B. Holton

J. T. Ireland

Active Participants in Symposia

PROFESSOR ALBERT DORFMAN

Milner Lecturer, Department of Paediatrics, University of Chicago, Chicago, U.S.A. 60637.

E. D. T. ATKINS

H. H. Wills Physics Laboratory, University of Bristol, Bristol.

A. J. BAILEY

Agricultural Research Council, Meat Research Institute, Bristol.

J. A. CIFONELLI

University of Chicago, Chicago, U.S.A. 60637.

GLYN DAWSON

Joseph P. Kennedy, Jr. Scholar, University of Chicago, Chicago, U.S.A. 60637.

M. F. DEAN

Kennedy Institute of Rheumatology, Hammersmith, London.

LARS ÅKE FRANSSON

Department of Physiological Chemistry (2), University of Lund, Lund, Sweden.

DOROTHY A. GIBBS

M.R.C. Unit, Northwich Park, Middlesex.

N. S. GORDON

Booth Hall Children's Hospital, Manchester.

M. E. GRANT

Department of Medical Biochemistry, University of Manchester, Manchester.

D. A. HALL

Department of Medicine, Leeds University, Leeds.

J. B. HOLTON

Biochemistry Laboratory, Southmead Hospital, Bristol.

J. T. IRELAND

Biochemistry Laboratory, Alder Hey Children's Hospital, Liverpool.

J. F. KENNEDY
The Chemical Department, University of Birmingham, Birmingham.

STANFORD T. LAMBERG
University of Chicago, Chicago, U.S.A. 60637.

P. W. LEWIS
Biochemistry Laboratory, Birmingham Children's Hospital, Birmingham 16.

R. O. MCKERAN
M.R.C. Unit, Northwich Park, Middlesex.

REUBEN MATALON
Joseph P. Kennedy, Jr. Scholar, University of Chicago, Chicago, U.S.A. 60637.

HELEN MUIR
Kennedy Institute of Rheumatology, Hammersmith. London.

P. C. H. NEWBOLD
Department of Medicine, Cambridge University, Medical School, Cambridge.

CHARLES A. PENNOCK
Research Floor, Bristol Royal Infirmary, Bristol.

R. J. POLLITT
M.R.C. Unit for Metabolic Studies in Psychiatry, Middlewood Hospital, Sheffield.

N. R. RAINE
Biochemistry Laboratory, Birmingham Children's Hospital, Birmingham 16.

J. SABATER
Instituto Provincial de Bioquimica Clinica, Barcelona, Spain.

INGRID SJÖBERG
Department of Physiological Chemistry (2), University of Lund, Lund, Sweden.

JURGEN SPRANGER
Universitat Kinderklinik, Keil, Germany.

ALLEN C. STOOLMILLER
University of Chicago, Chicago, U.S.A. 60637.

WALTER M. TELLER
Department fur Kinderheilkunde, Ulm, Germany.

JERRY N. THOMPSON
University of Chicago, Chicago, U.S.A. 60637.

R. W. E. WATTS

M.R.C. Unit, Northwich Park, Middlesex.

PAUL WHITEMAN

Hospital for Sick Children, Great Ormond Street, London.

ULRICH WIESMANN

Department of Paediatrics, University of Berne, Switzerland.

Contents

LABORATORY ASPECTS OF THE MUCOPOLYSACCHARIDES
Including diagnosis and screening

INBORN ERRORS
AND SKIN

Inborn errors of skin

P. C. H. Newbold

In three-day old rats, of average total weight 10 g each, the skin and dermis together weigh 950 mg, whereas the liver is 460 mg, the kidneys together are 100 mg, and the spleen is only 30 mg. Throughout life the skin is the largest metabolic organ of the body, although it is not possible to provide comparable data for man. The structure of the skin is shown in diagram form in Fig. 1. Fat comprises the bulk of the deepest layer of the cutis, and the dermis consists of blood vessels, nerves and accessory structures such as sweat glands, in a matrix of connective tissue. The shaded portion is the epidermis, synthesizing protein until

TABLE I   *Loss of keratinized material per m² per year in a 28-year-old-man*

Scalp hair	11·4
Facial hair	9·8
Body hair	8·3
Finger ⎤ Toe ⎦ nails	2·02
Desquamating epidermis	116·14
Total	147·66 g

it is shed as dead squames. Table I indicates that salvage is extremely efficient, as only a small loss of protein occurs in normal circumstances. It is not altogether surprising therefore that the skin is usually a mirror of metabolic disease, rather than a primary organ of involvement (Newbold, 1973). Lipid, connective tissue, and amino-acid disorders will be discussed separately.

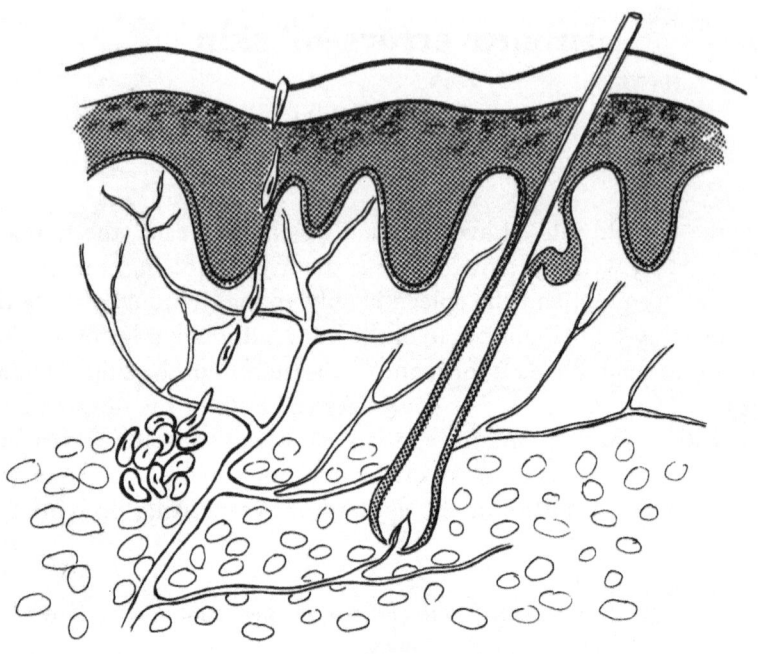

FIG. 1   Diagram of the skin as a metabolic organ.

Lipids

Xanthelasma was described in 1835, and there has been sustained clinical interest in xanthomata since that date. Recent advances in technique and chemistry have added a rational chemical background to this interesting field (Fredrickson and Levy, 1972). The lesions and the types of hyperlipoproteinaemias are summarized in Table II. Type 1 is due to decreased tissue lipoprotein lipase, the homozygote is involved, but the phenotype is probably produced by more than one mutation. Type 2 shows hyper-beta lipoproteinaemia and homozygous and heterozygous forms are known, although the fundamental biochemical defect has not yet been defined. Premature vascular disease and polyarthritis are important, and arcus senilis is usually present. Type 3 is broad beta disease, accompanied by decreased glucose tolerance, premature vascular disease and hyperuricaemia. It is uncommon, and neither its chemistry nor its pattern of inheritance has been clari-

TABLE II *Xanthomata and hyperlipoproteinaemias*

TYPE 1	Eruptive, any site.
TYPE 2	Xanthelasma, others according to severity and duration, in 80 per cent.
	Tendinous in 50 per cent.
	Subperiosteal lesions occasionally.
TYPE 3	Planar lesions on palms.
	Tendinous in 20 per cent. Tubero-eruptive and subperiosteal lesions common.
TYPE 4	Eruptive lesions in 15 per cent.
TYPE 5	Eruptive, and tubero-eruptive in 45 per cent.
TENDINOUS	Mainly in 2, in 3 to lesser extent.
TUBEROUS	Mainly in 3, less in 2, rare in 1, 4 and 5.
PLANAR	Mainly in 2, palmar only in 3.
ERUPTIVE	Mainly in 1, 4 and 5, less often in 3.

fied. Type 4 is also linked with decreased glucose tolerance, and vascular disease, although the patients are thin and often show hyper-insulinaemia. Type 5 features both diabetes and hyperuricaemia, but no apparent excess of vascular disease. Xanthomata are important cutaneous markers of metabolic disease (Parker and Short, 1970), and because serious vascular hazards may be present, diagnosis should not be delayed as treatments are available (Lees and Wilson, 1971). Eruptive xanthomata disappear speedily when the plasma lipids are controlled, tuberous and tendinous lesions go more slowly, and xanthelasma rarely if ever clears with treatment (Palmer and Blacket, 1972; Dean, 1973).

Tangier disease is of recessive inheritance, and there is deficiency of normal α-lipoproteins in plasma, while a small amount of abnormal high density lipoprotein is present. Cholesterol esters are widely deposited throughout the body, producing amongst other lesions the well-known orange tonsils. They are also deposited in the skin, both in papules and in areas which look normal (Waldorf, Levy and Fredrickson, 1967).

Lipoid proteinosis is a rare recessive disorder, most frequently seen in South Africa (Scott and Findlay, 1960). The child is unable to cry, and later has a hoarse whisper. Crops of sores and ulcers involve the mouth, and infiltration of the mucous membranes of tongue, larynx, and vocal cords follows. The tongue and lips are thickened, and scars and irregular plaques are present. Recurrent infections are important, as are bullae and pustules which predispose to scars (Grosfeld, Spaas, van de Staak and Stadhouders, 1965). Light sensitivity occurs in some patients (Calnan and Shuster, 1962), and histology indicates a hyaline deposit similar to that found in porphyria cutanea tarda and erythropoietic protoporphyria. Skin lesions mainly involve the face, neck, shoulders, and the backs of the hands and fingers. Treatment consists mainly of speedy attention to infections, but the long term prognosis is good. The chemical nature of the deposit is uncertain, and reports range from normal lipids only (Heyl and DeKock, 1964), to galactolipids (Wood, Urbach and Beerman, 1956) and mucopolysaccharides (Moynahan, 1966). It seems likely that there is considerable variety in the deposits, even before they are modified by infection.

Fabry's disease is an X-linked recessive with lack of α-galactosyl hydrolase, so that trihexosyl ceramide accumulates. This can involve

TABLE III   *Tissues with increased neutral glycosphingolipids in Fabry's disease*

NERVOUS SYSTEM	Autonomic ganglia
	Brachial plexus
	Brain
	Brain stem
	Thalamus
ORGANS	Heart
	Kidney
	Liver
	Lungs
	Intestines
	Tonsils
VESSELS	Aorta
	Renal artery
TISSUES	Smooth muscle
	Striated muscle
	Subcutaneous fat

most parts of the body, as indicated in Table III. The patients may present with severe pains in fingers and toes, accompanied by fever, or they may have vascular lesions and renal failure (Wallace, 1973). The skin lesions (angiokeratomata) are small, dark-red, flat telangiectases, which do not fade on pressure. These are most common around the mucosae of mouth, eyes and genitals, as well as the lips, back and buttocks. It is also clear that Fabry's disease can occur without skin lesions (Clarke, Knaack, Crawhall and Wolfe, 1971), although skin involvement is one of the commonest presentations. Deposits of the ceramides can also be found in eyelids and cornea, as well as the vasculature of the brain, kidneys and heart (Wallace, 1973). There is now optimism for treatment by infusions of purified enzyme (Brady *et al.*, 1973), whereas previous reports, even of renal transplantation, had not been successful.

Refsum's disease (see Fig. 2) is another syndrome due to deposits of abnormal metabolites, in this case of phytanic acid. It shows autosomal recessive inheritance, and constant features are retinitis pigmentosa, peripheral neuropathy, cerebellar ataxia, and raised CSF protein with normal cells. The cutaneous lesion is a minor and irregular component of the syndrome. It consists of variable ichthyosis, ranging from minor involvement of the extremities to widespread and atypical lesions (Fryer, Wincklemann, Ways and Swanson, 1971). Skin lesions improve when dietary restrictions are imposed on dairy products and chlorophyll, to reduce the intake of phytanic acid.

Connective tissue

Marfan's syndrome is an autosomal dominant condition, without a defined biochemical defect. Pectus excavatum, long thin limbs, and flat feet produce the typical appearance of the patients. There is ectopia lentis, with dislocation of the lens being upward and congenital (McKusick, 1972), and there are frequently secondary eye changes such as glaucoma. Cutaneous features are a minor component, but striae distensae have been reported over the thighs, chest and shoulders (McKusick, 1972). Elastosis perforans serpiginosa of Miescher has also been seen, but this occurs with cutis laxa, the Ehlers–Danlos syndrome, osteogenesis imperfecta, and Down's syndrome—amongst other associations (Meara, 1958; Smith, Malak, Goodman and McKusick, 1962; Korting, 1966). It is therefore not diagnostic of any single entity but

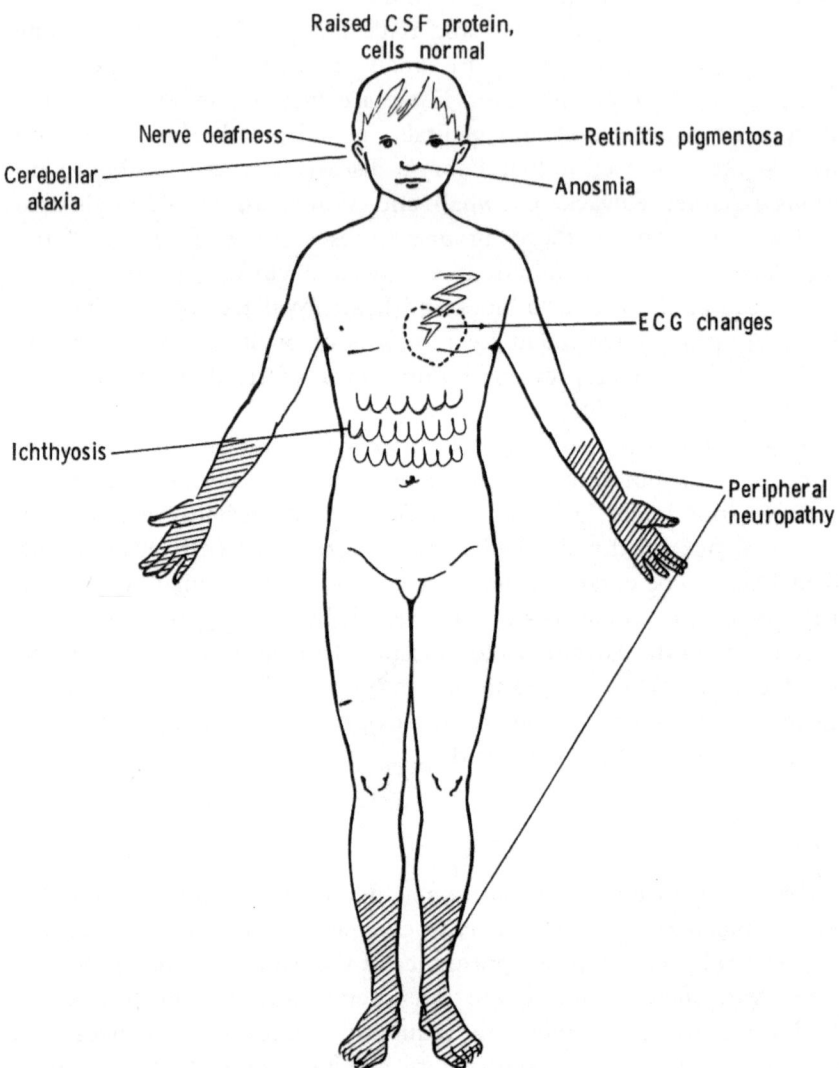

FIG. 2   Refsum's syndrome.

only of a dermal-epidermal interaction. There is decreased cross-linkage of collagen in these patients but the cause is not known (Grant and Prockop, 1972). Similar changes are seen with lathyrism, after β-aminopropiononitrile, as well as with penicillamine therapy for scleroderma (Harris and Sjoerdsma, 1966).

The Ehlers–Danlos syndrome consists of an overlapping group of disorders (McKusick, 1972). Hyperextensible joints and generalized fragility of tissues are the most important features, but hiatus hernia, diverticulosis, and intestinal perforation also occur. Fragile skin with easy bruising, and tissue-paper scars are seen, but these are of minor import besides the vascular lesions which can be fatal (Beighton, 1968; Imahori, Bannerman, Graf and Brennan, 1969). Generalized disturbance is also seen in cutis laxa, where aortic involvement can be fatal (Goltz, Hult, Goldfarb and Gorlin, 1965). The clinical syndrom; is shown in Fig. 3, and inheritance is probably an autosomal dominant with incomplete penetrance. The aetiology may be excess elastase activity producing damage to the elastic fibres (Goltz *et al.*, 1965), and there seems to be a link also with low copper levels, as copper regulates the elastase activity (Chadfield and North, 1971).

Pseudoxanthoma elasticum is an interesting and well-studied autosomal recessive disorder (McKusick, 1971). Angioid streaks are seen in the fundus, but they are also seen with Paget's disease of the bone, and with familial hyperphosphataemia. Yellowish pebbly, xanthoma-like thickenings of the skin are especially common in the creases of the face and neck, the axillary folds, and in the umbilical and inguinal regions. The elastic fibres are fragmented, and show calcification in the deeper layers of the corium, while reactive perforating elastosis is sometimes seen (Smith *et al.*, 1962). The appearances are clusters or rings of papules with a central horny plug, on the neck, cheeks or limbs. In addition there are widespread mucosal lesions from lips to bowel, bladder, and genitals. Renal hypertension from renal artery involvement can occur, and calcification of peripheral arteries can lead to reduced pulses. The clinical picture is so bizarre, accompanied by unlikely and repeated haemorrhages, that hysteria and malingering can be suspected.

Pigmentary System

The pigmentary system is an important functional component of the skin. All aspects of melanosome formation and melanocyte function are

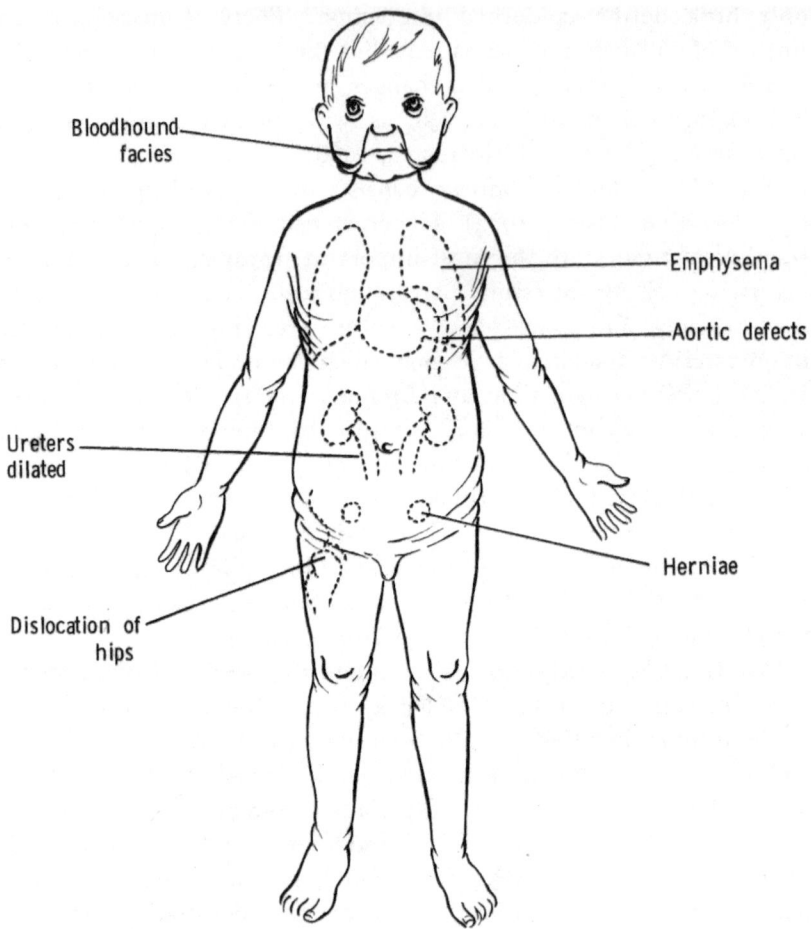

Bloodhound facies

Emphysema

Aortic defects

Ureters dilated

Herniae

Dislocation of hips

FIG. 3   Cutis laxa.

likely to be under genetic control, although details have not yet been worked out (Quevedo, 1973). With the recessive oculo-cutaneous albinism, both tyrosinase-negative and tyrosinase-positive forms occur (Fitzpatrick, Quevedo, Szabo and Seiji, 1971). The major clinical interest is the severe photosensitivity of albinos, and their associated risk of basal and squamous cell epitheliomata, and malignant melanomata. Increased risk of skin cancer is also the major consequence of xeroderma pigmentosum, an autosomal recessive disorder with a reduced capacity for excision repair of ultraviolet damage to DNA (Cleaver, 1973). The recessive alcaptonuria produces more widespread pathology, due to accumulation of homogentisic acid. Virchow described the grey-blue skin pigmentation in 1866, and the sclera and conjunctiva of the eyes are usually the first parts of the body to be pigmented. Pigment is also seen over tendons, and in cartilages, while a typical pattern of arthritis can develop in chronic cases (Pomeranz, Friedman and Tunick, 1941). Studies of the pigment systems and of photobiology are likely to explain many aspects of pre-cancer and neoplastic transformation, besides the light sensitivity of the porphyrias.

Amino-acids

Phenylketonuria is one of the best-known of all genetic disorders. The mental damage can be included within brackets in Fig. 4 as it is preventable. There is reduction in the colour of skin, hair and eyes, with a consequent risk of sunburn (Braun-Falco and Geissler, 1964). In addition, dermatitis is found in about half of the patients. This may be true atopic eczema (Fleisher and Zeligman, 1960), seborrhoeic dermatitis, or autosensitization eruptions (Efron and Gallagher, 1971), or else too ill-defined and irregular to classify. These skin changes are due to the toxic effects of phenylalanine and its decomposition products in the skin, and they respond to dietary restriction of phenylalanine.

Hartnup disease also features a rash which involves the exposed areas of the body, and which is worse in summer. The skin lesions are pellagra-like because they are due to nicotinamide deficiency consequent upon the abnormal tryptophan metabolism. However, the cerebellar ataxia, mental changes and specific amino-aciduria are more dramatic components of the syndrome (Baron, Dent, Harris, Hart and Jepson, 1956). It is possible that the skin lesions which have been observed in tyrosinosis may be explicable by such a vitamin deficiency (Zaleski, Hill and Kushniruk, 1973).

Homocystinuria is one of the most fascinating metabolic disorders known. Lack of cystathionine synthetase leads to the accumulation of homocystine, which is partially offset by the re-methylation of homocysteine, to methionine (Carey, Fennelly and Fitzgerald, 1968). Hence there is increased demand for folate co-enzymes and folate depletion may result in these patients. There is some suggestive evidence linking this deficiency with low I.Q. in some patients (Carey *et al.*, 1968; Butterworth, Krumdieck and Baugh, 1971). However, the increased thrombotic tendency, and the organic brain syndrome which can result

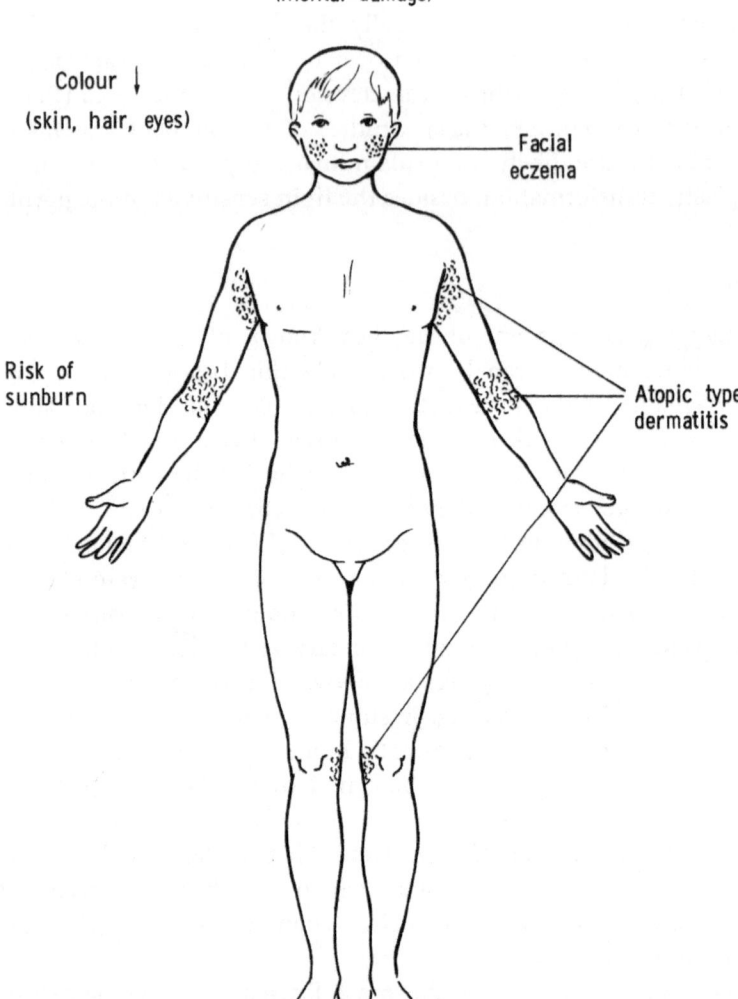

FIG. 4   Phenylketonuria.

(Dunn, Perry and Dolman, 1966) are also possible causes of mental damage. Vascular changes also produce the malar flush and the livedo reticularis of trunk and limbs, which are the major cutaneous signs. In addition, reduction in colour of skin, hair and eyes, unusually fragile hair, and telangiectases around scars have been reported (Price, Vickers and Brooker, 1968). The disease is extremely variable, which makes it extremely difficult to compare results from different centres or countries.

We are unlikely to be missing many cases of inborn errors of amino-acid metabolism, so it is safe to conclude that skin involvement is relatively trivial in these diseases. On the other hand, as the cause of most of the common skin disorders is not known, future studies may add psoriasis, lichen planus, and even acne vulgaris, to the list of inborn errors of skin. This is in addition to the benefit from genetic studies of the skin and its disorders, which have a very promising future (McKusick, 1973).

Acknowledgements

I thank Mrs Moira Sheldon of Addenbrooke's Hospital for her able help with the illustrations. I also acknowledge financial support from the Elmore Fund of the University of Cambridge, and from the Medical Research Council.

REFERENCES

BARON, D. N., DENT, C. E., HARRIS, H., HART, E. W. & JEPSON, J. B. (1956) *Lancet*, ii, 421.
BEIGHTON, P. (1968) *British Medical Journal*, 3, 656.
BRADY, R. O., TALLMAN, J. F., JOHNSON, W. G., GAL, A. E., LEAHY, W. R., QUIRK, J. M. & DEKABAN, A. S. (1973) *New England Journal of Medicine*, 289, 9.
BRAUN-FALCO, O. & GEISSLER, H. (1964) *Medizinische Welt*. 2, 1941.
BUTTERWORTH, C. E., KRUMDIECK, C. L. & BAUGH, C. M. (1971) *Alabama Journal of Medical Sciences*, 8, 30.
CALNAN, C. D. & SHUSTER, S. (1962) *Proceedings of the Royal Society of Medicine*, 55, 957.
CAREY, M. C., FENNELLY, J. J. & FITZGERALD, O. (1968) *American Journal of Medicine*, 45, 26.
CHADFIELD, H. W. & NORTH, J. F. (1971) *Transactions of St John's Hospital Dermatological Society*, 57, 181.
CLARKE, J. T. R., KNAACK, J., CRAWHALL, J. C. & WOLFE, L. S. (1971) *New England Journal of Medicine*, 284, 233.
CLEAVER, J. E. (1973) *Journal of Investigative Dermatology*, 60, 374.
DEAN, F. D. (1973) *British Journal of Dermatology*, 88, 191.
DUNN, H. G., PERRY, T. L. & DOLMAN, C. L. (1966) *Neurology*, 16, 407.
EFRON, M. L. & GALLAGHER, W. F. (1971) In *Dermatology in General Medicine*. Ed. T. B. Fitzpatrick *et al.* New York: McGraw-Hill.
FITZPATRICK, T. B., QUEVEDO, W. C. Jr., SZABO, G. & SEIJI, M. (1971) In *Dermatology in General Medicine*, Ed. T. B. Fitzpatrick *et al.* New York: McGraw-Hill.
FLEISHER, T. L. & ZELIGMAN, I. (1960) *Archives of Dermatology*, 81, 898.
FREDRICKSON, D. S. & LEVY, R. I. (1972) In *The Metabolic Basis of Inherited Disease*, 3rd Edition. Eds. J. B. Stanbury, J. B. Wyngaarden & D. S. Fredrickson. New York: McGraw-Hill.

FRYER, D. G., WINCKLEMANN, A. C., WAYS, P. O. & SWANSON, A. G. (1971) *Neurology*, **21**, 162.

GOLTZ, R. W., HULT, A. M., GOLDFARB, M. & GORLIN, R. J. (1965) *Archives of Dermatology*, **92**, 373.

GRANT, M. E. & PROCKOP, D. J. (1972) *New England Journal of Medicine*, **286**, 291.

GROSFELD, J. C. M., SPAAS, J., VAN DE STAAK, W. J. B. M. & STADHOUDERS, A. M. (1965) *Dermatologica*, **130**, 239.

HARRIS, E. D. & SJOERDSMA, A. (1966) *Lancet*, **ii**, 996.

HEYL, T. & DEKOCK, D. (1964) *Journal of Investigative Dermatology*, **42**, 333.

IMAHORI, S., BANNERMAN, R. M., GRAF, C. J. & BRENNAN, J. C. (1969) *American Journal of Medicine*, **47**, 967.

KORTING, G. W. (1966) *Archives fur klinische und Experimentelle Dermatologie*, **224**, 437.

LEES, R. S. & WILSON, D. E. (1971) *New England Journal of Medicine*, **284**, 186.

MCKUSICK, V. A. (1971) In *Dermatology in Central Medicine*. Ed. T. B. Fitzpatrick *et al.* New York: McGraw-Hill.

MCKUSICK, V. A. (1972) In *Heritable Disorders of Connective Tissue*, 4th edition. St. Louis: C. V. Mosby.

MCKUSICK, V. A. (1973) *Journal of Investigative Dermatology*, **60**, 343.

MEARA, R. A. (1958) *Transactions of St. John's Hospital, Dermatological Society*, **40**, 72.

MOYNAHAN, E. J. (1966) *Proceedings of the Royal Society of Medicine*, **59**, 1125.

NEWBOLD, P. C. H. (1973) *Journal of Medical Genetics*, **10**, 101.

PALMER, J. & BLACKET, R. (1972) *Lancet*, **i**, 66.

PARKER, F. & SHORT, J. M. (1970) *Journal of Investigative Dermatology*, **55**, 71.

POMERANZ, M. M., FRIEDMAN, L. J. & TUNICK, I. S. (1941) *Radiology*, **37**, 295.

PRICE, J., VICKERS, C. F. H. & BROOKER, B. K. (1968) *Journal of Mental Deficiency Research*, **12**, 111.

QUEVEDO, W. C. Jr. (1973) *Journal of Investigative Dermatology*, **60**, 407.

SCOTT, F. P. & FINDLAY, G. H. (1960) *South African Medical Journal*, **34**, 189.

SMITH, E. W., MALAK, J. A., GOODMAN, R. M. & MCKUSICK, V. A. (1962) *Bulletin of the John Hopkins Hospital*, **111**, 235.

WALDORF, D. S., LEVY, R. I. & FREDRICKSON, D. S. (1967) *Archives of Dermatology*, **95**, 161.

WALLACE, H. J. (1973) *British Journal of Dermatology*, **88**, 1.

WOOD, M. G., URBACH, F. & BEERMAN, H. (1956) *Journal of Investigative Dermatology*, **26**, 263.

ZALESKI, W. A., HILL, A. & KUSHNIRUK, W. (1973) *British Journal of Dermatology*, **88**, 335.

DISCUSSION
(of paper by Dr Newbold)

Bickel (Heidelberg). How many cases of the rather ill defined tyrosinosis have shown skin changes? If only one, is it permitted to generalize from this one case to call it a symptom of the disease?

Newbold. I have had only one case and two others have been reported. I think that by pointing this out we might find enough cases to say if it is a symptom or not, at the present I really don't know.

Komrower (Manchester). I am doubtful if we are missing any cases of tyrosinosis, we have screened 250,000 babies looking for this condition, and not found it. I am sure there are a number of people with a similar experience to myself, I think it is an extremely rare disorder, in this country. The other thing I would like to say is that we have had a good experience of homocystinuria and have never seen the skin lesions. Perhaps however we have never looked but I must ask my colleagues if we are missing these skin lesions.

Blaskovics (Los Angeles). With regard to ectodermal abnormalities and tyrosine metabolism, Dr Neil Buist of Portland, Oregon, recently reported in the *Lancet* that lens opacities could be associated with high serum tyrosine levels. I have read references in Monroe's *Protein Metabolism* that similar eye lesions were induced in rats when they were fed high tyrosine containing diets.

Sinclair (London). Some interesting and encouraging reports have appeared recently about the use of renal transplantation in the treatment of Fabry's disease where it has been claimed that plasma levels of the so-called Fabry enzyme increased, but not to normal levels, and there is marked improvement in the symptomatology, especially the relief of pain and the non-occurrence of fevers.

Dorfman (Chicago). In respect to the reports of therapy of Fabry's disease, I believe there is some difference of opinion in the literature.

Dr Hall (Leeds). I would like to comment on cutis laxa. A few years ago we had a case in which we observed no changes in elastase inhibitor levels, elastase levels or plasma copper concentrations: thus showing differences from the classical situation mentioned by Dr Newbold. However this could have been due to the fact that the case was one of late onset—39 years of age.

From one point of view the most important fact in this case was the way in which the lesions developed progressively from neck to abdomen.

An examination of skin from these two extremes at death six years after onset showed marked differences in apparent age of the dermis from these two sites. The patient demonstrated an age gradient in his own body, and it was possible to carry out longitudinal ageing studies on one subject using the tissues from the abdomen as controls for the apparently 'older' neck tissues.

INBORN ERRORS
AND HAIR

2

Inherited conditions affecting the proteins of hair

R. J. Pollitt

Hair in classical inborn errors of metabolism

Hair abnormalities attracted attention quite early in the study of inborn errors of metabolism. The frequent occurrence of blonde hair in phenylketonuria is an obvious feature, and abnormal hair has been reported in argininosuccinic aciduria, citrullinaemia, argininaemia, homocystinuria, tyrosinaemia, Hartnup disease, and others. Before the mechanism of protein synthesis was clearly understood, it was considered possible that excess of an amino acid in tissue fluids could result in the synthesis of abnormal proteins with excess of that particular amino acid, and various proteins from phenylketonurics were analysed with this in mind (Block, Jervis, Bolling and Webb, 1940). It is now obvious that with a few exceptions (such as the substitution of unnatural fluoro analogues for the correct amino acid) the composition of proteins cannot be changed in this way. Hair is a peculiar tissue, however, and interest in its composition in inborn errors of metabolism has continued. This is partly because of direct clinical observation of hair texture and colour changes during treatment in a number of these conditions, and perhaps also because of possible analagies with the selective accumulation of some trace metals.

Hair is a complex mixture of proteins which, as will be discussed later, can be present in variable proportions. Small changes in overall amino acid composition with nutritional status of the individual, site of sampling, and with the degree of weathering or exposure of the hair to harmful chemicals have been reported. Difficulties in obtaining complete hydrolysis without considerable losses of certain amino acids also add to uncertainty in analysis, so that the range of 'normal' results is quite large and there is a degree of conflict within the literature. The most comprehensive series has been published by Van Sande (1970) who collected hair specimens from various sources but performed the analyses in his own laboratory with an adequate number of controls. Even here the age of the hair (the time it had been on the scalp) could not be controlled. A number of slight changes in amino acid composition were found, particularly in the hair of phenylketonurics and homocystinurics, but these were too small to be of diagnostic use and their significance is unclear. However, the status of the hair in argininosuccinic aciduria and homocystinuria has attracted special attention.

Roughly half the patients with argininosuccinic aciduria have fragile hair associated with trichorrhexis nodosa, the hair breaking off leaving brush-like ends. This apparently straightforward observation has provided the basis for considerable confusion. The excretion of argininosuccinic acid in the urine of two children with monilethrix was reported (Grosfeld, Mighorst and Moolhuysen, 1964) and the summary of this paper contained the statement that 'like trichorrhexis nodosa, monilethrix seems to be an inborn error of metabolism'. A short time later, five patients with 'aminogenic alopecia' associated with argininosuccinic aciduria were described by Shelley and Rawnsley (1965). The 'argininosuccinic acid' in the monilethrix patients was shown to be largely glutamic acid (Efron and Hoefnagel, 1966), and the status of the aminogenic alopecia cases remains obscure, but considerable effort has been expended in showing that trichorrhexis nodosa is more usually associated with chemical or physical insults to the hair shaft than with an inborn error of metabolism (Chernosky and Owens, 1966; Rauschkolb, Chernosky, Knox and Owens, 1967). The wheel has now come full circle in that Papa, Mills and Hanshaw (1972) have suggested that the incidence of trichorrhexis nodosa in argininosuccinic aciduria and other conditions associated with mental subnormality may be simply due to the fact that 'such affected children are particularly exposed to physical factors which might precipitate the trichorrhexis nodosa. The repetitive head rolling, rubbing, picking and banging which may be seen in mentally retarded infants would suffice.' This extreme view is unlikely to command support and it must be recognized that, while trichorrhexis nodosa is a widespread, almost universal, phenomenon certain patients show hair fragility associated with trichorrhexis nodosa or similar defects to a quite disproportionate degree. The cause of this in argininosuccinic aciduria is obscure, though arginine deficiency has often been suggested, and arginine supplementation coincided with improvement in one case (Hockey, 1972). Argininosuccinic acid was absent from the hair of the two cases examined by Van Sande (1970), one described by Levin (1967) and one of Lewis and Miller (1970).

In homocystinuria the hair is often fine and sparse but with essentially normal composition. The recent demonstration of traces of combined homocysteine in hair from two children with this condition (Woodhouse and Rajkotwala, 1973) is unexpected and of considerable theoretical interest, though it cannot at present be explained satisfactorily.

Cystine-deficient hair in mentally retarded sibs

Though the chemical examination of hair in the classical inborn errors of metabolism has so far proved disappointing, there are inherited conditions where the chemistry of the hair is significantly affected. The overall composition of the hair protein is altered grossly in the condition described by Pollitt, Jenner and Davies (1968) in a brother and sister with mental and physical retardation. The hair was short and brittle and showed trichorrhexis nodosa, pili torti and variable diameter, though not so regularly as to be described as monilethrix. The cuticular scale pattern was almost completely absent, the surface of the hair presenting an irregular ropy appearance. Under polarized light the birefringence was irregular. The cystine content of this hair was only half that of normal, and threonine, serine and proline were markedly reduced. This suggested that the hair was deficient in the high-sulphur group of proteins that are thought (by some) to form the matrix between the helical low-sulphur microfibrils. In wool, where this has been studied in great detail, the proportion of high sulphur protein is rather variable, and in particular a high molecular weight protein of very high cystine content is only synthesized in quantity when the diet is specially supplemented by abomasal feeding (Gillespie and Reis, 1966). In man, a protein of comparable molecular weight and cystine content is normally present in hair (Pollitt and Stonier, 1971), but in malnutrition states such as Kwashiorkor the contents of this and a number of other high-sulphur proteins are reduced, suggesting some degree of dietary control of synthesis (Gillespie, 1967).

Detailed examination of the proteins extracted from the hair of the mentally retarded patients showed that the defect extended very widely —not only was the proportion of high-sulphur protein reduced but also the amino acid compositions of the remaining high-sulphur proteins and of the low sulphur proteins were abnormal (Pollitt and Stonier, 1971). The number of distinct proteins that can be extracted from wool is very large indeed. Many of those originally thought to be homogenous show microheterogeneity—that is they can be separated into several proteins that differ from each other in only short sequences of amino acids. Presumably in our patients each of these separate proteins is affected either qualitatively or quantitatively.

The structure of wool protein and its synthesis at the different levels in the follicle are the subjects of very divergent views. It is not surprising then that no completely satisfactory explanation of the defect in our patients' hair is possible at this stage. The most likely theory is that the second stage of keratin synthesis—a process which occurs some way up the follicle and results in increased sulphur content—is in some way defective. The overall composition of our patients' hair would then resemble that of the freshly synthesized hair at the base of the follicle. The third stage in keratinization—the formation of the S-S-bridges between the cysteine residues—has occurred in our patient, however, as the free S-H content of the patients' mature hair is normal. In agreement with this theory, certain structures in the cuticular cells of our patients' hair are more characteristic of the hair root than the mature hair (Robson and Sikorski 1968).

Other conditions with abnormal hair

Two further patients with extremely brittle hair showing almost complete absence of cuticular structure have been discovered (Brown Gerdes and Johnson, 1971). Both the hair samples had an extremely low cystine content and the amino acid analysis of the sample, reported in detail, is very similar to that of our patient (Brown, Belser, Crounse and Wehr, 1970). The breaking points in these hairs were much cleaner than in our patients, however, and the phenomenon is described as trichoschisis; whether this indicates a fundamentally different biochemical condition is uncertain. Only one of the patients was mentally retarded. A tendency to trichoschisis and abnormal birefringence patterns is also seen in the Marinesco–Sjögren syndrome (Porter, 1971), but no detailed study of this has been made. Possibly a number of other syndromes of this type may show abnormal hair protein, but there are formidable methodological difficulties in establishing strict chemical homology between these hair defects.

A sex-linked condition of retarded growth, progressive neuro-degeneration and early death associated with short sparse hair of wiry texture was described by Menkes *et al.* in 1962. Biochemical studies have revealed an abnormality in brain lipid (O'Brien and Sampson, 1966) and defective terminal oxidation in the mitochondria (French, Sherard, Lubel, Brotz and Moore, 1972). The hair showed essentially a normal composition except for an unusually high proportion of cysteine residues still in the unoxidized-SH form (Danks *et al.*, 1972). A high sulphydryl content had previously been noted in 'steely wool' produced by sheep suffering from nutritional copper deficiency (Gillespie, 1964), and it appears that the basic abnormality in kinky hair disease is an inability to absorb copper from the gut. Studies on parenteral copper administration to these patients are proceeding in several centres.

Abnormal sulphur content of the hair has been described in a case of hydrotic ectodermal dysplasia (Brown *et al.*, 1971), but in the hydrotic ectodermal dysplasia first described by Clouston and currently being investigated by Gold and Scriver (1971, 1972) the sulphur content is normal. There was, however, a low cystine yield from this latter hair on hydrolysis, but after oxidation a normal yield of cysteic acid. This was originally interpreted as indicating a high proportion of cysteine, but the -SH content turned out to be only slightly raised. It app ars that this missing cysteine may be involved in thioether links of some sort, possibly with melanin precursors. There are also indications that other aspects of keratin structure may be affected in this condition.

Summary

Studies of hair protein appear to have little to offer in the classical inborn errors of metabolism. In a number of other inherited conditions where hair morphology and composition are affected, a clearer understanding of the hair defect may be helpful, and both ultrastructural and chemical investigations are appropriate. Interpretation of the chemical results is hindered by the extreme complexity of the extractable proteins, by methodological difficulties in their investigation, and by lack of general agreement as to the relationship between the extracted proteins and the intact keratins. Nevertheless, investigation of the hair defects appears one of the most promising approaches to unravelling the large number of trichoneurocutaneous syndromes now known.

REFERENCES

BLOCK, R. J., JERVIS, G. A., BOLLING, D. & WEBB, M. (1940) *Journal of Biological Chemistry*, **134**, 567.

BROWN, A. C., BELSER, R. B., CROUNSE, R. G. & WEHR, R. (1970) *Journal of Investigative Dermatology*, **54**, 496.

BROWN, A. C., GERDES, R. J. & JOHNSON, J. (1971) *Scanning Electron Microscopy*, p. 369. Chicago: I.T.T. Research Institute.

CHERNOSKY, M. E. & OWENS, D. W. (1966) *Archives of Dermatology*, **94**, 577.

DANKS, D. M., STEVENS, B. J., CAMPBELL, R. E., GILLESPIE, J. M., WALKER-SMITH, J., BLOOMFIELD, J. & TURNER, B. (1972) *Lancet*, **i**, 1100.

EFRON, M. L. & HOEFNAGEL, D. (1966) *Lancet*, **i**, 321.

FRENCH, J. H., SHERARD, E. S., LUBEL, H., BROTZ, M. & MOORE, C. L. (1972) *Archives of Neurology*, **26**, 229.

GILLESPIE, J. M. (1964) *Australian Journal of Biological Science*, **17**, 282.

GILLESPIE, J. M. (1967) In *Symposium on Fibrous Proteins (Canberra)*, p. 362. Edited by R. G. Crewther. London: Butterworth.

GILLESPIE, J. M. & REIS, P. J. (1966) *Biochemical Journal*, **98**, 969.

GOLD, R. J. M. & SCRIVER, C. R. (1971) *Birth Defects: Original Article Series*, **VII (8)**, 91.

GOLD, R. J. M. & SCRIVER, C. R. (1972) *American Journal Human Genetics*, **24**, 549.

CROSFELD, J. C. M., MIGHORST, J. A., MOOLHUYSEN, T. M. G. F. (1964) *Lancet*, **ii**, 789.

HOCKEY, A. (1972) Referred to in *Mental Retardation, an Atlas of Diseases Associated with Physical Abnormalities*, p. 7. Edited by L. B. Holmes *et al*. New York: Macmillan and Co.

LEVIN, B. (1967) *American Journal of Diseases of Childhood*, **113**, 162.

LEWIS, P. D. & MILLER, A. L. (1970) *Brain*, **93**, 413.

MENKES, J. H., ALTER, M., STEIGLEDER, G. K., WEAKLEY, D. R. & SUNG, J. H. (1962) *Pediatrics*, **29**, 764.

O'BRIEN, J. S. & SAMPSON, E. L. (1966) *Journal of Neuropathology and Experimental Neurology*, **25**, 523.

PAPA, C. M., MILLS, O. H. & HANSHAW, W. (1972) *Archives of Dermatology*, **106**, 888.

POLLITT, R. J., JENNER, F. A. & DAVIES, M. (1968) *Archives of Diseases of Childhood*, **43**, 211.

POLLITT, R. J. & STONIER, P. D. (1971) *Biochemical Journal*, **122**, 433.

PORTER, P. S. (1971) *Birth Defects: Original Article Series*. **VII (8)**, 69.

RAUSCHKOLB, E. W., CHERNOSKY, M. E., KNOX, J. M. & OWENS, D. W. (1967) *Journal Investigative Dermatology*, **48**, 260.

ROBSON, R. M. & SIKORSKI, J. (1968) *Journal Annali di Dermatologica Clinica e Sperimentale*, **22**, 340.

SHELLEY, W. B. & RAWNSLEY, H. M. (1965) *Lancet*, **ii**, 1327.

VAN SANDE, M. (1970) *Archives of Diseases of Childhood*, **45**, 678.

WOODHOUSE, J. M. & RAJKOTWALA, R. A. (1973) *Biochemical Society Transactions*, **1**, 469.

DISCUSSION
(of paper by Dr Pollitt)

Fowler (Manchester). I would like to comment on the hair of homo-cystinuric patients. Woodhouse and Rajkotwola (Leeds) found cysteine-homocysteine disulphide and homocystine in acid hydrolysates of hair from two patients with homocystinuria. We have examined hair from four patients with homocystinuria using an ion-exchange chromato-graphic system, in which the column effluent is reacted with ninhydrin and iodoplatinate. The presence of cysteine-homocysteine disulphide is confirmed but in smaller amounts than that found by Woodhouse. The amount was between 2 and 3 μmols/g hair compared to 16 and 36 μmol/g hair found by Woodhouse. However an additional compound was found which elutes in the position of leucine but is detectable due to its positive reaction with iodoplatinate. This additional compound was also found in normal hair and since it may be present as a shoulder on the leucine peak it could have been incorrectly identified as cysteine-homocysteine disulphide by Woodhouse. The amount of this compound is approximately 20–40 μmol/g hair.

It is possible that this unusual sulphur-containing compound may represent part of the 'missing sulphur' referred to by Dr Pollitt. We have confirmed the presence of homocysteic acid in performic acid oxidized hydrolysates of homocystinuric hair.

Wadman (Utrecht). I can mention that we had a young patient with hyperammonemia, caused by ornithine transcarbamylase deficiency, who had very few and short hairs. He had low plasma arginine and ornithine concentrations. We treated him by giving extra arginine and ornithine together with a normal protein load. This resulted in normali-zation of hyperammonemia and blood amino acids. Hair growth became completely normal.

3

Some aspects of the use of hair follicles for the biochemical study of inborn errors of metabolism

R. W. E. Watts, Dorothy A. Gibbs and R. O. McKeran

The root of a hair which has been plucked from the scalp is surrounded by three or four layers of cells which have been avulsed from the hair follicle (Fig. 1). Hairs begin to develop when the foetus is 5–6 weeks old. Each hair follicle develops from a small group of ectodermal cells which grows into the subjacent mesoderm, and there is an appreciable probability that this group of cells will in turn have been derived from a single cell. Under these circumstances the follicles would be clonal. The random inactivation of one X-chromosome in females (Lyon, 1962) together with the suggestion that hair follicle

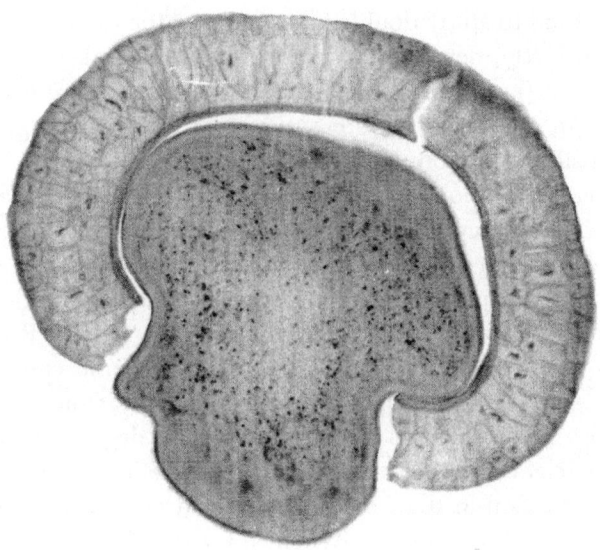

FIG. 1   Transverse section of a plucked hair follicle.

cells are clonal led to the prediction that the heterozygous carriers of a sex-linked enzyme variant would show two classes of hair follicles containing the normal and the abnormal enzyme respectively. Gartler, Gandini, Angioni and Argiolas (1969) studied the isoenzyme composition of hair follicles from a subject who was heterozygous for the fast and slow moving electrophoretic variants of D-glucose-6-phosphate: NADP+oxidore-ductase (EC 1.1.1.49) (glucose-6-phosphate dehydrogenase or G6PD). They found three classes of hair follicle, which contained: the fast migrating, the slowly migrating and both variants respectively. These results confirmed that it would be possible to use hair follicles to determine the genetic status of a subject who might be a carrier of a sex linked defect of an enzyme which is normally present in the cells around the root of a hair. They also indicated that sufficient hairs would have to be examined to allow for the imperfect cloning of the follicles.

Gartler, Scott, Goldstein, Campbell and Sparkes (1971), Silvers, Cox, Balis and Dancis (1972) and Francke, Bakay and Nyhan (1973) demonstrated hair follicle cell mosaicism for IMP: pyrophosphate phosphoribosyltransferase (EC 2.4.2.8) (hypoxanthineguanine phosphoribosyltransferase or HGPRT) in the mothers of patients with the Lesch Nyhan syndrome. Goldstein, Marks and Gartler (1971) also used the method to study double heterozygotes for G6PD and HGPRT deficiency, directly, demonstrating that for two X-linked loci, genes in the *cis* position (i.e. both on the same chromosome), are turned on or off together in a cell and its clone; conversely, when the genes are in the *trans* position only one gene or the other is expressed.

Seegmiller, Rosenbloom and Kelley (1967) recognized the association of very gross deficiency of erythrocyte HGPRT with the clinical features of the Lesch Nyhan syndrome (sex-linked choreoathetosis, spasticity, aggressiveness, compulsive self mutilation, mental retardation and the complication of gross uric acid overproduction). Kelley, Rosenbloom, Henderson and Seegmiller (1967) reported that some cases of severe gout, uric acid urolithiasis and sometimes minor neuropsychiatric abnormalities are associated with a less severe degree of erythrocyte HGPRT deficiency (termed partial HGPRT deficiency to distinguish it from the situation in the Lesch Nyhan syndrome which they termed complete HGPRT deficiency). Evidence for the existence of considerable genetic heterogeneity in these disorders is now accumulating (Kelley and Meade, 1971), and the validity of drawing this firm distinction between the so-called complete and partial HGPRT deficiency on the basis of different but very low levels of erythrocyte HGPRT has been questioned (Emmerson and Thompson, 1973).

Patients with the Lesch Nyhan syndrome do not reproduce so that one-third of the cases should arise from new mutations provided that the population is in genetic equilibrium (Harris, 1959). There is, therefore, an appreciable chance that the mothers of single cases of the Lesch Nyhan syndrome who have no affected male relatives will not be carriers. If the genetic status of the mother can be established with certainty it should be possible to make the genetic advice which she is given more reliable.

A patient with the Lesch Nyhan syndrome who had no affected relatives and whose parents sought genetic advice was recently referred to one of us (R.W.E.W.*). We measured the HGPRT and AMP: pyrophosphate phosphoribosyltransferase (EC 2.4.2.7.) (adenine phosphoribosyltransferase or APRT) activities by a modification of the method of Gartler *et al.* (1971) and expressed the results as ratio HGPRT activity/APRT activity. The APRT activity is increased in the Lesch Nyhan syndrome so that the use of this ratio improves the discrimination between high and low HGPRT results. It also provides a check on the viability of the hair follicle, and any follicles without measurable APRT activity are rejected. The results obtained for control subjects, the mother (Mrs H.) of the propositus, two mothers (Mrs B. and Mrs T.) of other clinically typical and biochemically proven cases of the Lesch Nyhan syndrome, another case of the Lesch Nyhan syndrome (son of Mrs T.) and a patient (A.R.) with the syndrome of incomplete HGPRT deficiency (severe gout from about puberty, uric acid overproduction, and mild mental retardation) are shown in Fig. 2. The following points emerge from an examination of the data:

1. The results for Mrs H. are all within the same range as those of the control subjects.
2. Mrs B. and Mrs T. both have follicles with abnormally low HGPRT/APRT ratios, and only Mrs T. yielded any follicles with HGPRT/APRT ratios within the normal range.
3. None of the follicles from the heterozygotes gave unmeasurably low results.

* Dr Margaret I. Griffiths of Birmingham University Department of Child Health and Birmingham Children's Hospital referred the patient who continues under her clinical care.

MEASUREMENT OF THE RATIO $\frac{HGPRT}{APRT}$ IN HAIR FOLLICLES
OF CONTROLS SUBJECTS., HETEROZYGOTES AND HEMIZYGOTES
FOR THE LESCH-NYHAN SYNDROME

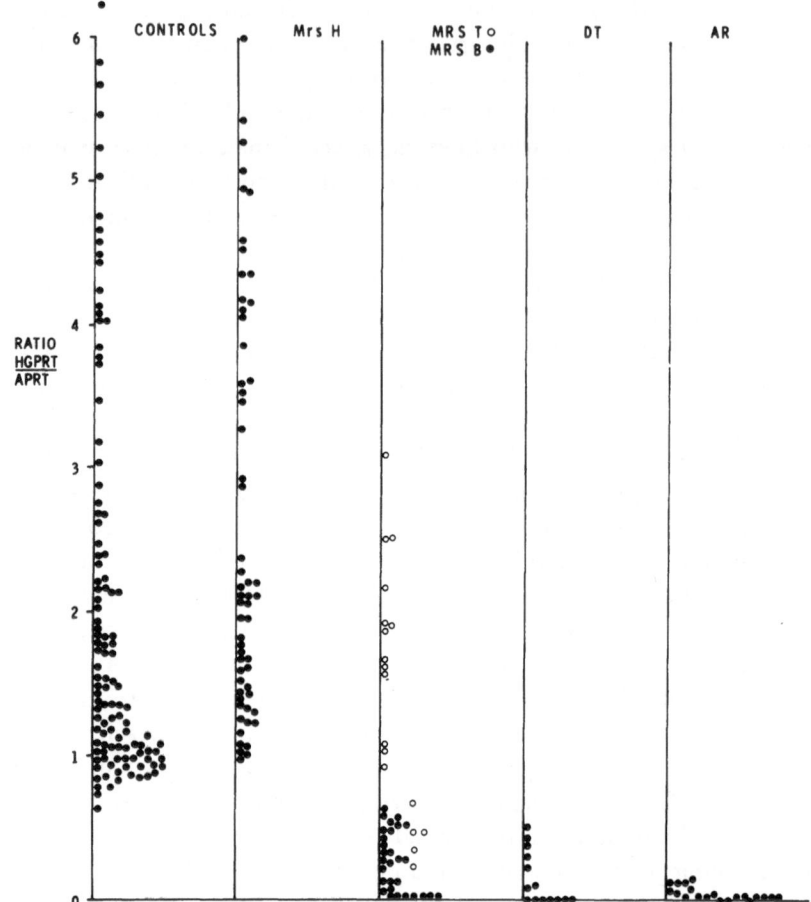

FIG. 2   HGPRT/APRT ratios for plucked hair follicles from: (i) control subjects; (ii) patient whose genotype was to be determined (Mrs H.); (iii) two mothers (Mrs B. and Mrs T.) who had both had one son with the Lesch Nyhan syndrome; (iv) a hemizygote for complete HGPRT deficiency (son of Mrs T.); (v) hemizygote for partial HGPRT deficiency (A.R.). The results on Mrs H. are compatible with the condition in her son having arisen because of a new mutation. '*Note added in proof:* This subject has recently conceived. Cells grown from a specimen of amniotic fluid revealed a normal female karyotype of 46 XX with prominent satellites on one no. 13–15 in each cell. It was shown that the cultured cells consist of a single population of HGPRT+ cells, indicating the presence of a non-carrier foetus. This is consistent with the present evidence that Mrs H. is not a carrier of the mutant gene which produces the Lesch Nyhan syndrome. (We are indebted to Dr Renata Lax for the karyotyping and to Dr Gregory Stewart who investigated the ability of the cultured cells to incorporate [3H]hypoxanthine.)'

4. Some of the follicles from the hemizygote (D.T.) contained small amounts of HGPRT.

5. The case of partial HGPRT deficiency gave results which were not distinguishable from those obtained from the patient with the Lesch Nyhan syndrome (i.e. complete HGPRT deficiency).

These findings illustrate the usefulness of hair follicles in studies of the genetic status of suspected carriers of X-linked recessive disorders. The results on Mrs H., Mrs B. and Mrs T. were independently confirmed by fibroblast culture techniques.

Fujimoto and Seegmiller (1970) were the first to report the presence of very low but detectable levels of HGPRT in fibroblasts of patients with the Lesch Nyhan syndrome. This was further investigated by Kelley *et al.*, (1971) who found very low levels of AGPRT in eleven cell lines obtained from different patients, they also found evidence for considerable heterogeneity in the mutations of the HGPRT molecule which cause the Lesch Nyhan syndrome. The presence of HGPRT protein in erythrocytes from cases of the Lesch Nyhan syndrome has been demonstrated immunochemically indicating that the mutation affects a structural gene (Rubin, Dancis, Yip, Nowinski and Balis, 1971; Arnold, Meade and Kelley, 1972).

Emmerson *et al.* (1973) developed an ultrasensitive assay for erythrocyte HGPRT and demonstrated very low levels of enzyme activity in eight members of five sibships. These investigators concluded that the severity of the clinical manifestations did not correlate with the red blood cell HGPRT level. The present results on the hair follicles of DT (classical Lesch Nyhan syndrome with unmeasurable erythrocyte HGPRT) and AR (juvenile gout and mild mental retardation with measurable residual erythrocyte HGPRT) indicate that similar considerations apply to hair follicle cells and corroborate the conclusion of Emmerson *et al.* (1973) that additional factors besides the actual level of HGPRT in red cells are important in determining the severity of the neuropsychiatric lesions and the urate abnormality. The recent observation that replacement blood transfusion with normal HGPRT containing blood cells did not detectably alter either the plasma and urine uric acid levels or the clinical state of a two and a half year old boy with the Lesch Nyhan syndrome is also compatible with this (Watts, McKeran, Andrews, Brown and Griffiths, 1973). The lack of correlation between blood cell HGPRT and the clinical state is understandable if the relatively high level of HGPRT in the central nervous system and especially in the basal ganglia is considered (Kelley, Green, Rosenbloom, Henderson and Seegmiller, 1969).

The presence of a preponderance of HGPRT containing fibroblasts in cultures prepared from heterozygotes for the Lesch Nyhan syndrome (Rosenbloom, Kelley, Henderson and Seegmiller, 1967) rather than the equal proportions of HGPRT positive and HGPRT negative cells expected on the basis of random inactivation of the X-chromosome in females (Lyon, 1962) was explained by metabolic co-operation* (Fujimoto *et al.*, 1970). Mosaicism was not demonstrated in skin epithelial cells by Frost, Weinstein and Nyhan (1970), and this was also explained by metabolic co-operation. The intermediate enzyme levels in the heterozygotes in the present studies cannot readily be explained on this basis because it needs cell to cell contact, and the individual hair follicles do not grow so closely to one another; incomplete cloning is therefore a better explanation.

The studies of G6PD deficiency and HGPRT deficiency which are reviewed in this paper illustrate the practicability of using hair follicle cells to study the carrier state in sex linked inborn errors of metabolism where the relevant enzymes are normally present in these cells. Examination of plucked hair follicles for O-diphenyl:O_2 oxidoreductase (EC 1.10.3.1) (catechol oxidase or tyrosinase) activity showed that two types of oculocutaneous albinism exist. They are both inherited in an autosomal recessive manner, but the hair follicles are tyrosinase positive in one variant and tyrosinase negative in the other (Fitzpatrick and Quevedo, 1972). It may be possible to extend this simple biopsy technique to the study of other autosomally inherited disorders in the future. Some apparently normal individuals who were selected as controls in our own investigations (McKeran, Andrews, Howell, Gibbs and Watts, 1973) had abnormally brittle hair which made it difficult to collect sufficient hair follicles, and this may limit the use of the technique especially in disorders such as argininosuccinic aciduria (Allan, Cusworth, Dent and Wilson, 1958) in which the hair is abnormally fragile. It should also be emphasized that investigators should aim to relate the activity of the enzyme under consideration to the activity of one or more metabolically unrelated enzymes, and to a parameter of the number of cells present. The measurement of DNA by

* Metabolic co-operation is the phenomenon whereby when cultured mammalian cells come into contact their individual metabolism is modified by the exchange of elaborated material (Subak-Sharpe, 1969).

a spectrophotofluorimetric method (Blackburn, Andrews and Watts, 1973) appears to be the most satisfactory reference to use for the latter purpose.

Addendum

Another case of the Lesch Nyhan syndrome arising from a new mutation has now been reported by Itiaba, Banfalvi, Crawhall and Mongeau (1973). These authors based their conclusions on the results of cultured studies with fibroblast lines derived from the mother and maternal female relatives of the propositus.

Acknowledgements

We are indebted to the following physicians who allowed us to study patients who were under their care: Professor E. G. L. Bywaters, Dr Margaret I. Griffiths, Dr R. Robson, Dr J. J. Bourke. The fibroblast cultures were made in Professor P. E. Polani's laboratory and we are most grateful to him for this help.

REFERENCES

ALLAN, J. D., CUSWORTH, D. C., DENT, C. E. & WILSON, V. K. (1958) *Lancet*, **i**, 182.

ARNOLD, W. J., MEADE, J. C. & KELLEY, W. N. (1972) *Journal of Clinical Investigation*, **51**, 1805.

BLACKBURN, M. J., ANDREWS, T. M. & WATTS, R. W. E. (1973) *Analytical Biochemistry*, **51**, 1.

EMMERSON, B. T. & THOMPSON, L. (1973) *Quarterly Journal of Medicine N.S.*, **42**, 423.

FITZPATRICK, T. B. & QUEVEDO, W. C. (1972) Albinism, Chapter 14. In the *Metabolic Basis of Inherited Disease*. Edited by J. B. Stanbury, J. B. Wyngaarden & D. S. Fredrickson. New York: McGray-Hill.

FRANCKE, U., BAKAY, B. & NYHAN, W. L. (1973) *Pediatrics*, **82**, 472.

FROST, P., WEINSTEIN, G. D. & NYHAN, W. L. (1970) *Journal of American Medical Association*, **212**, 316.

FUJIMOTO, W. & SEEGMILLER, J. E. (1970) *Proceeding of the National Academy of Sciences of the U.S.A.*, **65**, 577.

GARTLER, S. M., GANDINI, E., ANGIONI, G. & ARGIOLAS, N. (1969) *Annals of Human Genetics*, **33**, 171.

GARTLER, S. M., SCOTT, R. C., GOLDSTEIN, J. L., CAMPBELL, B. & SPARKES, R. (1971) *Science*, **172**, 572.

GOLDSTEIN, J. L., MARKS, J. F. & GARTLER, S. M. (1971) *Proceedings of the National Academy of Sciences of the U.S.A.*, **68**, 1425.

HARRIS, H. (1959) Some aspects of mendelian heredity in man. *Human Biochemical Genetics*, Ch. 24, p. 30. Cambridge: University Press.

ITIABA, K., BANFALVI, M., CRAWHALL, J. C. & MONGEAU, J.-G. (1973) *American Journal of Human Genetics*, **25**, 134.

KELLEY, W. N., GREEN, M. L., ROSENBLOOM, F. M., HENDERSON, J. F. & SEEGMILLER, J. E. (1969) *Annals of Internal Medicine*, **70**, 155.

KELLEY, W. N. & MEADE, J. C. (1971) *Journal of Biological Chemistry*, **246**, 2953.

KELLEY, W. N., ROSENBLOOM, F. M., HENDERSON, J. F. & SEEGMILLER, J. E. (1967) *Proceedings of the National Academy of Sciences of the U.S.A.*, **57**, 1735.

LYON, M. F. (1962) *American Journal of Human Genetics*, **14**, 136.

McKERAN, R. O., ANDREWS, T. M., HOWELL, A., GIBBS, D. A. & WATTS, R. W. E. (1973) *Clinical Science and Molecular Medicine*, **45**, 17.

ROSENBLOOM, F. M., KELLEY, W. N., HENDERSON, J. F. & SEEGMILLER (1967) *Lancet*, ii, 305.

RUBIN, C. S., DANCIS, J., YIP, L. C., NOWINSKI, R. C. & BALIS, E. R. (1971) *Proceedings of the National Academy of Sciences of the U.S.A.*, **68**, 1468.

SEEGMILLER, J. E., ROSENBLOOM, F. M. & KELLEY, W. N. (1967) *Science*, **155**, 1682.

SILVERS, D. N., COX, P., BALIS, M. E. & DANCIS, J. (1972) *New England Journal of Medicine*, **286**, 390.

SUBAK-SHARPE, J. (1969) Metabolic cooperation between cells. In *Homeostatic Regulators*. Edited by G. E. W. Wolstenholme. London: Churchill.

WATTS, R. W. E., MCKERAN, R. O., ANDREWS, T. M., BROWN, E. & GRIFFITHS, M. I. (1973) (unpublished data).

DISCUSSION
(of paper by Dr Watts)

Harkness (Edinburgh). Have you tried the effect of nucleotidase inhibitors in your enzyme assay to reducd product destruction.

Watts (London). We have used the ration of HG to APRtase to avoid these effects.

Harkness. This might not compensate for such destruction which would result in low values for activity because the activities of tissue nucleotidases for the substrates AMP, GMP and IMP vary considerably. The apparent activity of APRtase might thus be altered relative to that apparent for HGPRtase.

INBORN ERRORS OF
CONNECTIVE TISSUE

4

Morphological aspects of the Mucopolysaccharidoses

Jurgen Spranger

Clinical, roentgenographic and cytological aspects of the mucopoly-saccharidoses are of basic importance to the practicing physician, whose observations will frequently allow an accurate diagnosis on morphological grounds alone. They are valuable screening tools for the research-oriented clinician looking for 'atypical cases' in whom the application of modern and frequently complicated biochemical methods will be most rewarding. It is in these patients that new enzyme defects and metabolic pathways will be detected.

Clinical features

The clinical aspects of the systemic mucopolysaccharidoses have recently been discussed in detail (McKusick, 1972) (Spranger, 1972). They will not be extensively reviewed here. Some pertinent features are listed in Table I.

Mucopolysaccharidosis I–H

The Hurler disease (formerly mucopolysaccharidosis I) is usually manifested in later infancy. Some unspecific signs of the disease may be present before this time such as a slightly enlarged head or herniae (Fig. 2). The characteristic phenotype (Fig. 1) is usually not recognized before the end of the first year of life. A definitely Hurler-like appearance in an infant younger than six months is more compatiable with a diagnosis of GM_1 gangliosidosis or mucolipidosis II (I-cell disease) than with a mucopolysaccharidosis. Patients with Hurler disease rarely survive the fourteenth year of life but in many instances remain emotionally attached to their families until the end of their life.

TABLE I *Classification of the systemic mucopolysaccharidoses*

mildly present — absent   a.r. autosomal recessive   + present   (+) occasionally or
X.r. X-chromosomal recessive

Mucopoly-saccharidosis	Synonym	Dysmorphism	Mental retardation	Corneal opacities	Inheritance	Defective enzyme
I —H	Hurler	+	+	+	a.r.	α-Iduronidase
—S	Scheie	(+)	—	+	a.r.	α-Iduronidase
II —A	Hunter, severe	+	+	—	X.r.	Sulphoiduronate-sulphatase
—B	Hunter, mild	+	—	—	X.r.	
III—A	Sanfilippo A	(+)	+	—	a.r.	Heparan sulphate-N-sulphatase
—B	Sanfilippo B	(+)	+	—	a.r.	α-Glucosaminidase
IV	Morquio	+	—	(+)	a.r.	?
V	vacant					
VI—A	Maroteaux–Lamy severe	+	—	+	a.r.	N-acetylgalacto-samine-4-sulphatase
—B	Maroteaux–Lamy mild	(+)	—	+	a.r.	
VII	β-Glucuronidase defect	(+)	+	—	a.r.	β-Glucuronidase

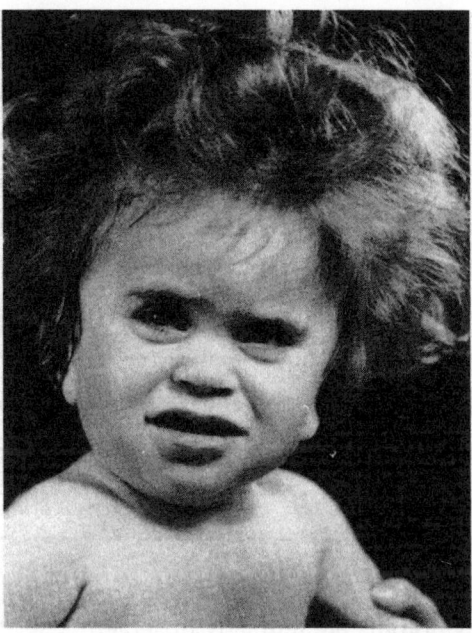

FIG. 1   Girl, age 2½ years with Hurler disease. Note abundant, coarse hair, coarse facies with depressed nasal bridge, full cheeks and large mouth.

Mucopolysaccharidosis I–S

The Scheie disease (formerly mucopolysaccharidosis V) and mucopolysaccharidosis I–H are caused by a defect of the same enzyme, α-iduronidase (Table I). The striking phenotypic differences between the two disorders may be due to different rest activities of the enzyme in various tissues. Patients with mucopolysaccharidosis I–S are of normal intelligence. Between the third and the sixth year of life joint contractures, herniae and corneal clouding are noted (Fig. 3). In the older child and in the adult the facial features become coarse but not Hurler-like. Cardiac defects, most notably aortic valve disease, may be prominent, and, in view of the co-existing joint contractures, an erroneous diagnosis of rheumatoid arthritis or rheumatic fever may be entertained for years.

Mucopolysaccharidosis II

The Hunter disease is caused by the hemizygous state of a mutant gene located on the X-chromosome. As a general rule, it is manifested

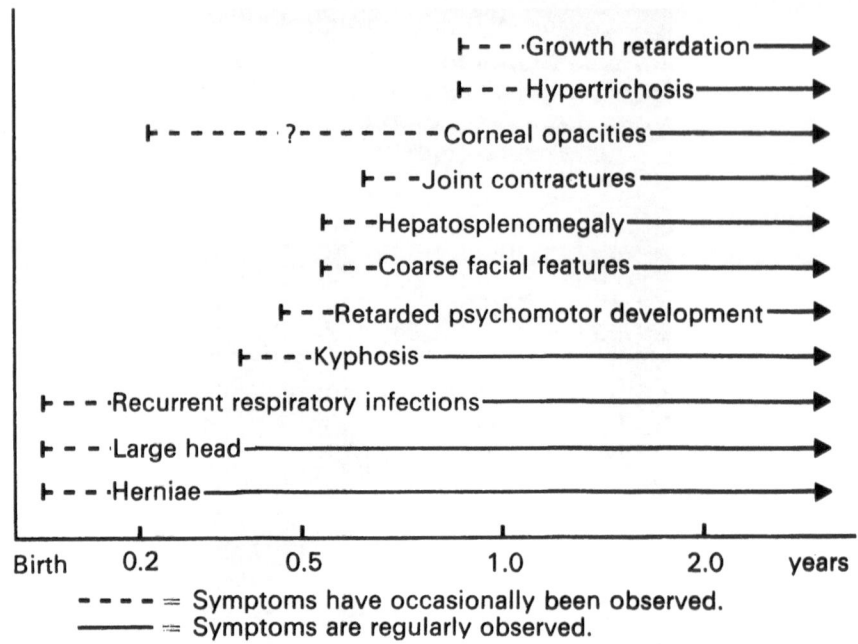

FIG. 2   Early clinical manifestations in mucopolysaccharidosis I–H.

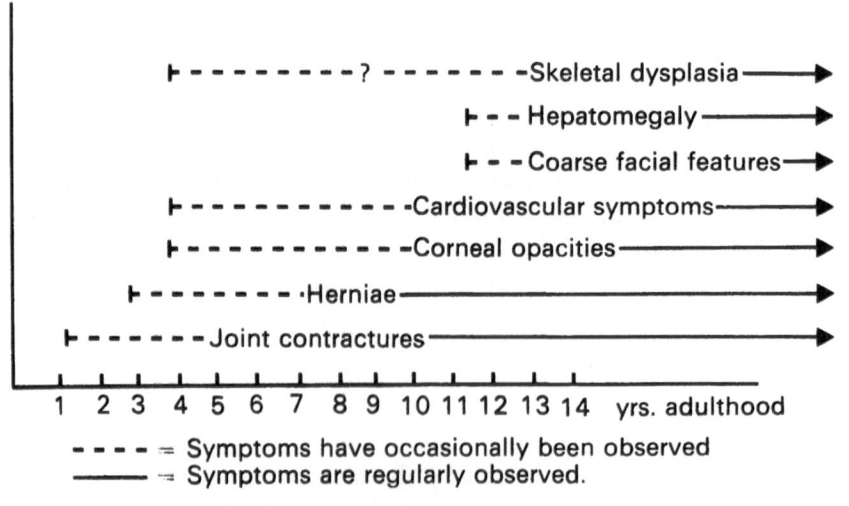

FIG. 3   Early clinical manifestations in mucopolysaccharidosis I–S.

in males only. A female with Hunter disease has recently been described (Milunsky and Neufeld, 1973). There are probably two allelic mutations. One causes a severe disease resembling mucopolysaccharidosis I–H (Fig. 4). Patients with this form frequently show a rapid mental and neurologic degeneration in the pre-pubertal phase and die in their early teens. Clinically they show many features of Hurler disease except corneal opacities. These cases may explain the discrepancy between the predicted and the observed incidence of the Hurler and Hunter diseases. According to the prediction, there should be more patients with Hunter than with Hurler disease (McKusick, 1970). Incidence figures had shown the reverse (Spranger, 1972; Lowry and Renwick, 1971). A recent re-evaluation of our personal cases shows a higher frequency of Hunter than of Hurler patients (Table II).

Patients with the milder form of mucopolysaccharidosis II are of normal or borderline intelligence. Available information suggests that neuronal storage occurs in the severe but not in the mild form (Spranger, 1972). Intelligence testing should take the impaired hearing into account which is regularly present in Hunter disease. A major complication occurring in both forms (as well as in mucopolysaccharidosis I–H and

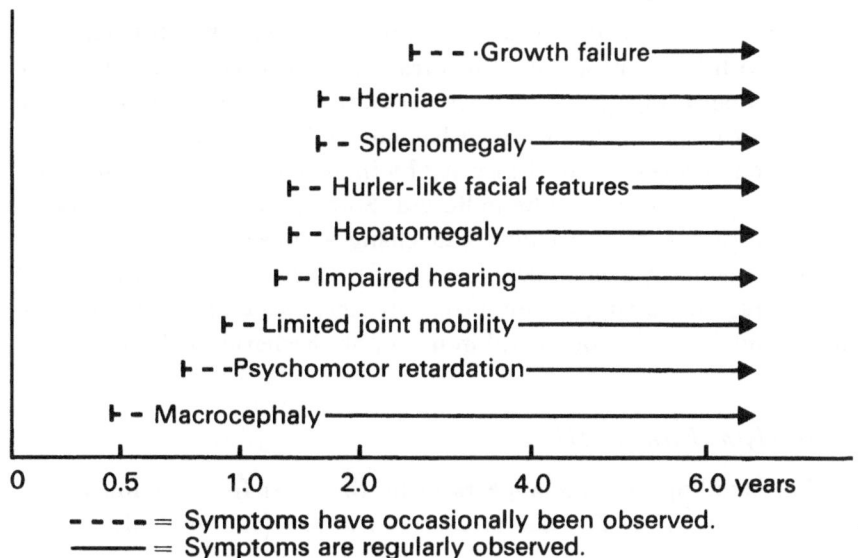

FIG. 4 Early clinical manifestations in severe form of mucopolysaccharidosis II. In the mild form, there is no psychomotor retardation and the Hurler-like deformities are usually noted after the fourth year of life.

TABLE II   *Patients with different mucopolysaccharidoses and mucolipidoses registered at the University of Kiel Children's Hospital between 1964 and 1972*

Mucopoly- saccharidosis type	Number	Per cent
I–H	24	16
I–S	2	1
II	33	21
III	46	30
IV	5	3
VI	9	6
VII	1	1
Mucolipidoses	14	9
Unclassifiable	20	13
	154	100

VI) is an increase of the intracranial pressure caused by obstruction of the spinal fluid pathways due to thickening and cyst formation of the leptomeninges (Fig. 5) (Neuhauser, Gricom, Gilles and Crocker, 1968). Attacks of unexplained bizarre behaviour and restlessness may be the expression of severe headache caused by increased intracranial pressure. Shunting procedures may be indicated. Some patients with mucopolysaccharidosis II have peculiar skin changes consisting of hard, non-tender, irregularly shaped papules (Fig. 6). They are apparently caused by a storage material, possibly proteoglycans, located between collagen fibres, and have been described in mucopolysaccharidosis II only.

Mucopolysaccharidosis III

The Sanfilippo disease appears to be the most frequent mucopolysaccharidosis. The disorder is caused by two (and possibly more?) non-allelic mutations leading to a defective degradation of mostly heparan sulphate. The two genotypes listed in Table I cannot be differentiated clinically. In our personal experience the sulphatase

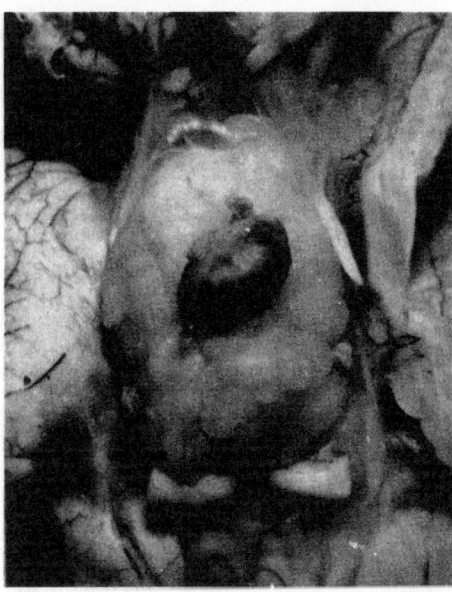

FIG. 5 Large leptomeningeal cyst located in the sella of a patient with Hurler disease. (From Neuhauser, E. *et al.*, 1966, by permission of author and publisher.)

defect is much more common than the glucosaminidase defect (Cantz, Gehler, Tolksdorf and Spranger, unpublished).

Isolated cases are usually not detected before the second year of life. First symptoms are most commonly behavioural problems such as sleep disturbances and motor hyperactivity (Fig. 7). The physical growth is accelerated rather than retarded. The clinical changes are comparatively mild (Fig. 8). Even in adolescence the physical appearance of a patient with Sanfilippo disease may be quite normal. In our experience, the most consistent clinical sign is the abundant and coarse scalp hair. The combination of behavioural problems and abundant scalp hair should be reason enough to order a screening test for abnormal mucopolysacchariduria.

Mucopolysaccharidosis IV

The Morquio disease has been clearly defined in recent years. (Maroteaux, Lamy and Foucher, 1963; Langer and Carey, 1966). It is characterized by the triad of particular skeletal changes, fine corneal opacities and increased urinary excretion of a keratan sulphate—chondroitin sulphate complex. Other manifestations are shown in Fig. 9. In contrast to spondyloepiphysial dysplasia congenita and other bone dysplasias, patients with Morquio disease are normal at birth.

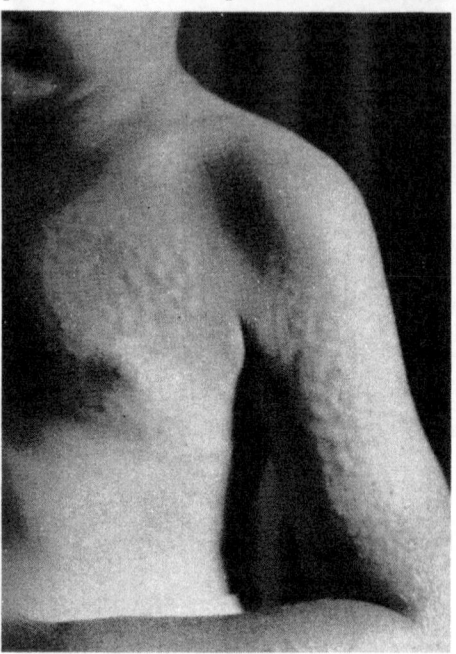

FIG. 6   Papular skin lesions in mucopolysaccharidosis II. (From Levin, S., 1960, by permission of author and publisher.)

The existence of a non-keratan sulphate-excreting form of mucopolysaccharidosis IV is claimed by some (McKusick, 1972). Possibly, this type is identical to the so-called "Dale variant", a particularly mild form of Morquio disease (Spranger, 1972). However, it should be noted that with the usual biochemical techniques, keratan sulphate is easily missed in the urine and that, even in patients with bona fide Morquio disease, the urinary excretion of keratan sulphate decreases with advancing age.

A preventable complication of Morquio disease is atlanto-occipital dislocation with spinal cord compression. The anatomic basis for this is a hypoplasia of the odontoid process in combination with an abnormal laxity may lead to death. First symptoms include an increased fatiguability and abnormal sensation of the upper extremities. Cervical fusion

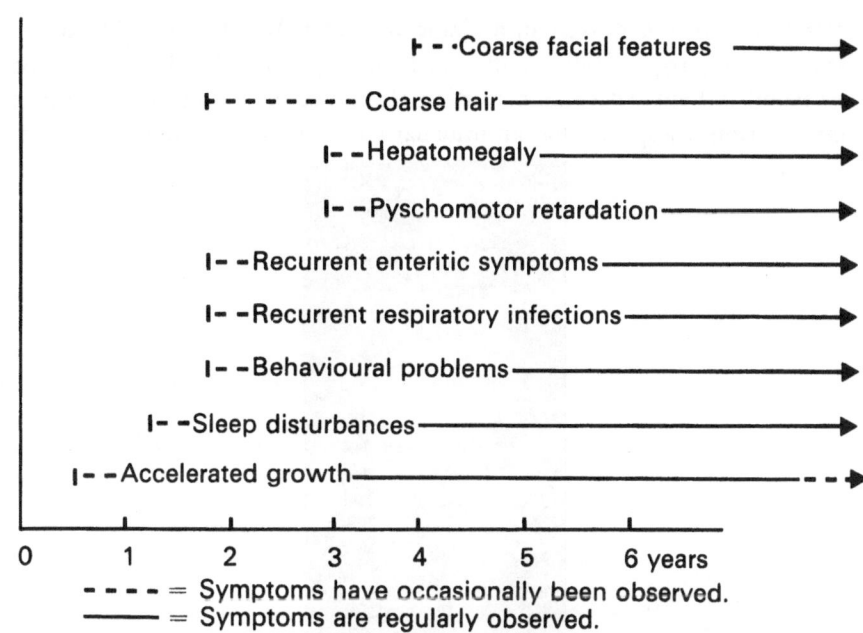

FIG. 7 Early clinical manifestations in mucopolysaccharidosis III.

has been recommended as a routine procedure (Kopits, Perovic, McKusick, Robinson and Bailey, 1972). Spinal cord compression may also occur at the site of the thoracolumbar gibbus which is present in many patients with Morquio disease.

Mucopolysaccharidosis VI

The Maroteaux–Lamy disease is characterized by a moderate to marked Hurler-like phenotype with excessive urinary excretion of dermatan sulphate and normal intelligence. Possibly, there are two allelic mutations, one causing a severe disesae with marked dysmorphism and severe skeletal changes, and another with milder abnormalities and a longer survival (McKusick, 1972; Spranger, 1972).

The disorder is usually recognized in the third to fourth year of life though some non-specific signs of the disease may be present earlier (Fig. 10).

Mucopolysaccharidosis VII

The disorder and its basic defect, a deficiency of β-glucuronidase activity, were recognized in a single patient (Sly, Quinton, McAlister and Rimoin, 1973; Hall, Cantz and Neufeld, 1973). We have observed a second patient with this condition (Cantz *et al.*). From the available information it appears that an unusual facies, hepatosplenomegaly and/

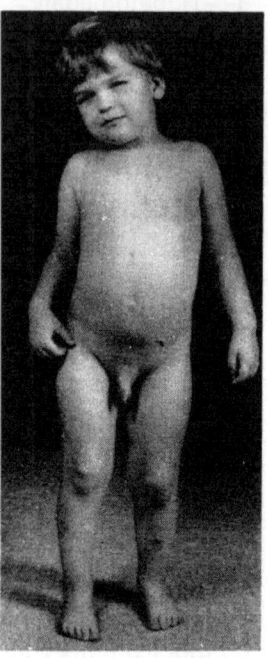

FIG. 8   Boy age 3 years with mucopolysaccharidosis IIIA. The only abnormality in this patient is the abundant and coarse scalp hair.

or hip dysplasia may be noted soon after birth. More specific signs of a Hurler-like condition appear towards the end of the first or in the second year of life when mental retardation, small stature and a Hurler-like facies become evident. In both patients, there was a marked protrusion of the sternum (Fig. 11). On slit-lamp examination, the corneae were clear during the first years of life. There were coarse leucocytic inclusions and the urinary excretion of acid mucopolysaccharides was slightly increased. In our patient, the urinary mucopolysaccharides had characteristics of a modified dermatan sulphate.

Other mucopolysaccharidoses

Numerous reports have described "new" mucopolysaccharidoses. There is little doubt that many more enzyme defects exist than is

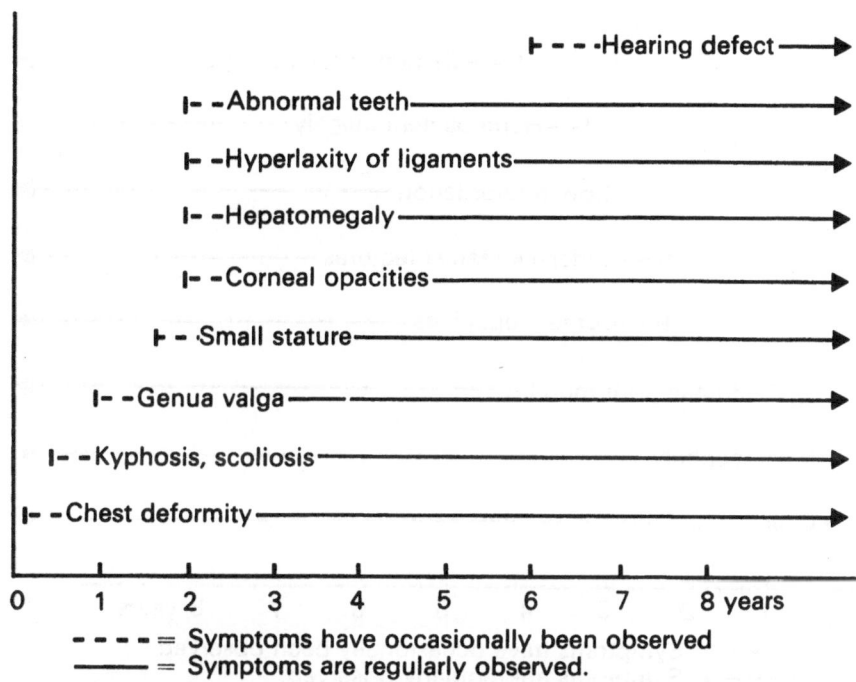

⊢ - - -Hearing defect ⟶

⊢ - -Abnormal teeth ⟶

⊢ - -Hyperlaxity of ligaments ⟶

⊢ - -Hepatomegaly ⟶

⊢ - -Corneal opacities ⟶

⊢ - ·Small stature ⟶

⊢ - -Genua valga ⟶

⊢ - -Kyphosis, scoliosis ⟶

⊢ - -Chest deformity ⟶

0   1   2   3   4   5   6   7   8 years

- - - - = Symptoms have occasionally been observed
———— = Symptoms are regularly observed.

FIG. 9   Early clinical manifestations in mucopolysaccharidosis IV.

presently known leading to conditions with distinctive clinical manifestations. Our personal files contain data from at least twenty patients with unclassifiable mucopolysaccharidoses or mucolipidoses. In four of them, ^{35}S incorporation studies in cultured fibroblasts, enzyme determinations and cross-correction experiments have ruled out the known mucopolysaccharidoses (Cantz *et al.*). The biochemical definition of these and other disorders or mucopolysaccharide metabolism is hampered by our incomplete knowledge of normal metabolic pathways, the lack of appropriate substrates for enzyme determinations and the difficulties involved in the biochemical analysis of glycosaminoglycans.

In the present context only a few unusual disorders will be mentioned.

Hurler–Scheie compound

McKusick, Howell, Hussel, Neufeld and Stevenson (1972) described four patients whose fibroblasts were deficient in the Hurler–Scheie corrective factor, i.e. α-iduronidase. The patients presented many

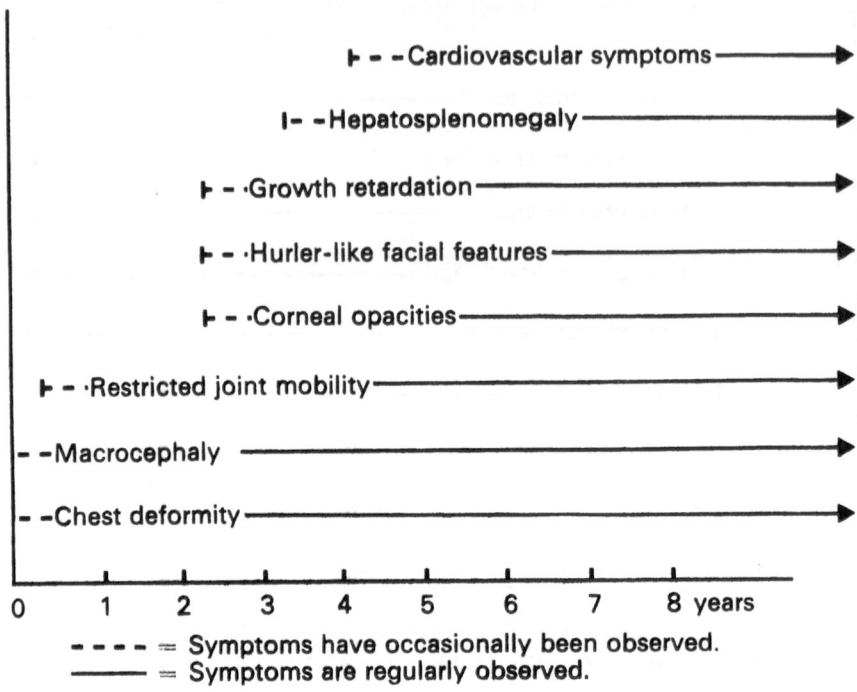

Cardiovascular symptoms ⟶

Hepatosplenomegaly ⟶

Growth retardation ⟶

Hurler-like facial features ⟶

Corneal opacities ⟶

Restricted joint mobility ⟶

Macrocephaly ⟶

Chest deformity ⟶

0   1   2   3   4   5   6   7   8 years

− − − − = Symptoms have occasionally been observed.
———— = Symptoms are regularly observed.

FIG. 10 Early clinical manifestations in severe form of mucopolysaccharidosis IV. In the mild form the clinical symptoms usually appear some years later and progress slower.

features of Hurler disease such as severe skeletal abnormalities, clouded corneae and hepatosplenomegaly but were of normal intelligence. The clinical changes developed slower than in true Hurler disease, and one patient was 22 years old at the time of publication. It was suggested that these four patients represent a genetic compound caused by a Hurler mutation of one gene and an (allelic) Scheie mutation of the second gene coding for α-iduronidase. Other possibilities such as homozygozity for an allele at the Hurler–Scheie locus differing from that in mucopolysaccharidoses I–H and I–S could not be ruled out. If the compound hypothesis were correct, the incidence of the Hurler–Scheie compound would be only slightly lower than that of the Hurler disease (1:112.000 vs. 1:100,000) (McKusick *et al.*, 1972).

Winchester type

Two siblings described by Winchester, Grossman, Lim and Danes,

1969) showed progressive osteolytic lesions in addition to a Hurler-like phenotype with gingival hypertrophy, macroglossy and peripheral corneal opacities. The patient's intelligence and the urinary excretion of acid mucopolysaccharides were normal. Increased amounts of acid mucopolysaccharides were found in stromal cells of the cornea and in cultured fibroblasts.

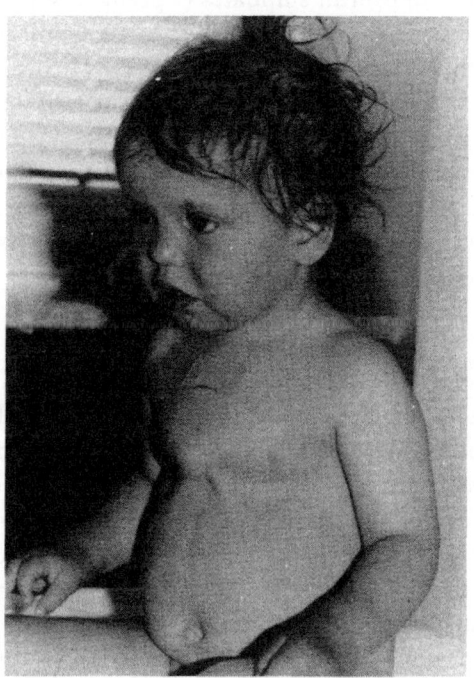

FIG. 11   Girl age 2 years with β-glucuronidase deficiency. The facial features are slightly coarse and the nasal bridge is depressed. There is marked sternal protrusion.

Mucopolysaccharidosis with athetosis

In two independent publications, seven patients were reported with a peculiar combination of Hurler-like clinical features and an extrapyramidal disorder (Maroteaux, 1973; Buscaino, 1968). The patients had a short-trunk type of dwarfism, corneal opacities and skeletal changes of dysostosis multiplex. Their intelligence was unimpaired, and there were no signs of visceral storage. Between the fifth and seventh year of life extrapyramidal signs developed with athetosis, sialorrhoea and dysarthria. Increased amounts of keratan sulphate were found in the urine, and metachromasia was present in cultured fibroblasts. Sulphate incorporation or enzyme studies were not reported.

Chondroitin sulphate mucopolysaccharidosis

Three patients have been described with excessive urinary excretion of predominantly chondroitin sulphates (Spranger and Schuster, 1971; Thompson, Nelson, Castor and Grobelny, 1971). Clinically, the patients were normal in their first years of life. Later, a Hurler-like phenotype developed with clinical and histologic evidence of visceral storage, corneal opacities, skeletal changes and leucocytic inclusions. The intelligence deteriorated after the tenth year of life. Recent studies of cultured fibroblasts showed an increased rate of S^{35} incorporation which was not corrected by any of the known corrective factors (Cantz *et al.*). No enzyme defect was detected.

Roentgenographic features

The roentgenographic changes in various mucopolysaccharidoses and mucolipidoses are called 'Dysostosis multiplex'. Dysostosis multiplex is characteristic in the sense that its presence strongly suggests intracellular storage of acid mucopolysaccharides, glycoproteins and/or glycolipids. It is uncharacteristic in the sense that it is found in a great number of conditions. In these, the degree of involvement varies and is of some diagnostic significance (Spranger and Schuster, 1969). Thus, severe skeletal changes are present in mucopolysaccharidosis I–H, moderate changes are present in mucopolysaccharidosis II and mild changes in mucopolysaccharidosis III. Some more specific skeletal abnormalities are found in mucopolysaccharidosis IV and in mucolipidosis III (Langer *et al.*, 1966; Melhem, Dorst, Scott and McKusick, 1973).

It is important to remember that most skeletal changes appear relatively late in the course of the mucopolysaccharidoses. Usually, they are not detected before the age of six months, though wide ribs, plump scapulae and dysplastic ilia have been noted already in the second month of life. The gross changes, particularly periosteal cloaking, which was formerly thought to be an early diagnostic sign of Hurler disease (Caffey, 1952) are more compatible with a diagnosis of GM_1 gangliosidosis or mucolipidosis II. Some of the characteristic features of fully manifested dysostosis multiplex are illustrated in Fig. 12. They are detailed elsewhere (Spranger, Langer and Wiedmann, 1974).

Hematologic aspects

Peripheral blood and bone marrow smears show abnormal intracellular inclusions in various cell types of many mucopolysaccharidoses and mucolipidoses. Clean preparations, proper staining technique and careful search are essential. The May–Grunwald–Giemsa stain has been most satisfactory (Hansen, 1972). Since the aspect, distribution and quantity of inclusions are different in the various conditions, they are of diagnostic significance. Some of the characteristic changes are summarized in Table III.

Ultrastructural changes

Electron microscopic studies have been performed in various mucopolysaccharidoses and mucolipidoses. They have consistently shown abnormal intracellular inclusions in a great number of tissues (Spranger, 1972). The intracellular inclusions are contained in vacuoles, i.e. in membrane bound structures, and consist mainly of a fibrillogranular material (probably proteoglycans), of different types of homogenous, opaque structure (probably neutral fat and other lipids), and of lamellar substances (probably gangliosides). In neurons, the latter have been called zebra bodies. The vacuolar inclusions indicate abnormal intralysosomal storage and are of considerable theoretical interest. In the routine work-up of patients with mucopolysaccharidoses they are dispensable.

Differential diagnosis

In infancy, a Hurler-like appearance may be found in hypothyroidism, Pompé disease or in the Wiedemann–Beckwith syndrome (Fig. 13). More frequently, a Hurler disease will be confused with a GM_1 gangliosidosis or a mucolipidosis II (so-called I-cell disease). It should be noted that up to the age of about 5 months, patients with Hurler disease are clinically comparatively inconspicuous. At this age, a Hurler

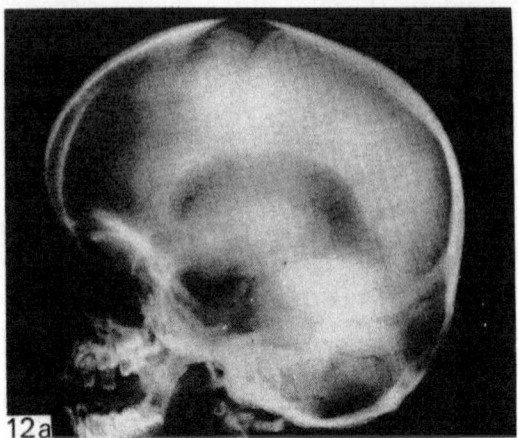

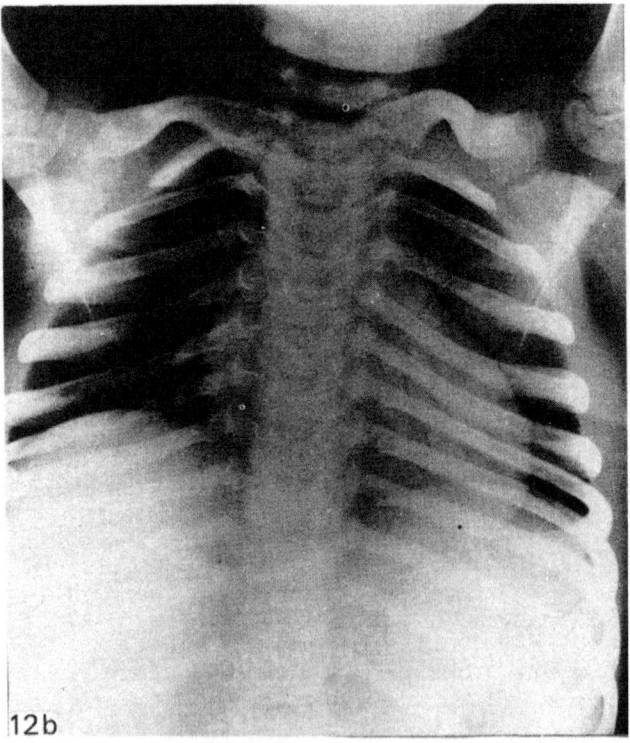

FIG. 12   Severe manifestations of dysostosis multiplex.
a. **Age 2 years.** Macrocephaly, J-shaped sella, ventricular dilatation.
b. **Age 4 years.** Thick clavicles, widening of the lateral and anterior portions of the ribs.

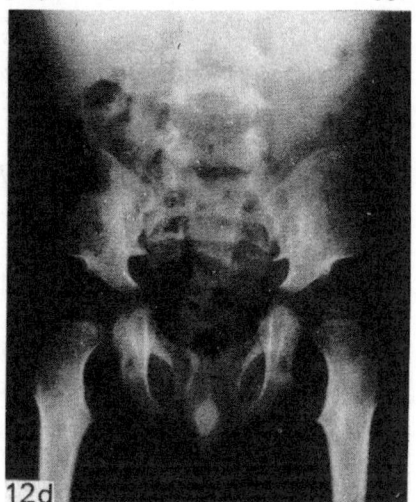

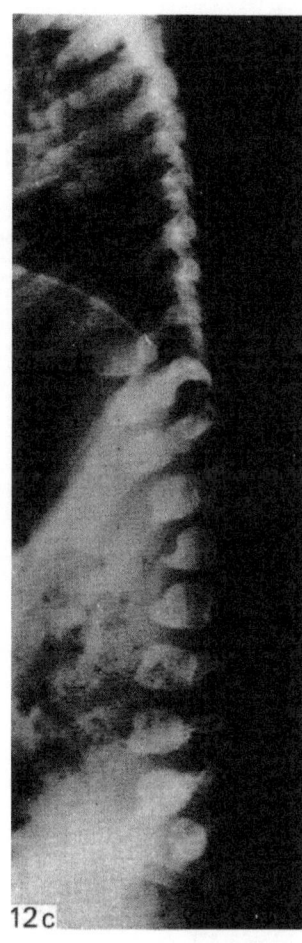

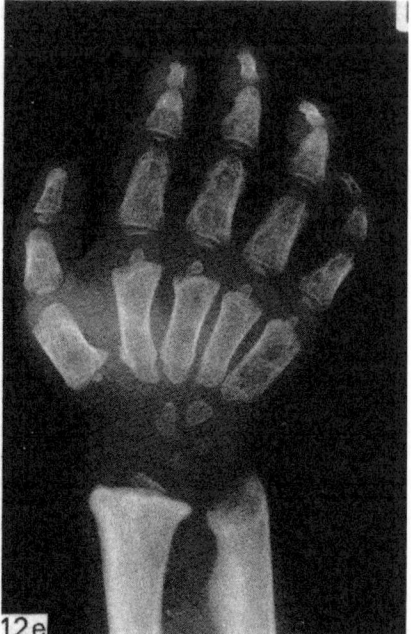

c. Age 4 years. Hook-shaped deformity of L-1 to L-3 with thoracolumbar gibbus. Ovoid (immature) aspect of the vertebral bodies.

d. Age 1½ years. Hypoplasia of the lower portions of the ilia; iliac flare; coxa valga.

e. Age 8 years. Flexion contractures (clawing) of the fingers. Shortening and diaphyseal expansion of the tubular bones; bullet-shape of the phalanges; proximal pointing of the metacarpals II–V; retarded ossification; deformity of distal ends of radius and ulna.

TABLE III   *Characteristic changes of blood and bone marrow cells in different mucopolysaccharidoses. Adapted from Hansen (1972)*

Mucopoly-saccharidosis	Peripheral blood
I–H	Lymphocytes: evenly distributed inclusions in large percentage of cells
I–S	Lymphocytes: fine and sparse inclusions in less than 10 % of cells
II	Same as mucopolysaccharidosis I–H
III	Lymphocytes: coarse inclusions confined to restricted plasma areas
IV	Granulocytes: one to three large, plaque-like inclusions in 50–90 % of cells
VI	Neutrophils and eosinophils: abundant coarse inclusions
VII	Similar to mucopolysaccharidosis VI
	Bone marrow
I–H	Reticulum cells: moderately coarse to thick inclusions ('Gasser cells')
I–S	Reticulum cells: sparse inclusions in occasional cell
II	Same as mucopolysaccharidosis I–H
III	Plasma cells: coarse, oddly shaped inclusions, occasionally surrounded by vacuoles ('Buhot cells')
IV	Reticulum cells: fine inclusions
VI	Neutrophils and eosinophils: abundant coarse inclusions
VII	Similar to mucopolysaccharidosis VI

phenotype is more compatible with a diagnosis of a GM_1 gangliosidosis or mucolipidosis II.

In later infancy and childhood, the mucopolysaccharidoses must be differentiated mainly from the mucolipidoses (Spranger and Wiedemann, 1970). Mucolipidoses are disorders which look like mucopolysaccharidoses but cannot be classified as such. Clinically they combine

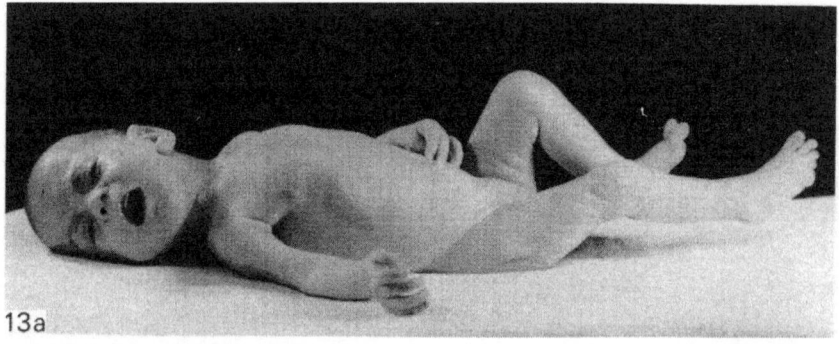

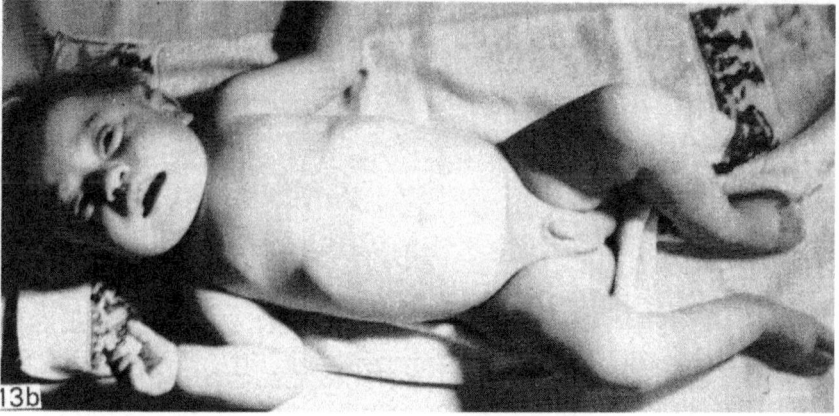

FIG. 13 Differential diagnosis of the mucopolysaccharidoses in infancy.
a. Patient with Hurler disease at the age of 6 weeks.
b. Patient with mucolipidosis II at the age of 6 months.

Hurler-like features which signs and symptoms usually found in the sphingolipidoses (such as rapid neurologic degeneration, cherry-red macuolar spots, vacuolized lymphocytes, etc.). Biochemically, the mucolipidoses are heterogenous (Table IV). In contrast to the muco- polysaccharidoses there is evidence of a primary defect of lipid or glycoprotein metabolism which may or may not be combined with primary defect of mucopolysaccharide metabolism. They are differen- tiated from the mucopolysaccharidoses by their pattern of morpho- logical finding, their natural course, the normal mucopolysacchariduria in most of them and by the appearance and lysosomal enzyme activities of cultured fibroblasts.

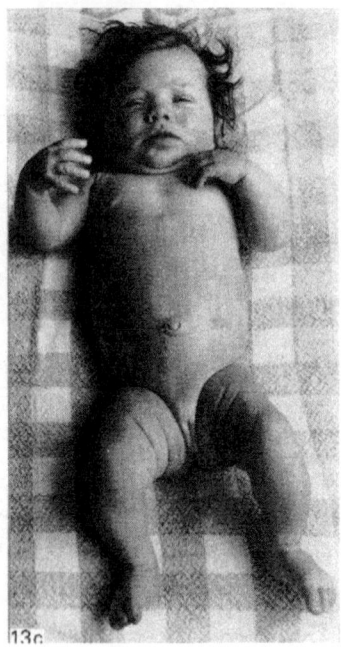 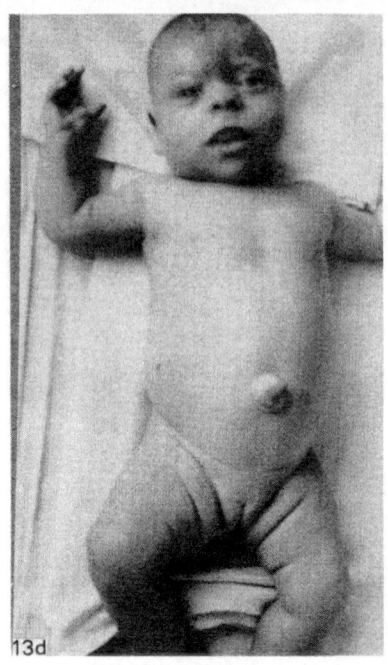

FIG. 13 *contd.*

c. Patient at the age of 6 months with hypothyroidism.

d. Patient at the age of 2 months with the Wiedemann–Beckwith syndrome of exomphalos, gigantism and macroglossy.

Summary

Some of the morphological aspects of the mucopolysaccharidoses are reviewed. Graphs are presented illustrating the early manifestations of different genotypes. In early infancy, marked Hurler-like changes are more compatible with a GM_1 gangliosidosis or a mucolipidosis II than with a mucopolysaccharidosis. The skeletal changes are relatively uniform in most mucopolysaccharidoses and are called dysostosis multiplex. Abnormal inclusions are found in peripheral leucocytes and in bone marrow cells and are of diagnostic significance. Ultrastructural studies show lysosomal storage but are dispensable in the routine diagnosis. The mucopolysaccharidoses must be differentiated mainly from the mucolipidoses, a group of disorders with a Hurler-like phenotype and primary involvement of lipid or glycoprotein metabolism.

TABLE IV   *Classification of the mucolipidoses*

Mucolipidosis	Storage substance	Defective enzyme
GM$_1$ gangliosidosis I	GM$_1$ ganglioside &	β-galactosidase
GM$_1$ gangliosidosis II	keratin sulphate	β-galactosidase
Sandhoff disease	sulphatide and acid mucopoly-saccharides	hexosaminidases A & B
Mucosulfatidosis	sulphatide and acid mucopoly-saccharides	arylsulphatases A & B
Fucosidosis	fucose-containing glycosphingolipid	α-fucosidase
Mannosidosis	mannose-containing glycopeptice	α-mannosidase
Mucolipidosis I (probably heterogenous)	?	?
Mucolipidosis II (probably heterogenous)	various lipids, incl. globoside, sulpha-tide; acid muco-polysaccharides	multiple lysosomal enzymes
Mucolipidosis III (possibly heterogenous)	?	probably multiple lysosomal enzymes

REFERENCES

BUSCAINO, G. A. (1968) Difficile inquadramento di una forma clinica di osteochondro-distrofia associata a disturbi neurologici di tipo extrapiramidale. Studio clinicobio-chimico in 4 fraternali. *Acta Neurologica* (Napoli), **25**, 34.

CAFFEY, J. (1952) Gargoylism (Hunter–Hurler disease, dysostosis multiplex, lipo-chondrodystrophy). *American Journal of Roentology*, **67**, 715.

CANTZ, M., GEHLER, J., TOLKSDORF, M. & SPRANGER, J. Unpublished observations.

HALL, C. W., CANTZ, M. & NEUFELD, E. F. (1973) A β-glucuronidase deficiency muco-polysaccharidosis: studies in cultured fibroblasts. *Archives of Biochemistry and Biophysics*, **155**, 32.

HANSEN, H. G. (1972) Haematological studies in mucopolysaccharidoses and muco-lipidoses. *Birth Defects: Original Article Series*, **8**, no. 3, part 14: 115.

KOPITS, S. E., PEROVIC, M. N., McKUSICK, V. A., ROBINSON, R. A. & BAILEY, J. A. (1972) Congenital atlantoaxial dislocation in various forms of dwarfism. *Journal of Bone and Joint Surgery*, **54-A**, 1349.

LANGER, L. O. & CAREY, L. W. (1966) The roentgenographic features of the KS mucopolysaccharidosis of Morquio (Morquio–Brailsford) disease. *American Journal of Roentogenology*, **97**, 1.

LEVIN, S. (1960) A specific skin lesion in Gargoylism. *American Journal of Diseases of Childhood*, **99**, 444.

LOWRY, R. B. & RENWICK, D. H. G. (1971) Relative frequency of the Hurler–Hunter syndromes. *New England Journal of Medicine*, **284**, 221.

McKUSICK, V. A. (1970) The relative frequency of the Hurler and Hunter syndromes. *New England Journal of Medicine*, **283**, 853.

McKUSICK, V. A. (1972) In *Heritable disorders of Connective Tissue*, 4th ed. St. Louis: Mosby.

McKUSICK, V. A., HOWELL, R. R., HUSSELLS, I. E., NEUFELD, E. F. & STEVENSON, R. E. (1972) Allelism, non-allelism and genetic compounds among the mucopolysaccharidoses. *Lancet*, **i**, 993.

MAROTEAUX, P., LAMY, M. & FOUCHER, M. (1963) La malade de Morquio. Etude clinique, radiologique et biologique. *Presse Médicale*, **71**, 2091.

MAROTEAUX, P. (1973) Un nouveau type de mucopolysaccharidose avec athétose et elimination urinaire de keratin-sulphate. *Presse Médicale*, **81**, 975.

MELHEM, R., DORST, J. P., SCOTT, C. I. & McKUSICK, V. A. (1973) Roentogen findings in mucolipidosis III (pseudo-Hurler polydystrophy). *Radiology*, **106**, 153.

MILUNSKY, A. & NEUFELD, E. F. (1973) The Hunter syndrome in a 46XX girl. *New England Journal of Medicine*, **288**, 106.

NEUHAUSER, E. B. D., GRISCOM, N. T., GILLES, F. H. & CROCKER, A. C. (1968) Arachnoid cysts in the Hurler-Hunter syndrome. *Annals of Radiology*, **11**, 453.

SLY, W. S., QUINTON, B. A., McALLISTER, W. H. & RIMOIN, D. L. (1973) Beta-glucuronidase deficiency: report of clinical, radiological and biochemical features of a new mucopolysaccharidosis. *Journal of Pediatrics*, **82**, 249.

SPRANGER, J. & SCHUSTER, W. (1969) Classifiable and non-classifiable mucopolysaccharidoses. *Annals of Radiology*, **12**, 365.

SPRANGER, J. & WIEDEMANN, H. R. (1970) The genetic mucolipidoses. *Humangenetik*, **9**, 113.

SPRANGER, J. & SCHUSTER, W. (1971) Chondoitin-4-sulphate mucopolysaccharidosis. *Helvetica pediatrica acta*, **26**, 387.

SPRANGER, J. (1972) The systemic mucopolysaccharidoses. *Ergebnisse der inner Medizin Kinderheilk*. N.F., **32**, 165. Berlin, Heidelberg, New York: Springer.

SPRANGER, J., LANGER, L. O. & WIEDEMANN, H. R. (1974) In *Bone Dysplasias*. An atlas on generalised disorders of skeletal development. Stuttgart, Philadelphia: Fischer, Saunders.

THOMPSON, G. R., NELSON, N. A., CASTOR, C. W. & GROGELNY, S. L. (1971) A mucopolysaccharidosis with increased urinary excretion of chondroitin-4-sulphate. *Annals of Internal Medicine*, **75**, 421.

WINCHESTER, P., GROSSMAN, H., LIM, W. G. & DANES, S. B. (1969). A new mucopolysaccharidosis with skeletal deformities simulating rheumatoid arthritis. *American Journal of Roengentology*, **106**, 121.

5

Glycosaminoglycans of foetal tissue in two cases of Hurler's syndrome

M. F. Dean and Helen Muir

The mucopolysaccharidoses are a group of connective tissue disorders, classified by McKusick (1966), in which specific recessively inherited enzyme deficiencies result in an inadequate catabolism of glycosaminoglycans (GAGs), leading to an excessive accumulation within the tissues and a greatly increased urinary excretion. In pregnancies where it is suspected that the foetus may have inherited one of these disorders, amniocentesis is often carried out in order to ascertain the GAG composition of the amniotic fluid as a diagnostic aid to prophylactic abortion. A number of instances have now been reported (Matalon, Dorfman, Nadler and Jacobson, 1970; Matalon and Dorfman, 1972a; Crawfurd *et al.*, 1973) in which qualitative and quantitative GAG abnormalities have been detected in the amniotic fluid of suspected cases, presumably due to excretion by the foetus. We have carried out further studies of foetal tissue from two cases of Hurler's syndrome in which GAG abnormalities have been detected following amniocentesis and, in both cases, the GAG abnormalities in the amniotic fluids reflected the abnormalities in the foetal tissues.

Experimental

Livers were removed from the foetuses immediately following abortion and stored at $-20°$ without a preservative. GAGs were extracted by homogenizing the tissue in a Sorvall omnimixer with 0·2 M sodium acetate, pH 6·8 at 4°, the tissue debris was removed by centrifugation and then re-homogenized. The pooled supernatant solutions were then filtered through a pad of 'Hyflo Supercel' (Hopkins and Williams, Chadwell Heath, Essex), GAGs were precipitated from the filtrate with 9-aminoacridine HCl and were converted to their soluble sodium salts by shaking with an aqueous suspension of Dowex-50 in the Na^+ form (Muir and Jacobs, 1967) with added sodium acetate buffer (30 g anhydrous sodium acetate $+15$ ml acetic acid in 100 ml water). The procedure was repeated a second time and the GAGs were finally precipitated in 80 per cent v/v ethanol, washed and dried in acetone.

Amniotic fluid was clarified by centrifugation and dialysed for 24 hours at 4° in Visking tubing, previously heated at 95° to reduce its porosity (Callanan, Carrol and Mitchell, 1957). After recentrifugation, GAGs were precipitated from the supernatant solution with 9-amino-acridine and converted to their sodium salts as described above. The total uronic acid concentration of part of this material was determined (Bitter and Muir, 1962), the remainder was incubated for 24 hours at 37° with 3,000 turbidity reducing units of testicular hyaluronidase (EC 3.2.1.35) and polymeric material was precipitated again with 9-aminoacridine. After reconversion to their sodium salts, the total uronic acid content of the remaining GAGs was determined. The amount of material depolymerised by hyaluronidase was equivalent to the combined amounts of chondroitin sulphate and hyaluronic acid in the sample, whilst the remaining GAGs consisted of dermatan and heparin sulphates.

The percentage composition of GAGs isolated from foetal liver was estimated from the glucosamine/galactosamine molar ratios and uronic acid content before and after incubation with testicular hyaluronidase and reprecipitation with 9-aminoacridine (Dean, Muir and Ewins, (1971). Glucosamine/galactosamine molar ratios were determined with a Locarte amino acid analyser after hydrolysis for three hours in 8 M HCl (Tsiganos and Muir, 1969).

The molecular size of the GAGs was determined by gel chromatography, carried out on a column (12 mm by 550 mm) of Sephadex G-200 packed with 0·2 M sodium acetate pH 6·8. Samples of 2 mg were dissolved in 1·0 ml of acetate, 0·85 ml fractions were eluted in 0·2 M sodium acetate and their uronic acid contents determined by an automated modification of the method of Bitter and Muir (1962).

Results and Discussion

Normal levels of GAGs in amniotic fluids have been found to be about 20 μg/ml (Matalon *et al.*, 1970; Danes, Queenan, Gadow and Cederqvist, 1970). However, values are subject to considerable variation, amounts between 5 and 110 μg/ml being recorded, and they are generally higher during the earlier stages of pregnancy and considerably elevated in cases of rhesus incompatibility (Danes *et al.*, 1970). Elevated amniotic fluid GAG values alone are a poor indication of abnormality, since a value of 30 μg/ml has been recorded in this laboratory in one normal case and a value of only 37 μg/ml in a case of Hurler's syndrome. In these instances, however, 85 per cent of the GAG isolated from the normal sample were degraded by hyaluronidase, but only 25 per cent of the GAGs from the abnormal sample. This illustrated the importance of qualitative analysis in the diagnosis of foetal abnormality in addition to the estimation of the total GAG content.

In the case of a patient 'O' the GAG content was found to be 60 μg/ml and, of this, 78 per cent was not depolymerised by hyaluronidase, i.e. consisted of dermatan and/or heparan sulphates. This elevated GAG content together with the high proportion of dermatan and/or heparan sulphates was considered to be sufficient evidence of abnormality for termination of pregnancy. This was confirmed by comparing the uptake of $^{35}SO_4$ by amniotic cells with the uptake by normal fibroblasts from cultures of foetal skin.

Further examination of the abortus from patient 'O' revealed a number of connective tissue abnormalities analogous to those found in affected children at later stages of the disease. Electron micrographs of this liver (Crawfurd *et al.*, 1973) showed that most cells contained electron translucent vacuoles like the lysosomal storage vacuoles described by Van Hoof and Hers (1964). However, the cells of the CNS showed no sign of such inclusions, nor of Zebra body formation, indicating that in the earliest stages of the disease there is little, if any, accumulation of GAG, or of gangliosides, in the CNS although, presumably, accumulation of partially degraded GAG has begun in the viscera.

Confirmation of the diagnosis was provided by the large amounts of readily soluble GAG extracted from the foetal livers, amounting to 500 μg of uronic acid/g wet weight in the case of patient 'O' and 553 μg of uronic acid/g wet weight in the case of patient 'W'. In contrast, extraction of homogenates of two normal foetal livers of about the same age with iso-osmotic sodium acetate, yielded only 38 μg and 19 μg of uronic acid/g wet weight. The GAGs from the abnormal foetal livers were of low molecular size as evidenced by their elution profiles on Sephadex G-200. They chromatographed primarily as a single retarded component (Fig. 1) with approximate molecular weights of 5,000 in the case of patient 'W' and of less than 5,000 in the case of patient 'O' (calculated from the data of Wasteson, 1969). In contrast, the small

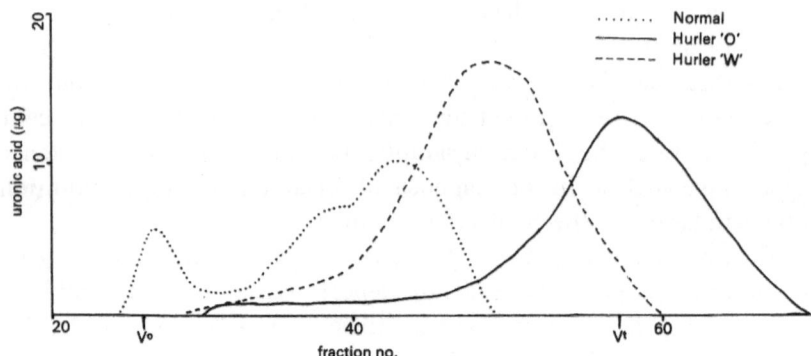

Fig. 1   Gel chromatography on Sephadex G-200 of glycosaminoglycans from two foetal livers in cases of Hurler's syndrome and from a normal foetal liver.

amount of readily soluble material extracted from normal foetal livers chromatographed as three components, one of which was eluted at the void volume of the column and the other two at volumes corresponding to molecular weights of approximately 16,000 and 7,000.

The percentage composition of the GAG isolated from each abnormal foetal liver is given in Table I. The high proportion of dermatan and

TABLE I   *Percentage composition of glycosaminoglycans from foetal livers in two cases of Hurler's syndrome*

	Chondroitin sulphates	*Dermatan sulphate*	*Heparan sulphate*
Hurler 'W'	23	31	46
Hurler 'O'*	9	29	62

* From Crawfurd *et al.*, 1973.

heparan sulphates in foetal tissue suggests that in these cases the deficient enzyme cannot be supplied by the maternal circulation, either because of a placental barrier, or because of a quantitative enzyme insufficiency in the maternal heterozygote.

In each case, heparan sulphate is the predominant GAG, followed by dermatan sulphate, with lesser amounts of chondroitin sulphate. In contrast, heparan sulphate represented only 5 per cent of the easily soluble GAGs in liver and spleen tissues from a 4-year-old boy with Hurler's syndrome (Dean *et al.*, 1971).

The predominant accumulation of heparan sulphate in foetal liver in these two examples of Hurler's syndrome is somewhat unexpected since it is now known that the basic defect is a deficiency in α-L-iduronidase (Bach, Friedman, Weismann and Neufeld, 1972; Matalon and Dorfman, 1972b) and, although iduronic acid residues are present in both dermatan sulphate and heparan sulphate, dermatan sulphate is the GAG primarily affected by this enzyme deficiency. It is possible that at this stage of foetal development the synthesis of dermatan sulphate is less than that of heparan sulphate in the visceral organs, so that an inability to degrade heparan sulphate assumes greater significance, whereas in older tissues partially degraded dermatan sulphate predominates due to the more profound effect of an α-L-iduronidase deficiency on its catabolism than on that of heparan sulphate.

Acknowledgements

We would like to thank the Medical Research Council for a grant to M.F.D. and the Arthritis and Rheumatism Council for their financial support. We gratefully acknowledge help provided by Dr P. F. Benson and Dr R. M. Forrester in supplying us with clinical material.

REFERENCES

BACH, G., FRIEDMAN, R., WEISMANN, B. & NEUFELD, E. F. (1972) *Proceedings of the National Academy of Sciences of the U.S.A.*, **69**, 2048.

BITTER, T. & MUIR, H. (1962) *Analytical Biochemistry*, **4**, 330.

CALLANAN, M. F., CARROLL, W. R. & MITCHELL, E. R. (1957) *Journal of Biological Chemistry*, **229**, 279.

CRAWFURD, M. D'A., DEAN, M. F., HUNT, D. M., JOHNSON, D. R., MACDONALD, R. R., MUIR, H. & PAYLING-WRIGHT, C. R. (1973) *Journal of Medical Genetics*, **10**, 144.

DANES, B. S., QUEENAN, J. T., GADOW, E. C. & CEDERQVIST, L. L. (1970) *Lancet* i, 946.

DEAN, M. F., MUIR, H. & EWINS, R. J. F. (1971) *Biochemical Journal*, **123**, 883.

MATALON, R., DORFMAN, A., NADLER, H. L. & JACOBSON, C. B. (1970) *Lancet* i, 83.

MATALON, R. & DORFMAN, A. (1972a) In *Antenatal Diagnosis*, p. 215. Ed. A. Dorfman, The University of Chicago Press.

MATALON, R. & DORFMAN, A. (1972b) *Biochemical and Biophysical Research Communications*, **47**, 959.

McKUSICK, V. A. (1966) In *Heritable Disorders of Connective Tissue*, 3rd ed., p. 325. St Louis: C. V. Mosby.

MUIR, H. & JACOBS, S. (1967) *Biochemical Journal*, **103**, 367.

TSIGANOS, C. P. & MUIR, H. (1969) *Biochemical Journal*, **113**, 885.

VAN HOOF, F. & HERS, H. G. (1964) *Comptes rendus hebdomadaires des séances de l'Académie des sciences*, **259**, 128.

WASTESON, A. (1969) *Biochimica et biophysica acta*, **117**, 152.

6

The mucolipidoses: with special reference to I-cell disease

Neil Gordon

The mucolipidoses bridge the gap between the mucopolysaccharidoses and the sphingolipidoses. Diagnosis of the mucopolysaccharidoses depends on the appearance of the patient and the finding of excess urinary MPS, but more recently identification of specific enzyme deficiencies has been possible. The diagnosis of the sphingolipidoses such as GM_2 gangliosidosis (Tay Sach's disease) and the sulphatidoses (Infantile metachromatic leukodystrophy) may sometimes be made on clinical grounds, but often depends on establishing the presence of a specific enzyme deficiency. Where the appearance of the child and X-ray findings are suggestive of gargoylism but there is no urinary excess of MPS, then mucolipidosis is a strong possibility. Exceptionally in juvenile sulphatidosis, and possibly in type II GM_1 ganglisidosis, there is however an excess of urinary MPS.

Spranger and Wiedmann (1970) have recently reviewed the conditions categorized as mucolipidoses.

GM_1 gangliosidosis, Types I and II. The affected infant is gargoyle-like in appearance, with hepatosplenomegaly, multiple contractures of the joints and often a cherry red spot at the maculae. The child fails to thrive and rarely survives after the age of 2 years. Generalized dysplasia of the bones similar to that found in Hurler's syndrome is found on X-ray examination.

There is a generalized accumulation of a keratan sulphate-like MPS and the lymphocytes are frequently vacuolated, although the urine has no excess of MPS. The isoenzymes β-galactosidase A, B and C are deficient (O'Brien, 1969).

Type II GM_1 gangliosidosis cases have an abnormal storage of GM_1 ganglioside in the brain and of MPS in the viscera (Kint, 1968) but show none of the generalized features of gargoylism. There appears to be a deficiency of β-galactosidase B and C.

α-Fucosidosis is a rare condition characterized by mild gargoyle-like features and evidence of cerebral degeneration (Durand, Borrane and Della Cella, 1969). An accumulation of fucose-rich MPS arises as the result of interference with the degradation of fucose-containing glycolipids due to the absence of α-fucosidase. Survival past the age of 6 years is rare.

Mannosidosis is an even rarer condition arising from the storag of mannose-containing glycoproteins due to a lack of α-mannosidase (Ockerman, 1969). Features of gargoylism including hepatosplenomegaly are seen and the clinical course is one of fairly rapid deterioration.

Juvenile Sulphatidosis or, as it is sometimes referred to, the Austin type (Austin, 1965) has a later onset than that of the commoner form of metachromatic leucodystrophy, deterioration often not starting until the age of 2 years. The clinical features are a combination of those for metachromatic leucodystrophy and gargoylism including the bone changes of the latter condition. Death occurs before puberty. Features common to metachromatic leucodystrophy include raised cerebrospinal fluid proteins and reduction of nerve conduction velocities. Arylsulphatase A, B and C are lacking but in the infantile type only A appears to be affected.

Mucolipidosis I—Lipomucopolysaccharidosis

The classification of the mucolipidosis types I, II and III is still a very tentative one. In type I, symptoms of gargoylism are mild with only moderate mental retardation. Accumulation of MPS and glycolipids is probable but the urine shows no excess of MPS. Dysostosis multiplex, hepatosplenomegaly and cherry red maculae have been reported. Progress of the disease is slow with ataxia and hypotonia. Cultured lymphocytes stained with toluidine blue show inclusion bodies and nerve biopsy shows metachromatic myelin degeneration. There have been reports (Spranger and Wiedmann, 1970) of increased activity of the lysosomal enzymes, in particular β-galactosidase.

Mucolipidosis II (I-cell disease)

This condition takes its name from the striking granular inclusions seen in cultured fibroblasts (Lercy and De Mars, 1967). Both the clinical and X-ray signs of gargoylism are very marked and the lymphocytes are vacuolated. Severe mental retardation occurs and growth is retarded.

Death usually takes place at an early age from a respiratory infection. High forehead, epicanthic folds, flat antiverted nose, long upper lip, swollen gums and thickened skin are common features. X-ray changes are common including marked periosteal new bone formation, short plump arm bones, irregular metacarpal bones and bullet shaped phalanges. The distal end of the radius and ulna are tilted. The vertebral bodies are short and rounded with possible anterior breaking of D12 and L1. The ribs are broad and the cranial vault thickened (Leroy, Spranger, Fiengold, Opitz and Crocker, 1971). The urinary mucopolysaccharide pattern is normal. The stored material as far as present evidence goes seems to be acid mucopolysaccharides (dermatan sulphate and hyaluronic acid) and lipids (GM_2 ganglioside)—(Crome and Stern, 1972). Dorfman (1972) had found low values of a -L-iduronidase and other lysosomal enzymes, whilst Tandeur *et al.* (1971) found a decrease of liver β-galactosidase activity. Correction factor experiments on cultured fibroblasts suggest that the disease is caused by a deficiency of more than one enzyme.

Mucolipidosis III—Pseudopolydystrophy

These cases show mild mental retardation, with gargoyle-like features such as dwarfism, corneal opacity, slow progressive degeneration (Maroteaux and Lamy, 1960) and bony changes, particularly underdevelopment of the spine and pelvis but there is little evidence that they constitute a storage disease similar to those described earlier.

Case report

A child was admitted to Booth Hall Hospital, Manchester in 1969 with I-cell disease (Gordon, 1973). There was no family history of significance, and an older sibling was normal. The pregnancy and birth were uneventful. Multiple deformities were noted at birth and a dislocated hip was treated. When seen at $2\frac{1}{2}$ years, development was around 8 months and the child could not sit on her own. Cyanotic attacks had occurred during the previous year. Her appearance was highly suggestive of gargoylism. The bridge of the nose was flattened, with antiverted nostrils. The eyelids were puffy, and the eyebrows prominent. The tongue was abnormally large. The cheeks were highly coloured and the skin coarse. There was a prominent abdomen and marked kyphoscoliosis. The right thumb could not be extended or abducted. Both hips were held in 45° abduction due to contractures. There was a generalized hypotonia but the tendon reflexes were easy to elicit. The liver was slightly enlarged. The height was around the third percentile, and the D.Q. on the Griffiths mental development scale was 27.

X-ray examination confirmed a scoliosis, convex to the left. There was a widening of the interpeduncular space in the lumbar spine and the posterior borders of the lumbar vertebrae were concave. The proximal ends of the femora were constricted. The metacarpal and phalangeal cavities were widened, and the cortices were narrow and thin. There was tapering of the lower ends of the radius and ulna.

The E.E.G. showed a non specific dysrhythmia. The analysis of the urine was normal with no excess of MPS. There were abnormal vacuoles in about 30 per cent of the mononuclear cells in the blood. Bone marrow taps were dry and fibroblast cultures were unsuccessful. While further investigations were being planned the child died of pneumonia. Permission for autopsy was refused.

Summary

From family studies it would appear that the mode of inheritance of the mucolipidoses is an autosomal recessive one. The appearance of the children affected by most of these conditions is suggestive of a mucopolysaccharidosis. Although examination of the urine shows no evidence of such a disorder, other investigations may strongly support such a diagnosis. However, in I-cell disease for example, the evidence of lipid storage is less conclusive (Tandeur *et al.*, 1971). In I-cell disease there is also a bewildering number of possible enzyme disturbances. Some of these have already been mentioned, such as the low level of α-L-iduronidase, a gross deficiency of β-D-galactosidase and α-L-fucosidase as well as a lessened activity of other enzymes. Perhaps the explanation is a defect in the lysosomal membrane with leakage of enzymes (Wiesmann, Lightbody, Vasella and Herschkowitz, 1971), or lack of a common recognition site which allows the molecule to re-enter the cell (Wiesmann, this symposium).

A simple explanation for the combination of a disorder of mucopolysaccharide and lipid metabolism would be the involvement of an enzyme for the degradation of both classes of substance. In GM_1 gangliosidosis it has been demonstrated, using liver biopsy material, that a deficiency of β-galactosidase, apart from its role in sphingolipid metabolism, is responsible for an accumulation of a keratin-like substance, since it is also concerned in the cleavage of galactose from a mucopolysaccharide (MacBrinn *et al.*, 1969).

The mucolipidoses seem to offer a particularly interesting sphere for biochemical research, but until this has been done the clinician must hold the responsibility for diagnosis. Therefore, whenever the appearance of a child has even the suggestion of gargoylism combined with a variety of other anomalies, investigations should be directed towards demonstrating a possible disorder of both mucopolysaccharide and sphingolipid metabolism.

REFERENCES

AUSTIN, J. H. (1965) Mental retardation. Metachromatic Leucodystrophy. *Medical Aspects of Mental Retardation*. Ed. C. C. Carter. Springfield: Thomas (III).

CROME, L. & STERN, J. (1972) *Pathology of Mental Retardation*. Eds. L. Crome & J. Stern. London: Churchill-Livingstone.

DORFMAN, A. (1972) The molecular basis of the mucopolysaccharidoses: Current status of knowledge. *Triangle*, **11**, 43.

DURAND, P., BORRANE, C. & DELLA CELLA, G. (1969) Fucosidosis. *Journal of Paediatrics*, **75**, 665.

GORDON, N. (1973) I-cell disease—mucolipidosis II. *Post Graduate Medical Journal*, **49**, 359.

KINT, J. S., DACREMONT, G. & VLIENTINCK, R. (1968) Type II GM$_1$ gangliosidosis. *Lancet*, **ii**, 1080.

LEROY, J. G. & DEMARS, R. J. (1967). Mutant enzymatic and cytological phenotypes in cultured human fibroblasts. *Science*, **157**, 804.

LEROY, J. G., SPRANGER, J. W., FIENGOLD, M., OPITZ, J. M. & CROCKER, A. C. (1971) I-cell disease. A clinical picture. *Pediatrics*, **79**, 360.

MACBRINN, M. C., OKADA, S., HO, M. W., HU, C. C. & O'BRIEN, J. S. (1969) Generalised gangliosidosis: impaired cleavage of galactose from a mucopolysaccharide and a glycoprotein. *Science*, **163**, 946.

MORATEAUX, P. & LAMY, M. (1960) La pseudopdydotrphie de Hurler. *Presse Medicale*, **71**, 2889.

O'BRIEN, J. (1969) Generalised gangliosidoses. *Journal Paediatrics*, **75**, 167.

OCKERMAN, P. A. (1969) Mannosidosis: Isolation of oligosaccharide material from brain. *Journal of Pediatrics*, **75**, 361.

SPRANGER, J. W. & WIEDEMANN, H. R. (1970) The genetic mucolipidoses. *Humangenetik*, **9**, 113.

TANDEUR, M., VAMES-HIRWITZ, E., MOCKEL-POHL, S., DEREUME, J. P., CREMER, N. & LOEB, H. (1971), Clinical, biochemical and ultrastructural studies in a case of chondrodystrophy presenting the I-cell phenotype in tissue culture. *Pediatrics*, **79**, 336.

WEISMANN, U. N., LIGHTBODY, J., VASELLA, F. & HERSCHKOWITZ, N. N. (1971) Multiple lysosomal enzyme deficiency due to enzyme leakage? *New England Journal of Medicine*, **284**, 109.

DISCUSSION
(of papers by Professor Spranger, Drs Muir & Dean and Dr Gordon)

Sinclair (London) on the *Ultrastructure of Lymphocytes in the Genetic Mucopolysaccharidoses.* It has been reported (Belcher, 1972)[*] that 18–39 per cent of lymphocytes in patients with the genetic mucopolysaccharidoses show metachromatic changes in the cytoplasm after staining with toluidine blue at pH 2.

Electron microscopic examination of such lymphocytes involved examination of the lower layer of the buffy coat and embedding in araldite. Three changes were found in the vacuoles which are bound by a definitive membrane:

(1) The commonest findings were electron translucent larger type membrane bound structures (Fig. 1).

(2) Less frequently, finely granular electron dense or multivesicular like bodies were found (Fig. 2).

(3) Membranous whorls, or myelin figure-like structures, were also found (Fig. 3).

The highest concentration of these structures was found close to the Golgi zone and in some examples would appear to originate from it. The numbers of these vacuoles (20–30 per section of lymphocytes) was greater than those recognizable by metachromatic staining and light microscopy.

Weismann (Berne). We have been able to demonstrate a deficiency of a number of lysosomal enzymes in cultured fibroblasts from four cases of I-cell disease, together with an increased activity of the same enzymes in the culture medium. Correspondingly, three patients with the disease were shown to have an increased level of the enzymes in their extracellular fluids. We speculate that, in agreement with Dr Neufeld's findings, the primary cause of this disorder may be found in an inability of the lysosomal enzymes to stay within the lysosomal compartment, due to a recognition defect. It is postulated that the enzymes flow normally out of the cells, but they are unable to be pinocytosed into the cells to affect re-entry.

Gordon (Manchester). Could I ask Professor Spranger two questions,

[*] Belcher, R. W. 1972 *Archives of Pathology,* **93,** 1.

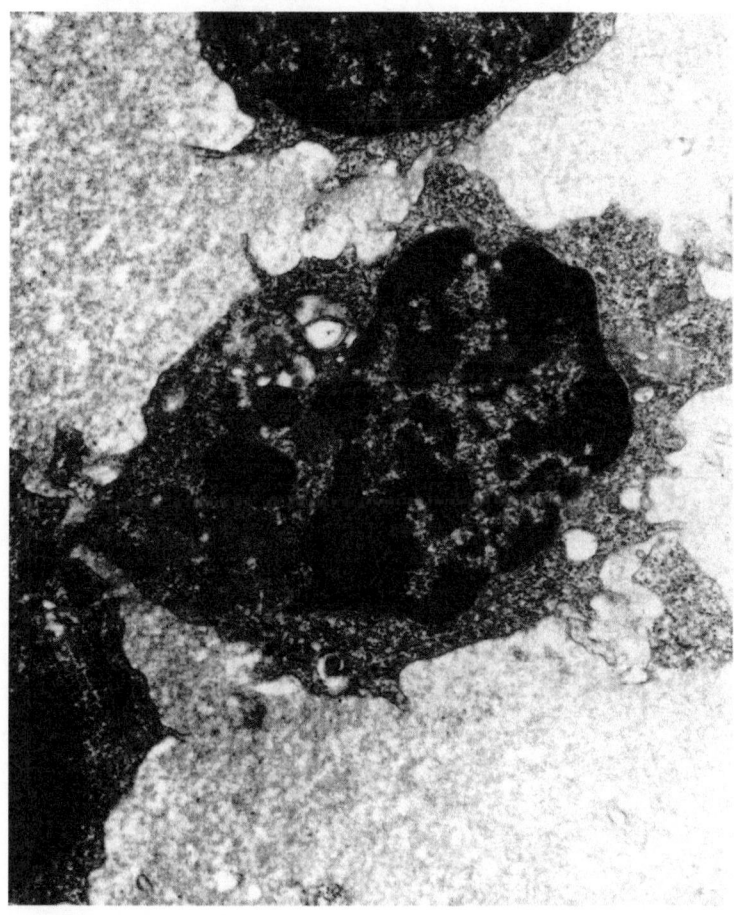

Fig. 1

firstly concerning the early appearances of infants with Hurler's syndrome. Do they look fairly normal in contrast to babies suffering from a mucolipidosis? The second question relates to Sanfilippo syndrome. We have recently seen three cases of this condition, all very severely affected. One died about the age of 12 years, another is just over 13 now and is unlikely to survive very much longer and the third case may not be quite so severely affected. However, the group that we have seen seem to have been almost more severely affected than Hurler's syndrome patients. I would like to ask whether the degree of severity

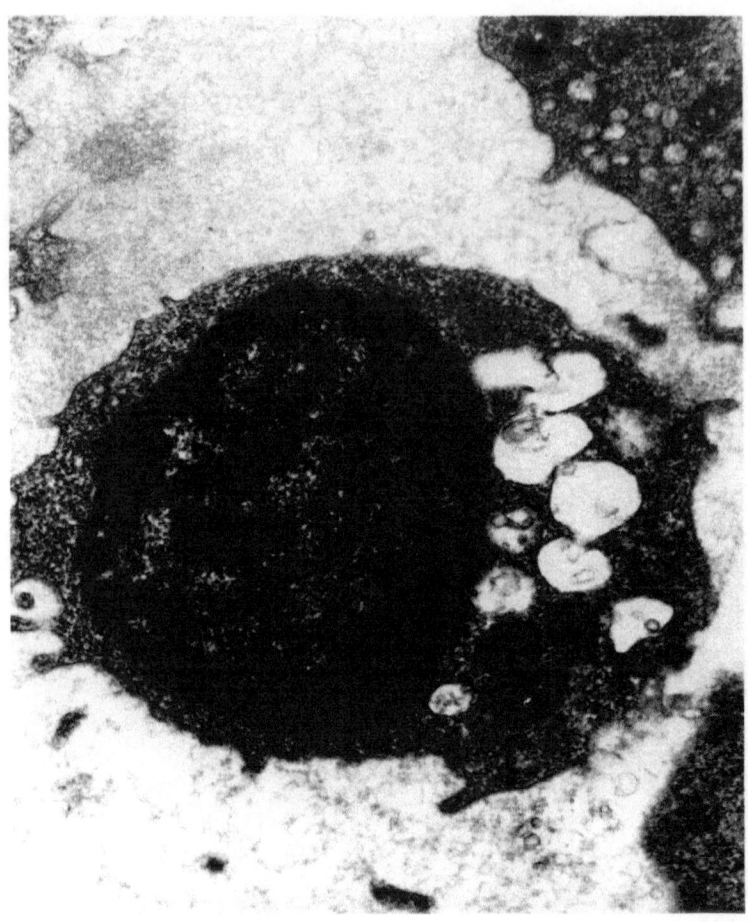

FIG. 2

in Sanfilippo syndrome may be linked up with different types of enzyme disorder?

Spranger. I have not been impressed by clinical changes in the young infant with Hurler disease. Our patients were detected by the radiologist who saw broad ribs and plump scapulae on routine X-ray film of the chest. A marked Hurler-like appearance in a young infant is, in my experience, more compatible with a diagnosis of GM_1 gangliosidosis or mucolipidosis II (I-cell disease) than with Hurler disease.

Gordon. We have just admitted a baby 3 months old who looks grossly

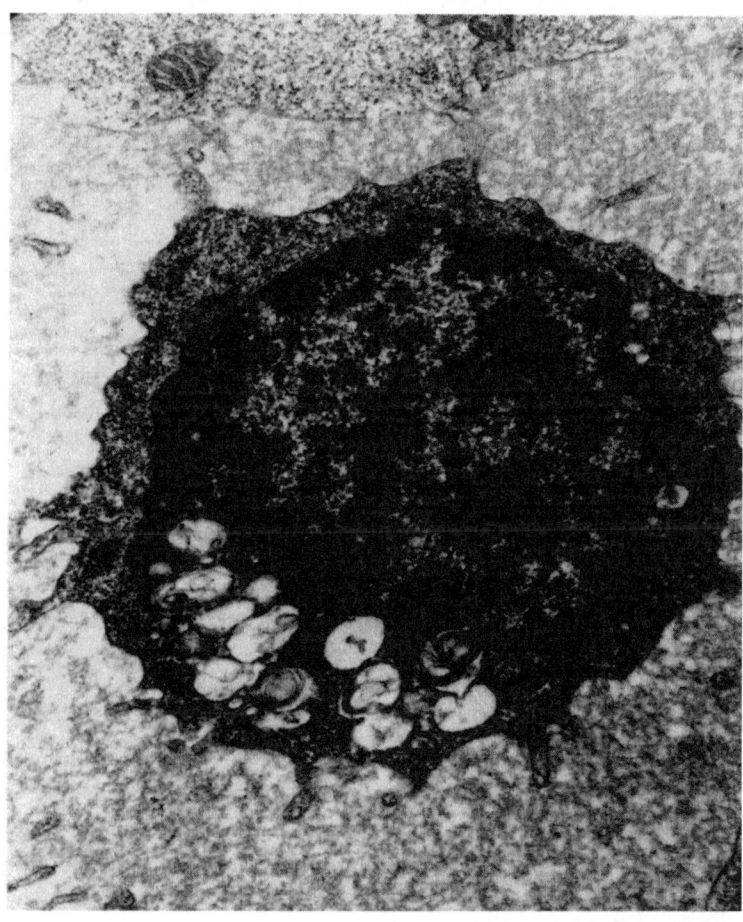

FIG. 3

abnormal and I have been told that there is an older child in the family who has been diagnosed as Hurler's syndrome. This baby then looks abnormal by the age of 3 months and is presumably a Hurler patient, although we haven't completed our tests yet.

Spranger. The results of these tests will be interesting. The infants whom I saw were not grossly abnormal. If radiographs are suggestive of Hurler disease, one must be careful not to overrate developmental variations which are commonly found in normal babies such as a depressed bridge of the nose, epicanthal folds or upturned nares. In

case of doubt, studies of the urinary mucopolysaccharides are indicated
even in the very young infant. I know of one patient with Hurler disease
who excreted excessive amounts of urinary acid mucopolysaccharides
on the first day of life. During and after an exchange transfusion, the
urinary mucopolysaccharides fell to normal levels and rose to the pre-
treatment levels several days later.

In answer to your second question, we did not find striking clinical
differences between Sanfilippo A and B patients, but we did not study
this systematically. I think that there is considerable variability in both
genopathies.

Muir (London). I just wanted to emphasize the normality of the
neonate, because the two foetuses which were aborted at 20 weeks
showed no abnormality of appearance or the skeleton. The liver was
perhaps slightly enlarged although it was full of easily soluble glycosaminoglycans of abnormal type. So you wouldn't perhaps expect the
neonate to look abnormal.

Green (Birmingham). I would like to ask Professor Spranger a
question about the size of the brain. I gather that in types I and II the
brain may be enlarged and this is a true increase of brain substance
(megaloencephalic). However, in type III the brain is small. Does this
mean that in types I and II there is excessive storage, but in type III
there is more degeneration than there is storage?

Spranger. I am afraid that I cannot answer your question. Apparently,
there is mucopolysaccharide and glycolipid storage in Sanfilippo disease
as in Hurler and infantile Hunter disease. One difference between the
conditions is that in mucopolysaccharidosis I and II there is considerable
mesenchymal storage which affects perivascular and leptomeningeal
structures. Leptomeningeal involvement apparently interferes with
cerebrospinal fluid circulation and is probably an important factor in the
development of the hydrocephalus which is present in many patients
with mucopolysaccharidosis I and II but which I have not yet seen in
mucopolysaccharidosis III. Why there should be loss of neuronal cells
in mucopolysaccharidosis III, but not in mucopolysaccharidosis I and
II, I cannot explain.

Green. Is the spinal cord enlarged too in some of the mucopolysaccharidoses, and would this possibly contribute to some of the damage
which can occur?

Spranger. Though the neurones in the spinal cord show storage phenomena, I cannot say whether the size of the cord itself is abnormal.

Teller (Ulm). This question is very difficult to answer, the first one too, because there are really no clear-cut series comparing different weights of the spinal cord and brain of one type versus the others. There are only single cases recorded at autopsy, but no comparison with normal brain, or indeed with other types of mucopolysaccharidosis. I think that's very hard to answer.

Komrower (Manchester). Could I ask Dr Muir if there were any histological changes found in the brain of the affected foetuses she described?

Muir. This is not my work, but an electronmicroscopist could find no abnormality whatever, absolutely none.

Harris (Sheffield). May I ask which bones do you think will show the earliest changes in the young infant?

Spranger. Recalling the beautiful work of Dr Caffey,* he showed marked changes in the long bones of patients with presumed Hurler disease. Comparing his films with newer data, I suspect that Dr Caffey's patients had a GM_1 gangliosidosis or mucolipidosis II (I-cell disease) rather than a mucopolysaccharidosis. In these disorders there is excessive new bone formation along the shafts of the long bones. In Hurler disease, the first changes are widened ribs and plump scapulae. They do not have the periosteal cloaking seen in the mucolipidoses.

Dr Muir's answer regarding the brain histology is very important. If the brain cells are normal *in utero*, early postnatal treatment will hopefully allow a normal development, once treatment becomes available.

Komrower. If anyone was able to examine a positive case, which was born in the last trimester of pregnancy and died in the neonatal period (or say was still-born) it would be interesting to know if there was a significant difference in cell development at that stage compared with what Dr Muir and her colleagues found in foetuses removed earlier in pregnancy. Whether, in fact, the last trimester has a greater significance here.

Teller. I would think this is the case because of the fact that you always get storage phenomena. You get storage phenomena in the fibroblasts cultured from amniotic fluid. I should like to follow this up on the foetus itself, but does anybody know exactly what I can answer to this remark of Dr Komrower's.

*Caffey, J. (1952) *American Journal of Roentgenology, Radium Therapy and Nuclear Medicine*, **67**, 715.

Spranger. I do not know of a positive case born in the last trimester and cannot answer Dr Komrower's question. It is difficult to compare fibroblast storage to neuronal storage. The brain of patients with different mucopolysaccharidoses contains considerable amounts of glycolipids in addition to glycosaminoglycans. Probably, this glycolipid storage is secondary. It may be caused by secondary, non-specific enzyme depression (for instance of acid β-galactosidase) which is induced by stored mucopolysaccharides. Since it is secondary, there is hope that it occurs late in the development of the disease.

Teller. May I ask Dr Spranger three short questions relating to his presentation. Firstly, you mentioned one patient with Sanfilippo's disease (mucopolysaccharidosis III) who had pigmented hair and you indicated that this related to the disease itself. Do you think that the storage phenomena in this disease can go as far as altering the cells, pigmentation of the hair follicle, etc.? Are not Sanfilippo patients usually dark haired?

Secondly, you presented this very striking picture showing the physical appearance of the patient with Maroteaux–Lamy syndrome and you mentioned that his intelligence was 75, or something like this. Is this a unique problem, or do you feel that, in the course of time, all Maroteaux–Lamy patients become mentally retarded? I always had the impression that they were relatively normal.

Thirdly, is it true that a skilled haematologist can diagnose the type of mucopolysaccharidosis by just looking at blood smears and marrow slides? As far as I can remember Hansen himself stated, in his article in the Birth Defects series, that he cannot make the diagnosis from haematological studies only.

Spranger. Taking the last question, Dr Hansen is a very modest man and if he states it like that it is just for the sake of modesty. He cannot differentiate between types I and II. Types II and VI present relatively specific changes. I have learned in the past to re-check my data if they are at variance with Dr Hansen's opinion. The haematologist's help is of even greater importance in the diagnosis and differentiation of the various mucolipidoses. Sometimes I am wrong and they are right, so I think that what he says in his paper is a question of modesty. They can do very well providing they have good smears and in many diseases they need bone marrow smears.

With regard to the first question, concerning the hair in mucopolysaccharidosis III, some of them are well pigmented but I am struck by the fact that many patients have this coarse blonde hair which was shown in the slide. That's not infrequent and there is always that negro baby who turned white. In I-cell disease the hair is not only blonde— one of the prominent findings is the very blonde, whitish-blonde hair— but it is also very fine.

The second question concerned the mental retardation in mucopolysaccharidosis VI. I think that their mental capacity is good but they are severely handicapped people, many of them are blind and many are deaf, so that if they don't get optimal care they appear retarded. If they get good care their mental development probably is normal.

Bickel (Heidelberg). Professor Spranger, you showed us the enormous range of different manifestations and appearances of these conditions. I think many clinicians here, and biochemists, will wonder how many cases they miss and when one should start to suspect one has one of these cases. How highly do you value the Berry screening test, which is so simple and which we do regularly in our own laboratory?

Spranger. I am very pleased with the Berry test.* We use a modification of the original test† and in this form it is very reliable. It is the first thing we do.

Bickel. You went so far as to say that if you get a negative Berry test you start to look at your columns again, is that right?

Spranger. That is correct.

Sinclair. I wonder if I may ask Professor Spranger what his experience of the cardiovascular and pulmonary changes are in patients with mucopolysaccharidosis?

Spranger. The cardiovascular and pulmonary aspects are of particular importance in patients with a good general prognosis, for instance in the adult form of Hunter disease, in mucopolysaccharidoses I–S and VI. In these patients, cardiac failure is a leading cause of death. Haemodynamic abnormalities are mostly the result of valvular incompetence caused by nodular mucopolysaccharide inclusions along the free edges of the valves. The mitral, aortic, tricuspid and pulmonary valves are involved, in this order of frequency. Systemic hypertension is commonly found and is the result of an elevated systemic vascular resistence. Pulmonary complications result from a relatively rigid thorax, obstructed airways and chronic inflammation.

* Berry, H. and Spinanger, J. (1960) *Journal of Laboratory and Clinical Medicine*, **55,** 136.
† Spranger, J. and von Germar, R. (1967) *Mucopolysaccharid-Svchtest, Pädiatrische Praxis*, **6.** 659.

Harper (Cardiff). I was most interested in Dr Dean's and Professor Muir's account of the prenatal diagnosis of Hurler's syndrome. I should like to mention our recent experience in Wales with a family in which a previous sib had been diagnosed as having Sanfilippo syndrome.

We were able to study amniotic fluid and foetal material with the help of a number of colleagues, including Drs Wusteman, Logan and Whiteman, who are here today. Amniotic fluid was analysed in three laboratories using different methods and all agreed in showing large amounts of heparan sulphate, which was also present in the foetal liver. Electron-microscopy studies also showed abnormal inclusions in the liver. Studies using S^{35} on cultured cells were also abnormal and cells sent to Dr Neufeld for cross correction studies showed that this was Sanfilippo type A. Dr Kresse in Germany was able to show complete absence of heparan sulphate sulphaminohydrolase in the cultured cells, so that all the different lines of evidence suggested that the foetus was affected.

I feel that it is important, wherever possible, to use more than one method to establish a prenatal diagnosis, because although an error may be made if one relies on one technique alone, this is unlikely if multiple sources of evidence agree with each other.

Teller. That was a very interesting comment and I am glad that you presented this evidence that one can also pick up the Sanfilippo type A by these means.

Dorfman (Chicago). I would like to make a comment on the use of the amniotic fluid chemical method as a single means of diagnosis. We have given this up because of two unfortunate experiences where the analyses were normal and the infants turned out to be affected. We now insist on doing both sulphate uptake and enzyme studies before we accept diagnosis. I don't mean that it is never abnormal. Part of it is age, and I think it is understandable in that urine contributes very little to amniotic fluid before about the 14th week of gestation. After the 14th week it begins to rise and the urine problem is contributing much more. We had one case where the amniotic fluid was normal at 14 weeks and acted distinctly abnormal at 20 weeks. I agree with what Dr Dean had to say, that qualitative studies were better. We used more specific analyses for heparan sulphate, which is quite easily done and is more valuable. But I would, at least from my experience, caution against using simply chemical analysis for prenatal diagnosis. I think this is dangerous.

Dean (London). May I ask Professor Dorfman whether his two cases

were qualitatively abnormal or merely quantitatively abnormal?
Dorfman. No, they were qualitatively perfectly normal but they turned out to be infants with Hurler disease. They were both done at 14 weeks. We were conscious of the dangers of this at the time, but for reasons beyond our control, no later specimens were ever submitted.

Whiteman (London). We have had amniotic fluid from the abortus of a 21-week-old foetus. We showed an excess of dermatan sulphate in the liquor, but only a very small proportion of heparan sulphate. In fact, it would seem that a more thorough qualitative analysis is possibly necessary if one is to attempt to make a prenatal diagnosis by these means.

7

Structure and Biosynthesis of collagen

Michael E. Grant

Connective tissues, the supporting structures of the body include cartilage, ligaments, tendons, fascia, joint capsules, the subepidermal portions (corium) of the skin, important elements of the heart valves, aorta and small blood vessels and, finally, bone. In general, these tissues comprise cellular and fibrous constituents embedded in the extra-cellular matrix of so-called ground substance. The major components of such tissues are the fibrous proteins, collagen and elastin, and the interfibrillar mucopolysaccharides or proteoglycans; and the relative proportions of these components govern the properties of the different connective tissues. For example, tendon, a tissue requiring high tensile strength and little elasticity, is comprised of over 80 per cent collagen (Table I), whereas cartilage, which is required to be more resilient to pressure than other tissues, has a high content of mucopolysaccharides and contains approximately 50 per cent collagen (Table I).

TABLE I   *Collagen, elastin and acid mucopolysaccharide contents of some tissues**

Tissue	Collagen	Elastin	Mucopoly-saccharides
		(g/100 g dry wt.)	
Liver	4	<1	
Lung	10	3–7	
Aorta	12–24	28–32	6
Ligamentum nuchae	17	75	
Cartilage	46–64		20–37
Cornea	68		5
Achilles tendon	86	5	<1
Mineral-free cortical bone	88		1

* Values taken from literature and originally tabulated by Grant and Prockop (1972) have been approximated to nearest whole number.

The variations in the compositions and the interactions between the components are further revealed by electron microscopy of the various connective tissues, and although the collagen in most tissues is chemically similar (see below) the diameters of the collagen fibrils as well as their spatial orientation relative to each other vary greatly from tissue to tissue. In tendon, the collagen fibrils, which have diameters in the range 300–1,300 Å, are all laid down in parallel bundles along the axis of the tendon whereas the collagen of the cornea is laid down in a very regular network in which the fibrils (all approximately 300 Å in diameter) are in successive layers at right angles to one another. In cartilage, the collagen forms a highly irregular arcade in which it is difficult to see distinct fibrils and in basement membranes, such as the lens capsule, of which collagen comprises some 70 per cent of the dry weight, there is little evidence of any fibrillar structure.

The critical function of collagen is to give strength to, and to maintain the structural integrity of, the various tissues and organs. Consequently, the biological importance of collagen in the individual organism and phylogenetic series is tremendous. Collagen represents approximately 30 per cent of the total protein of the human body and, therefore, any direct or indirect effects which tend to alter the structure and strength of the collagen fibres are likely to have significant repercussions for the organism. In order to appreciate how such modifications, both genetic and non-genetic, can occur during the biosynthesis of collagen, it is necessary to undertake a brief examination of the structure of the collagen fibril (for detailed reviews see Ramachandran, 1967; Bailey, 1968; Gallop, Blumenfeld and Seifter, 1972).

Structure of the collagen fibril

The gross physical strength of collagen is a consequence of (*a*) the molecular structure of the basic unit of the collagen fibril, tropocollagen, (*b*) its packing arrangement in the collagen fibril and (*c*) the subsequent formation of cross-links between the tropocollagen monomers in the fibrils. It is the cross-linking which gives rise to the rigidity of the fibres and their marked insolubility, and it is the specific alignment of the tropocollagen monomers in the fibrils which give rise to the characteristic cross-striations seen when most connective tissues are fixed and stained for electron microscopy. The most prominent cross-striations in collagen fibrils are about 680 Å apart (Fig. 1) and this periodicity is

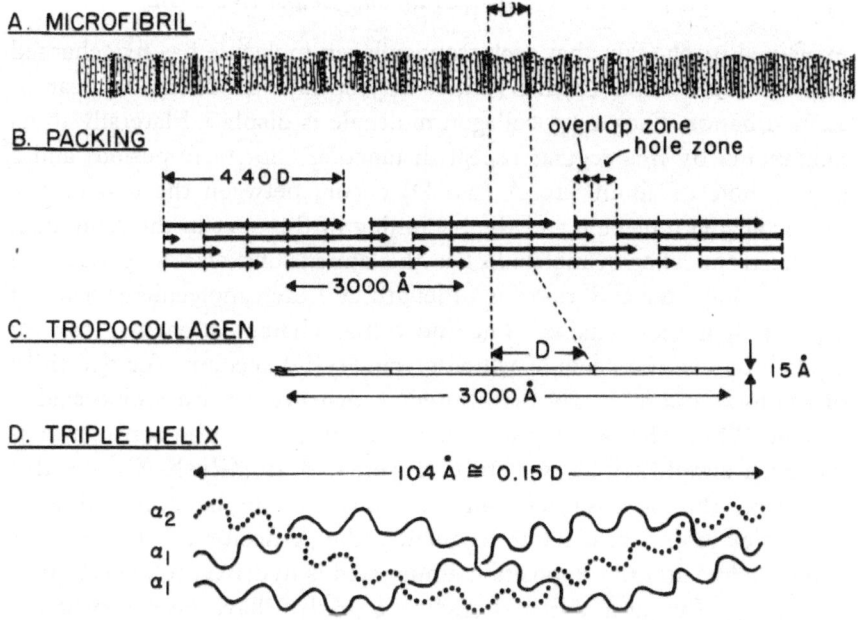

A. MICROFIBRIL

B. PACKING

overlap zone
hole zone

|← 4.40 D →|

← 3000 Å →

C. TROPOCOLLAGEN

|← D →|

← 3000 Å →

15 Å

D. TRIPLE HELIX

|← 104 Å ≅ 0.15 D →|

α_2
α_1
α_1

E. TYPICAL SEQUENCE IN α_1 AND α_2 CHAINS

–Gly–Pro—Y—Gly–Pro-Hypro-Gly–X—Hypro-Gly–X— Hylys–Gly–X—Y—

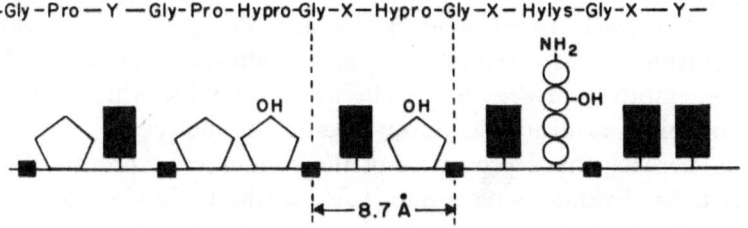

OH   OH   NH$_2$
                         -OH

|←—8.7 Å—→|

FIG. 1   Diagrammatic representation of collagen structure. (Reproduced from Grant
and Prockop (1972) with the permission of the publisher.)
A shows a stained collagen fibril exhibiting characteristic cross striations with a regular
repeat period (D) of approximately 680 Å.
B is a two-dimensional representation of the packing arrangement of tropocollagen
molecules in the fibril. The drawing indicates the lateral displacement of tropocollagen molecules, but not the three-dimensional geometry of the fibril.
C represents the collagen fibril monomer, tropocollagen, which has five highly charged
regions each approximately 680 Å (D) apart which under appropriate conditions
appear as darkly stained bands and account for the repeat period (D) in the fibril.
D indicates that each tropocollagen molecule consists of three polypeptides, two with
identical amino acid sequences (α_1 chains) and one with a slightly different amino
acid sequence (α_2 chain). Each α chain is coiled in a tight left-handed helix with a
pitch of 9·5 Å, and the three chains are coiled around each other in a right-handed
'super-helix' with a pitch of about 104 Å.
E shows that glycine occurs in every third position throughout most of the polypeptide
chains, and there are large amounts of proline and hydroxyproline in the other two
positions.

explained by the fact that each tropocollagen molecule has five charged regions 680 Å apart which (under appropriate conditions appear as stained bands. Each tropocollagen molecule is displaced laterally to its neighbours by this regular repeat distance of 680 Å (D period) and a gap or hole of about 410 Å (0·6 D) occurs between the end of one tropocollagen molecule and the beginning of the next in the same line.

The tropocollagen molecule has the dimensions of a long thin rod 15 Å in diameter and 3,000 Å in length and each molecule consists of three polypeptide chains. The individual chains (α-chains) contain about 1,050 amino acids of which glycine (Gly) accounts for one-third of the total and is evenly distributed so that every third amino acid is glycine. Thus, the polypeptide chains of collagen can be considered as having a simple triplet structure represented as $(Gly-X-Y)_n$. In this structure, the 'X-positions' and 'Y-positions' can be occupied by a variety of amino acids, but frequently the X-position amino acid is proline (Pro) and the Y-position amino acid is hydroxyproline (Hypro). Hydroxyproline and also hydroxylysine (Hylys) have been considered specific to collagen but there is good evidence for a small amount of Hypro in elastin (Foster, Bruenger, Gray and Sandberg, 1973), and both Hypro and Hylys are present in the CLq component of complement (Yonemasu, Stroud, Niedermeier and Butler, 1971; Calcott and Müller–Eberhard, 1972; Reid, Lowe and Porter, 1972). A further distinguishing feature of the amino acid composition of tropocollagen from interstitial collagens is the absence of cysteine which eliminates the possibility of disulphide cross-links in the molecule.

The stereochemical properties of the amino acids, Pro and Hypro, direct the individual polypeptide chains of the molecule into a coiled conformation which is a modification of the poly-L-proline II helix. This minor helix has a residue repeat distance of 2·91 Å and has 3·3 amino acid residues per turn. Although the amino acid content of collagen is not sufficient to stabilize a single polypeptide chain in the helical conformation, the presence of Gly (the smallest amino acid since it has no side chain) in every third position permits the super-coiling of three polypeptide chains about a common axis (Fig. 1). This triple helical conformation having a pitch of about 100 Å is stabilized by hydrogen bonds between HN-groups of Gly in one chain and a O—C group of Pro, or some other amino acid, in the X-position of a second chain (Traub, 1969; Traub, Yonath and Segal, 1969).

The three α-chains have their ends in at least approximate alignment

(Kang, Nagai, Piez and Gross, 1966) and, although the helicity extends throughout most of the molecule, there are regions involving 10–15 amino acids, at both the NH_2— and —COOH termini, which are non-helical. These regions, termed telopeptides, are susceptible to proteolysis whereas the triple helix is resistant to most proteolytic enzymes and in the native form is digested only by specific collagenases (Seifter and Harper, 1971). However, when tropocollagen is heated above 37°, there occurs the triple helix transition to random coils (gelatin) which are readily digested by non-specific proteolytic enzymes. In most body collagens, denaturation of tropocollagen yields two chains of one type, designated α_1, and one of another type, designated α_2. The α_1 and α_2 chains are almost identical but their amino acid compositions differ enough for the chains to be separable by carboxymethyl cellulose chromatography and other techniques.

Collagen having the composition $(\alpha_1)_2 \, \alpha_2$ is found in tissues such as bone, skin and tendon and has been termed Type I collagen or, more colloquially, 'collagen vulgaris'. This terminology was introduced following biochemical studies on cartilage collagen which revealed that cartilaginous structures contain a genetically distinct α-chain (Miller and Matukas, 1969). The collagen has been designated type II collagen. Further studies have shown that the $\alpha_1(II)$ chain is the predominant collagen chain in cartilage and that the chain composition of the majority of the collagen in these tissues may be characterized as $[\alpha_1(II)]_3$ (Trelstad, Kang, Igarashi and Gross, 1970; Miller, 1971; Strawich and Nimni, 1971). Evidence has also been presented suggesting that another genetically distinct α-chain may occur in embryonic skin and it has tentatively been described as a type III collagen (Miller, Epstein and Piez, 1971; Trelstad, Kang and Gross, 1972; Veis, 1972). More definite evidence for a fourth type of α_1 chain present in basement membrane collagen has been presented by Kefalides (1971, 1972) and he has proposed that this collagen, characterized from anterior lens capsule, has the composition $[\alpha_1(IV)]_3$. As the collagens from other tissues and different species are more closely examined, it seems likely that further differences will appear and the nomenclature will become increasingly confused unless a more meaningful connotation for the various collagens can be introduced.

The significance of the variations in primary structure, and whether the collagen monomer is comprised of three identical chains, three different chains or two α_1 plus one α_2 chain, is not understood. In considering possible physiological roles for the genetically distinct collagen in cartilage, it has been suggested that the process of endochondral bone formation would require that cartilage and bone collagens be degraded by mutually exclusive mechanisms because of the close proximity of resorbing cartilage and newly forming osteoid tissue (Robertson and Miller, 1972). In support of this thesis, evidence was reported indicating that human gingival and rabbit polymorphonuclear leukocyte collagenases, which were active against type I collagen, did not cleave the cartilage type II collagen (Robertson and Miller, 1972). However, more recent work has suggested that human skin collagenases will degrade type II chick and human cartilage collagen but the degradation occurs at a slower rate than for the type I collagen (Woolley, Glanville, Lindberg, Bailey and Evanson, 1973; also Woolley, personal communication). Similar results have been obtained with this human skin collagenase acting on soluble procollagens secreted by embryonic chick tendon and cartilage cells (Dehm and Prockop, 1971, 1973), the type I tendon precursor being cleaved more readily than the type II cartilage procollagen (Grant, Harwood and Woolley, unpublished work).

Synthesis of the collagen fibril

It is generally believed that proteins destined for export by the cell are synthesized on membrane-bound ribosomes whereas proteins which remain intracellularly are usually synthesized on free cytoplasmic ribosomes (see Palade, 1966; Campbell, 1970). There is no evidence to suggest that collagen biosynthesis does not fit into this scheme, and the translation of the collagen mRNA's and the assembly of the polypeptide chains is considered to follow the general system of protein synthesis in eukaryotic cells. However, in view of the distinctive amino acid composition, amino acid sequence and triple-helical structure of collagen, as well as the fact that tropocollagen under physiological conditions forms insoluble fibrils, it is not surprising that the intracellular synthesis of the molecule involves several unique biochemical steps.

Post-translational modifications of the primary structure. From the size of the polysomes which synthesize collagen it appears that the synthesis of each chain requires a separate monocistronic mRNA (Lazarides and Lukens, 1971). Although Hypro accounts for about 10 per cent of the collagen molecule and Hylys for about 0·5–4 per cent, depending on the origin of the collagen (Table II), the mRNA's carry no codons for these two hydroxyamino acids. Therefore, hydroxyproline and Hylys are not introduced into the molecule by the usual steps of polypeptide assembly but are synthesized by hydroxylation of Pro and lysine (Lys) residues which have already been incorporated into polypeptide chains (Fig. 2). The recent controversy concerning the

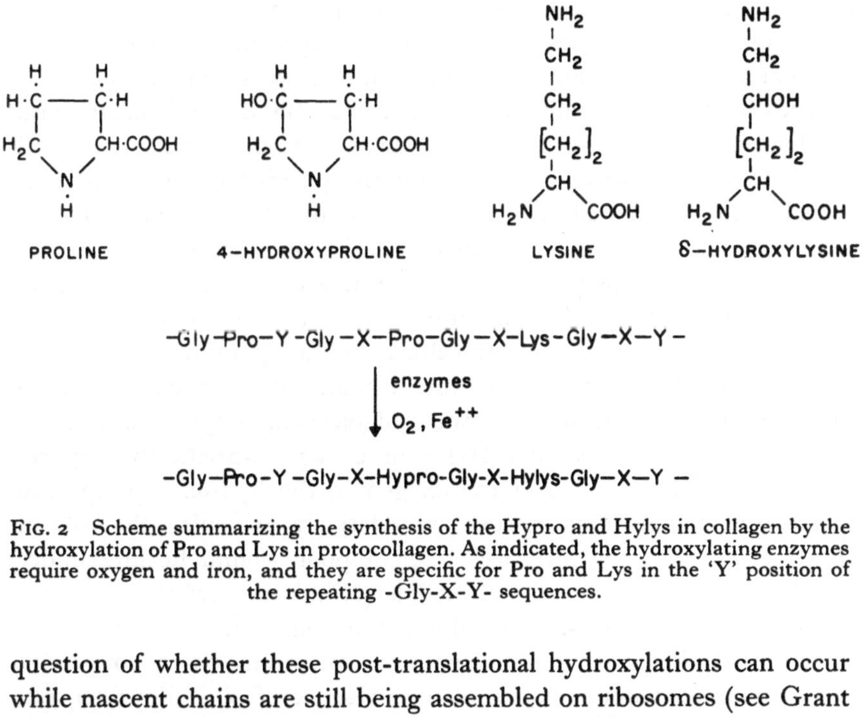

$$-Gly-Pro-Y-Gly-X-Pro-Gly-X-Lys-Gly-X-Y-$$

$$\downarrow \text{enzymes}$$

$$O_2, Fe^{++}$$

$$-Gly-Pro-Y-Gly-X-Hypro-Gly-X-Hylys-Gly-X-Y-$$

FIG. 2 Scheme summarizing the synthesis of the Hypro and Hylys in collagen by the hydroxylation of Pro and Lys in protocollagen. As indicated, the hydroxylating enzymes require oxygen and iron, and they are specific for Pro and Lys in the 'Y' position of the repeating -Gly-X-Y- sequences.

question of whether these post-translational hydroxylations can occur while nascent chains are still being assembled on ribosomes (see Grant *et al.*, 1972) has been largely resolved, and most laboratories now agree that some, if not all, hydroxylations occur at the ribosomal stage (Lazarides, Lukens and Infante, 1971). The fact that collagen has an unusually long synthesis time (Vuust and Piez, 1972), and that the rate at which amino acids are incorporated into peptide linkage is only about one-third of the rate observed in *E. coli* or in reticulocytes, now explains the apparent discrepancies concerning the site of proline hydroxylation (Rosenbloom and Prockop, 1969; Miller and Udenfriend, 1970; Lane, Rosenbloom and Prockop, 1971).

Two separate enzymes are required for the synthesis of Hypro and Hylys and both enzymes exhibit similar cofactor requirements. The prolyl hydroxylase has been studied the most extensively, for this enzyme is more readily solubilized, extracted and purified from connective tissues (Halme, Kivirikko and Simons, 1970; Rhoads and Udenfriend, 1970; Berg and Prockop, 1973a). Studies carried out predominantly in the respective laboratories of Drs Kivirikko, Prockop and Udenfriend have indicated that both enzymes require molecular oxygen, ferrous iron, α-ketoglutarate and a reducing agent such as ascorbate (for review see Grant and Prockop, 1972). In the hydroxylation reaction, the synthesis of 1 mole of Hypro or Hylys involves a stoichiometric conversion of α-ketoglutarate to succinate and CO_2 (Rhoads and Udenfriend, 1968; Kivirikko, Shudo, Sakakibara and Prockop, 1972). The role of ascorbate is not fully understood and ascorbate is not a specific cofactor for the purified enzyme, but it is probably the functional reducing agent required for enzyme activity in intact cells and tissues (for review see Barnes and Kodicek, 1972). On this basis it seems probable that the defective wound healing seen in scurvy is explained by inhibition of the two hydroxylases which subsequently results in an intracellular build up of unhydroxylated collagen and distortion of the protein synthesizing machinery (Ross and Benditt, 1964; Harwood, Grant and Jackson, 1973). Also, because the synthesis of Hypro and Hylys in collagen specifically requires molecular O_2 as a source of the oxygen in the hydroxyl group, and because most connective tissues are relatively avascular, the role of O_2 in these reactions may well explain poor wound healing under hypobaric conditions in animal models (Niinikoski, 1969).

When the hydroxylases are inhibited by elimination of oxygen or chelation of the iron, protein synthesis can continue in connective tissues incubated under N_2 or in the presence of α,α^1-dipyridyl, but instead of synthesizing Hypro and Hylsy and secreting a normal collagen, an accumulation of non or underhydroxylated collagen occurs (Hurych and Chvapil, 1965; Juva, Prockop, Cooper and Lash, 1966). This Hypro and Hylys-deficient collagenous material was described as 'protocollagen' by Prockop and co-workers and was shown to be an excellent substrate for both prolyl and lysyl hydroxylases (Kivirikko and Prockop, 1967). Because protocollagen was obtained only under artificial conditions, it has been considered by some workers not to be a natural precursor of collagen. However, Prockop *et al.* (1973) have argued that, since inhibition of hydroxylation by anaerobiosis is reversed on admitting oxygen to cartilage tissue incubated *in vitro* (Juva *et al.*,

1966), and because many connective tissues are relatively anaerobic and may be subjected to intermittent ischaemia, protocollagen may be a 'normal' intermediate in collagen synthesis.

The studies carried out with connective tissue systems in which the hydroxylations were inhibited have proved most useful in providing an understanding of the role of the hydroxylation process in collagen biosynthesis and the role of Hypro and Hylys in the collagen structure. Recent work in which fibroblasts in tissue culture (Ramaley and Rosenbloom, 1971), and more particularly the freshly isolated matrix-free cells from embryonic chick tendons (Dehm and Prockop, 1971, 1972; Jimenez, Dehm, Olsen and Prockop, 1973; Jimenez, Harsch and Rosenbloom, 1973), were incubated in the presence of α, α^1-dipyridyl have confirmed earlier radiographic studies (see Grant and Prockop, 1972) which suggested that unhydroxylated protocollagen was not secreted by cells. It is now clear that complete inhibition of the hydroxylases results in an intracellular accumulation of fully assembled collagen polypeptides deficient in both Hypro and Hylys which can be considered as true protocollagen, i.e. the amino acid sequence coded in the collagen mRNA's. This protocollagen is not secreted as such and the small portion of material that is secreted is apparently small peptides of degraded protocollagen (Ramaley *et al.*, 1971; Jimenez, Dehm, Olsen and Prockop, 1973). This failure to secrete protocollagen may be attributed to the great affinity of the prolyl hydroxylase for its substrate (Juva and Pročkop, 1969) or the failure of protocollagen to assume a triple helical conformation under physiological conditions (Berg and Prockop, 1973b; Jimenez *et al.*, 1973).

Considerably less information is available about the lysyl hydroxylase but, just as the amino acid sequence required for hydroxylation of Pro is -X-Pro-Gly-, the sequence analyses of the primary structure of collagen suggest that the lysyl hydroxylase preferentially hydroxylates Lys in the sequence -X-Lys-Gly-. However, the requirements for this sequence for the hydroxylation of Lys do not appear to he absolute, for Lys residues in the non-helical telopeptides of both α_1 and α_2 chains of some collagens have been found to be hydroxylated to a varying extent (Piez *et al.*, 1968; Barnes, Constable, Morton and Kodicek, 1971a, b; Stoltz, Furthmayr and Timpl, 1973). Incomplete hydroxylation of both Lys and also Pro in the respective sequences -X-Lys-Gly- and -X-Pro-Gly- has also been observed in several but not all of the triplets that have been sequenced to date (Bornstein, 1967a,b; Butler,

1968; Fietzek, Kell and Kuhn, 1973; Fietzek, Wendt, Kell and Kuhn, 1973). This microheterogeneity of collagen appears to be a direct consequence of the lack of template to direct the introduction of the hydroxyl groups into the molecule (see Grant and Prockop, 1972) but it should be noted that, although the content of Hylys is variable (Table II), all mammalian collagens, with the exception of basement membrane collagens (Kefalides, 1973), appear to contain 90-100 Hypro residues/1,000 amino acids.

The role of Hypro in terms of collagen structure has been the subject of considerable speculation but within the last year it became possible to provide experimental evidence for some of the proposals. The isolation and purification of protocollagen from chick tendon cells incubated in the presence of α, α^1-dipyridyl (Jimenez, Dehm, Olsen and Prockop, 1973) has permitted a direct comparison of hydroxylated and unhydroxylated collagen. The results demonstrate conclusively that Hypro stabilizes the collagen triple helix, for triple helical protocollagen has a much lower melting temperature than its hydroxylated equivalent (Berg and Prockop, 1973b) and is consequently more susceptible to proteolysis (Jimenez *et al.*, 1973; Uitto and Prockop, 1973). Studies on synthetic peptides having the structure $(\text{Gly-Pro-Pro})_n$ and $(\text{Gly-Pro-Hypro})_n$, where n=5 and also n=10, which have the ability to form triple helices, support this concept of Hypro stabilizing the triple helix (Sakakibara *et al.*, 1973). Because of this critical role of Hypro in maintaining the collagen triple helix at physiological temperature, one might anticipate that a mutation resulting in any deficiency in prolyl hydroxylase would be likely to have lethal consequences.

The role of Hylys in collagen structure has been the subject of considerable research since it became apparent that the small amount of carbohydrate found in most interstitial collagens is accounted for by galactose (Gal) and glucosylgalactose (Glc-Gal) in the unique O-glycosidic linkage to the hydroxyl group of Hylys (Butler and Cunningham, 1966; Spiro, 1967) and, also, since it was discovered that Hylys had a major role to play in the cross-linking of collagen fibrils (see Dr Bailey's paper in this symposium for a detailed assessment of this aspect of collagen structure.

The glycosylation of Hylys residues in collagen is of necessity a post-translational modification which has been shown to involve two enzymes, UDP–galactosyl transferase and UDP–glucosyl transferase, both of which require Mn^{++} and appear to be associated with membrane fractions of cells (Bosmann and Eylar, 1968a, b; Spiro and Spiro, 1971a, b). These enzymes have not yet been well characterized, but sequence studies of peptides including glycosylated Hylys residues indicate that most of the Hylys-Gal-Glc is found in sequences having the following general structure:

-Gly-X-Hylys (Gal-Glc)-Gly-X-Arg-.

To date seven sequences of this nature, all containing arginine in the third position of the triplet following the glycosylated Hylys, have been described from both vertebrate (Morgan, Jacobs, Segrest and Cunningham, 1970) and invertebrate tissues (Isemura, Ikenaka and Matsushima, 1972). Thus it may be that the presence of arginine in this position determines whether Hylys in the previous triplet will be glycosylated by the two transferases. However, in studies carried out on anterior lens capsule collagen which is particularly rich in Hylys-Gal-Glc (Table II) the amount of arginine in these peptides does not correlate with the degree of glycosylation of Hylys (Kefalides, 1972).

The role of the carbohydrate moieties in collagen structure have not been specifically defined, but the amount of glycosylated Hylys found in different tissue collagens (Table II) is known to vary from approximately one glycosylated Hylys/1,000 amino acid residues in scleral and tendon collagen to over thirty glycosylated Hylys residues/1,000 amino acid residues in basement membrane collagens (Spiro, 1969; Schofield, Freeman and Jackson, 1972). Since Hylys has such an important role to play in the cross-linking process (Tanzer, 1973), it has been suggested that glycosylation of Hylys might be an intermediate step in a cross-linking process or, alternatively, a means of inhibiting cross-linking of those particular Hylys residues. However, there can be little doubt that the sugars projecting out from the surface of the tropocollagen molecule will help to determine the geometric size and shape of the fibrils that are eventually formed (Morgan *et al.*, 1970; Grant and Prockop, 1972), and an inverse relationship between the amount of sugar associated with the collagen molecule and the diameter of fibrils found in the tissue has been proposed (Grant, Freeman, Schofield and Jackson, 1969).

To date, no disease has been described in which either of the glycosyl transferases are missing but, if discovered, such a genetic lesion may provide some of the answers to the role of Hylys-Gal and Hylys-Gal-Glc residues in collagen structure. Such mutations are not likely to be

TABLE II   *Contents of glycosylated hydroxylysines in several mammalian collagens**

	Total Hylys res/1,000	Substituted Hylys res/1,000	Distribution of carbohydrate units	
			Hylys-Gal-Glc %	Hylys-Gal %
Rabbit sclera	6·4	1·0	56	44
Bovine skin	8·7	2·2	54	46
Bovine tendon	12·6	1·4	64	36
Human heart valve	7·9	4·8	70	30
Rabbit cornea	10·4	5·9	60	40
Bovine cartilage	28·0	14·0	—	—
Bovine glomerular basement membrane	22·3	17·1	97	3
Bovine anterior lens capsule	36·7	32·6	94	6

* Values taken from Spiro (1969), Schofield *et al.*, (1972) and Strawich and Nimni (1971).

lethal, for recently a genetic defect resulting in the virtual absence of Hylys biosynthesis was described in patients who have been identified as having a variant of the Ehlers–Danlos syndrome (Pinnell, Krane, Kenzora and Glimcher, 1972) and have since been shown to have a marked deficiency in the lysyl hydroxylase (Krane, Pinnell and Erbe, 1972). These reports describe the first true collagen disease in man and chemical analysis of the collagen from the tissues of these patients revealed less than one residue of Hylys per tropocollagen molecule. Since all the sugar in collagen from higher organisms is attached to the molecule through the hydroxyl group of Hylys, the data indicate that there was a significant number of molecules which did not contain any glycosylated Hylys. In spite of this absence of Hylys or glycosylated Hylys there appeared to be no defect in collagen secretion and, consequently, the theory that the glycosylation of proteins is a prerequisite for secretion (Eylar, 1966) must put this 'sugar-tag' hypothesis in further doubt (see Winterburn and Phelps, 1972).

A further role of the carbohydrate side chains of collagen has been proposed following studies of the molecular basis of platelet adhesion to collagen which suggested that a platelet membrane–collagen complex is mediated through a membrane-bound glucosyl transferase (Jamieson, Urban and Barber, 1971; Barber and Jamieson, 1971). Further work by Chesney, Harper and Colman (1972) has supported this concept and indicated that multiple sites involving carbohydrate side chains may be necessary for platelet aggregation by collagen, and that the tertiary structure and degree of cross-linking may control the accessibility to these sites.

Secretion of a triple helical precursor of collagen. The synthesis and assembly of multichain proteins is one of the many fascinating aspects of protein synthesis (Williamson, 1969) and the assembly of the unique collagen triple-helix has attracted considerable attention and speculation. Recent work has indicated that the synthesis of the α_1 and α_2 chains requires separate monocistronic mRNA's (Lazarides and Lukens, 1971) and that the α_1 and α_2 chains are assembled simultaneously (Vuust *et al.*, 1972). However, at the moment there is no conclusive evidence whether the triple-helix forms while the chains are being synthesized on ribosomes or at some later stage. Either of these possibilities poses several problems, and the fact that α-chains obtained from extracellular collagen do not readily form triple-helices *in vitro*, and also that tropocollagen forms insoluble fibrils under physiological conditions, has made it difficult to understand how the cell assembles the molecules. In considering these problems, Speakman (1971) advanced the hypothesis that collagen is synthesized as a precursor with terminal segments having structures which facilitate rapid association. Speakman termed these hypothetical extensions 'registration peptides' and he proposed that they could be removed enzymatically after the three appropriate α chains were brought together to allow the rest of the molecule to coil into the in-register triple-helix.

Evidence for such a precursor came from three or more approaches. Tissue cultured fibroblasts probably provided the first suggestions that the initial collagen synthesized and secreted had properties different from tropocollagen (Fessler and Smith, 1970; Layman, McGoodwin and Martin, 1971) but the first definitive evidence for a precursor, which has been termed procollagen, came from studies carried out on connective tissues from cattle in Belgium which were found to have a recessive genetic defect resulting in an extremely fragile skin (Lenaers,

Nusgens, Ansay and Lapière, 1971; Lenaers, Ansay, Nusgens and Lapière, 1971). This condition, which is known as dermatosparaxis, was reported some years ago (Hanset and Ansay, 1967) and has since been encountered in cattle in Texas (O'Hara, Read, Romane and Bridges, 1970). More recently a similar disease has been described among sheep in Norway (Helle and Ness, 1972). In both the afflicted cattle and sheep, the disease manifests itself at birth or soon after by the fact that the skin readily tears with mild trauma. Multiple wounds arising in this manner lead to secondary infections which, in the case of the Norwegian sheep, proved lethal within the first week or two of life.

The collagen extracted from dermatosparactic skin contains a significant quantity of abnormal polypeptides (pro–α_1 and α_2 chains) which were shown to be α_1 and α_2 chains prolongated by an extra peptide at their N-terminal extremity (Lenaers, Ansay, Nusgens and Lapière, 1971). At approximately the same time, Bellamy and Bornstein (1971) presented evidence for procollagen, the biosynthetic precursor of collagen, using isotopic labelling in studies of rat calvaria in culture; and Jimenez, Dehm and Prockop (1971), using freshly isolated matrix-free embryonic chick tendon cells, demonstrated that the first collagen polypeptides synthesized and secreted had molecular weights of approximately 125,000 daltons. Limited cleavage of the secreted procollagen with pepsin resulted in a molecule with polypeptides resembling α chains in molecular size and chromatographic properties (Bellamy et al., 1971; Jimenez et al., 1971; Uitto, Jimenez, Dehm and Prockop, 1972). The results suggested that the secreted procollagen was triple helical but the extra peptides were non-helical and likely to have an amino acid composition significantly different from the collagenous-Gly-X-Y-triplet structure.

Electron microscopy of segment-long-spacing aggregates of the procollagen secreted by embryonic tendon cells (Fig. 3) reveals an extension of about 130 Å at the NH_2-terminal end (Dehm et al., 1972) which was similar to the extensions seen when procollagen from dermatosparactic skin was similarly examined in the electron microscope (Stark, Lenaers, Lapière and Kuhn, 1971). Characterization of the NH_2-terminal extensions, or registration peptides, has proceeded rapidly and there now seems general agreement that these peptides are atypical with respect to collagen because they contain some cysteine, or cystine, and probably some tryptophan, an amino acid not found in tropocollagen (Lenaers, Nusgens, Ansay and Lapière, 1971; Dehm,

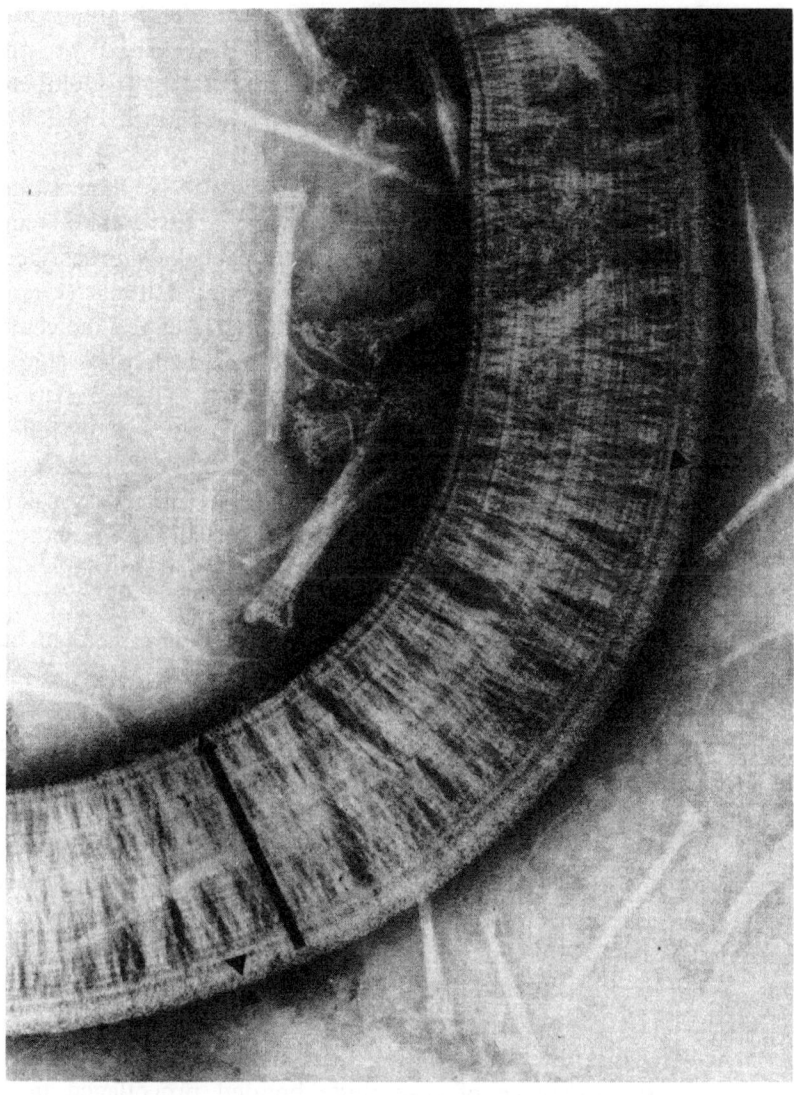

FIG. 3 Segment-Long-Spacing (SLS) Aggregate of Procollagen. [Photograph kindly provided by Dr Bjorn R. Olsen, Dept. of Biochemistry, Rutgers Medical School, New Jersey, U.S.A.] Procollagen secreted by embryonic chick tendon cells was dissolved in acetic acid and then dialysed against a solution of ATP, which in a non-specific reaction makes the collagen form aggregates. In the aggregates the individual molecules are in parallel alignment with the ends in register and not staggered as they are in the native fibril (Fig. 1). The aggregates were stained with 1 per cent potassium phosphotungstate (pH 7·0) and then examined in the electron microscope. The arrow indicates the length of the tropocollagen molecule and the amino-terminal extension of about 130 Å is seen in the procollagen SLS. (Magnification × 180,000.)

Jimenez, Olsen and Prockop, 1972; Bornstein, von der Mark, Wyke, Ehrlich and Monson, 1972; Uitto *et al.*, 1972; Burgeson, Wyke and Fessler, 1972; Tsai and Green, 1972; Furthmayr *et al.*, 1973; Goldberg, Epstein and Sherr, 1972; Dehm *et al.*, 1973; von der Mark and Bornstein, 1973).

Measurements of the molecular weights of the pro–α polypeptides from various tissues have ranged from 101,000 to 125,000 daltons and the highly glycosylated basement membrane procollagen has been estimated to comprise polypeptides of 140,000 daltons (Grant, Kefalides and Prockop, 1972). More recent estimates of the molecular weight of the tendon procollagen, based on amino acid analyses, suggest that each chain is about 110,000 (Uitto *et al.*, 1972). These variations in published molecular weights for the pro–α chains may simply reflect differences in the accuracy of the various techniques employed. However, one cannot yet rule out the possibility that NH_2-terminal extensions vary in the procollagens from different tissues or that different methods of isolation may result in some loss of part of the extensions (see Prockop *et al.*, 1973; Bornstein and Monson, 1973).

The role of these additional sequences in the collagen precursor has been discussed by Grant and Prockop (1972), Bornstein (1972) and Schofield and Prockop (1973) and it is clear that the extensions make the physical properties of the polypeptide chains different from α-chains. The proposal of Speakman (1971), that registration peptides might serve to align the chains and accelerate helix formation, can be considered initially. There is, as yet, no information available comparing the rates of renaturation of pro–α chains and α-chains respectively. However, the finding of cysteine incorporation into the NH_2-terminal extensions (Dehm, Jimenez, Olsen and Prockop, 1972; Uitto *et al.*, 1972; Tsai *et al.*, 1972; von der Mark *et al.*, 1973) raises the possibility of disulphide bonding between pro-α chains, which could promote alignment of chains thereby initiating helix formation. There is good evidence for the existence of disulphide bonded procollagen being secreted by cells (Dehm *et al.*, 1972; Burgeson *et al.*, 1972; Smith, Byers and Martin, 1972; Goldberg and Sherr, 1973) and recent studies on the synthesis of collagen by embryonic chick lens cells suggest that the formation of disulphide bonds among the precursor polypeptide chains of lens capsule procollagen may be of considerable importance in promoting the formation of the triple helix (Grant, Schofield, Kefalides and Prockop, 1973).

A second function for procollagen might be that the additional sequences modify the fibrogenic properties of collagen. It is well known that tropocollagen molecules aggregate spontaneously under physiological conditions. Such aggregation would result in precipitation of collagen fibrils and would not be desirable at the site of synthesis. For this reason, it would be logical to place the additional sequences at the NH_2-terminal end which is synthesized first. In fact, there is good evidence to suggest that procollagen is completely soluble under conditions which lead to the precipitation of collagen fibres (Dehm, Jiminez, Olsen and Prockop, 1972; Bornstein, 1972) and, for this reason, Prockop and co-workers have tended to consider the precursor as a 'transport' form of collagen (Jimenez *et al.*, 1971; Dehm and Prockop, 1972). However, whether the extra peptides in procollagen serve in some manner in the intracellular translocation and secretion of the protein is highly speculative. Nevertheless, it is clear from the electron microscopic studies on the dermatosparactic tissues of both cattle (Hanset *et al.*, 1967; O'Hara *et al.*, (1970) and sheep (Fjølstad and Helle, in preparation) that the additional peptides inhibit the formation of uniform fibres and of fibres capable of producing the normal cross-links (Bailey and Lapière, 1973).

Formation of collagen fibrils

As discussed above, collagen is an insoluble crystalloid under physiological conditions and the self assembly of tropocollagen into fibrils can be readily demonstrated *in vitro*. Until recently, the problem of how the fibroblast synthesizes and secretes the apparently insoluble tropocollagen has been well-discussed but ill-understood. The discovery of the heritable dermatosparactic condition in cattle and subsequent observations indicating that the first collagen synthesized and extruded by connective tissue cells is larger than tropocollagen, seems to have resolved this problem. Many questions remain on the exact details of the intracellular processing of the procollagen, its secretion, its extracellular transport to the site of fibril formation and the control of these processes. However, it is clear that before fibril formation occurs the NH_2-terminal extensions are removed enzymatically (Bellamy and Bornstein, 1971; Jimenez *et al.*, 1971). The exact site of cleavage of the procollagen is not known and although the possibility of the intracellular or cell membrane-mediated conversion of procollagen to tropocollagen has been postulated (Ehrlich and Bornstein, 1972), much of the available evidence suggests an extracellular conversion (Jimenez *et al.*, 1971; Kerwar, Kohn, Lapière and Weissbach, 1972; Goldberg *et al.*, 1973).

The nature of the enzyme or enzymes bringing about the cleavage of the collagen fibril precursor is under investigation in several laboratories and the demonstration of an extract of connective tissues having neutral procollagen peptidase activity has been reported (Lapière, Lenaers and Kohn, 1971; Bornstein, Ehrlich and Wyke, 1972). This activity is absent in the Belgian cattle with dermatosparaxis (Lenaers, Ansay, Nusgens, and Lapière, 1971) and preliminary studies carried out on some patients which present with joint dislocation, torn ligaments and fragile skin, suggests that a similar human disease may occur (Lichtenstein and Martin, personal communication).

The possibility that the procollagen to tropocollagen conversion may involve more than one cleavage performed by one or more enzymes has been proposed (Veis, Anesey, Garvin and Dimuzio, 1972; Goldberg *et al.*, 1973; Bornstein *et al.*, 1973). Intermediates in this conversion may have a role to play in fibrillogenesis, for Veis and co-workers have been able to extract from denatured acid soluble rat and bovine skin collagens, polypeptides (α_h chains), slightly larger than normal α-chains but smaller than pro-α chains (Veis *et al.*, 1972; Veis, Anesey, Yuan and Levy, 1973), which have heightened aggregative properties (Clark and Veis, 1972). Thus it is conceivable that the NH_2-terminal extensions of procollagen may serve a structural role extracellularly and the presence of cysteine in these peptides may also promote the covalent association of collagen and non-collagenous proteins (Burgeson *et al.*, 1972; Kefalides, 1973).

Once formed, tropocollagen spontaneously aggregates into fibrils as a result of interactions of polar and non-polar side groups of adjacent molecules. These interactions must be highly specific to produce the precisely overlapped array seen in most collagen fibrils (Fig. 1). and unlike most globular proteins the side chains of the collagen molecule are on the outside of a rigid structure with the result that interactions can only be intermolecular. Accordingly, collagen fibrils are readily dissolved by moderate changes in pH or salt concentration and have a very low tensile strength unless they are cross-linked. Thus, weak non-convalent interactions are sufficient to form fibril, but convalent cross-links are necessary to prevent its disruption by slippage of molecules past one another when under tension. It is clear that defects that result in either too little or too much cross-linking may have considerable significance (see Bailey—this symposium).

Earlier reference was made to the variation in connective tissue architecture and the possible role of glycosylated Hylys in directing fibril formation (see Grant and Prockop, 1972). Therefore, subtle differences in the chemical structure of tropocollagen may account for differences in the appearance and geometry of collagen fibrils formed in various tissues, but it must be remembered that fibril formation *in vivo* occurs in the extracellular phase of connective tissues that contain serum proteins, proteoglycans and perhaps other tissue specific glycoproteins. Glycosaminoglycans and proteoglycans have marked effects on the rate at which collagen fibrils are formed *in vitro* (Obrink, 1973) and it seems likely that they may play a physiological role in collagen fibrillogenesis (Jackson and Bentley, 1968).

REFERENCES

BAILEY, A. J. (1968) In *Comprehensive Biochemistry*, Vol. 26B, p. 297. Eds. M. Florkin & E. H. Stotz. Amsterdam: Elsevier Publishing Co.

BAILEY, A. J. & LAPIÈRE. C. M. (1973) *European Journal of Biochemistry*, **34**, 91.

BARBER, A. J. & JAMIESON, G. A. (1971) *Biochimica et biophysica acta*, **252**, 533.

BARNES, M. J., CONSTABLE, B. J., MORTON, L. F. & KODICEK, E. (1971a) *Biochemical Journal*, **125**, 433.

BARNES, M. J., CONSTABLE, B. J., MORTON, L. F. & KODICEK, E. (1971b) *Biochemical Journal*, **125**, 925.

BARNES, M. J. & KODICEK, E. (1972) *Vitamins and Hormones*, **30**, 1.

BELLAMY, G. & BORNSTEIN, P. (1971) *Proceedings of the National Academy of Sciences of the United States of Americ*, **68**, 1138.

BERG, R. A. & PROCKOP, D. J. (1973a) *Journal of Biological Chemistry*, **248**, 1175.

BERG, R. A. & PROCKOP, D. J. (1973b) *Biochemical and Biophysical Research Communication*, **52**, 115.

BORNSTEIN, P. (1967a) *Journal of Biological Chemistry*, **242**, 2572.

BORNSTEIN, P. (1967b) *Biochemistry*, 6, 3082.

BORNSTEIN, P. (1972) In *The Comparative Molecular Biology of Extracellular Matrices*, p. 309. Ed. H. Slavkin. New York: Academic Press.

BORNSTEIN, P., EHRLICH, H. P. & WYKE, A. W. (1972) *Science*, **175**, 544.

BORNSTEIN, P., VON DER MARK, K., WYKE, A. W., EHRLICH, H. P. & MONSON, J. M. (1972) *Journal of Biological Chemistry*, **247**, 2808.

BORNSTEIN, P. & MONSON, J. M. (1973) *Abstracts Ninth International Congress of Biochemistry*, Stockholm, p. 423.

BOSMANN, H. B. & EYLAR, E. H. (1968a) *Biochemical and Biophysical Research Communications*, **30**, 89.

BOSMANN, H. B. & EYLAR, E. H. (1968b) *Biochemical and Biophysical Research Communications*, **33**, 340.

BURGESON, R. E., WYKE, A. W. & FESSLER, J. H. (1972) *Biochemical and Biophysical Research Communications*, **48**, 892.

BUTLER, W. T. (1968) *Science*, **161**, 796.

BUTLER, W. T. & CUNNINGHAM, L. W. (1966) *Journal of Biological Chemistry*, **241**, 3882.

CALCOTT, M. A. & MÜLLER-EBERHARD, H. J. (1972) *Biochemistry*, **11**, 3443.

CAMPBELL, P. N. (1970) *Federation of European Biochemical Societies Letters*, **7**, 1.

CHESNEY, C. M., HARPER, E. & COLMAN, R. W. (1972) *Journal of Clinical Investigation*, **51**, 2693.

CLARK, C. C. & VEIS, A. (1972) *Biochemistry*, **11**, 494.
DEHM, P., JIMENEZ, S. A., OLSEN, B. R. & PROCKOP, D. J. (1972) *Proceedings of the National Academy of Sciences of the United States of America*, **69**, 60.
DEHM, P. & PROCKOP, D. J. (1971) *Biochimica et biophysica acta*, **240**, 358.
DEHM, P. & PROCKOP, D. J. (1972) *Biochimica et biophysica acta*, **264**, 375.
DEHM, P. & PROCKOP, D. J. (1973) *European Journal of Biochemistry*, **35**, 159.
EHRLICH, H. P. & BORNSTEIN, P. (1972) *Nature (New Biology)*, **238**, 257.
EYLAR, E. H. (1966) *Journal of Theoretical Biology*, **10**, 89.
FESSLER, J. & SMITH, L. A. (1970) In *Chemistry and Molecular Biology of the Intercellular Matrix*, Vol. 1, p. 457. Ed. E. A. Balazs. New York: Academic Press.
FIETZEK, P. P., KELL, I. & KUHN, K. (1973) *Federation of European Biochemical Societies Letters*, **26**, 66.
FIETZEK, P. P., WENDT, P., KELL, I. & KUHN, K. (1973) *Federation of European Biochemical Societies Letters*, **26**, 74.
FOSTER, J. A., BRUENGER, E., GRAY, W. R. & SANDBERG, L. B. (1973) *Journal of Biological Chemistry*, **248**, 2876.
FURTHMAYR, H., TIMPL, R., STARK, M., LAPIÈRE, C. M. & KUHN, K. (1973) *Federation of European Biochemical Societies Letters*, **28**, 247.
GALLOP, P. M., BLUMENFELD, O. O. & SEIFTER, S. (1972) *Annual Review of Biochemistry*, **41**, 617.
GOLDBERG, B., EPSTEIN, E. H. JR. & SHERR, C. J. (1972) *Proceedings of the National Academy of Sciences of the United States of America*, **69**, 3655.
GOLDBERG, B. & SHERR, C. J. (1973) *Proceedings of the National Academy of Science of the United States of America*, **70**, 361.
GRANT, M. E., FREEMAN, I. L., SCHOFIELD, J. D. & JACKSON, D. S. (1969) *Biochimica et biophysica acta*, **177**, 682.
GRANT, M. E., KEFALIDES, N. A. & PROCKOP, D. J. (1972), *Journal of Biological Chemistry*, **247**, 3545.
GRANT, M. E. & PROCKOP, D. J. (1972) *New England Journal of Medicine*, **286**, 194, 242, 291.
GRANT, M. E., SCHOFIELD, J. D., KEFALIDES, N. A. & PROCKOP, D. J. (1973) *Journal of Biological Chemistry*, **248**, 7432.
HALME, J., KIVIRIKKO, K. I. & SIMONS, K. (1970) *Biochimica et biophysica acta*, **198**, 460.
HANSET, R. & ANSAY, M. (1967) *Annales de médecine vétérinaire*, **7**, 451.
HARWOOD, R., GRANT, M. E. & JACKSON, D. S. (1973) *Biochemical Society Transactions*, **1**, 1217.
HELLE, O. & NESS, O. (1972) *Acta veterinaria Scandinavica*, **13**, 443.
HURYCH, J. & CHVAPIL, M. (1965) *Biochimica et biophysica acta*, **97**, 361.
ISEMURA, M., IKENAKA, T. & MATSUSHIMA, Y. (1972) *Biochemical and Biophysical Research Communications*, **46**, 457.
JAMIESON, G. A., URBAN, C. L. & BARBER, A. J. (1971) *Nature (New Biology)*, **234**, 5.
JACKSON, D. S. & BENTLEY, J. P. (1968) In *Treatise on Collagen*, Vol. 2A, p. 189. Ed. B. S. Gould. New York: Academic Press.
JIMENEZ, S. A., DEHM, P. & PROCKOP, D. J. (1971) *Federation of European Biochemical Societies Letters*, **17**, 245.
JIMENEZ, S. A., DEHM, P., OLSEN, B. R. & PROCKOP, D. J. (1973) *Journal of Biological Chemistry*, **248**, 720.
JIMENEZ, S. A., HARSCH, M. & ROSENBLOOM, J. (1973) *Biochemical and Biophysical Research Communications*, **52**, 106.
JUVA, K. & PROCKOP, D. J. (1969) *Journal of Biological Chemistry*, **244**, 6486.
JUVA, K., PROCKOP, D. J., COOPER, G. W. & LASH, J. W. (1966) *Science*, **152**, 92.
KANG, A. H., NAGAI, Y., PIEZ, K. A. & GROSS, J. (1966) *Biochemistry*, **5**, 509.
KEFALIDES, N. A. (1971) *Biochemical and Biophysical Research Communications*, **45**, 226.
KEFALIDES, N. A. (1972) *Biochemical and Biophysical Research Communications*, **47**, 1151.
KEFALIDES, N. A. (1973) *International Review of Connective Tissue Research*, **6**, 63.
KERWAR, S. S., KOHN, L. D., LAPIÈRE, C. M. & WEISSBACH, H. (1972) *Proceedings of the National Academy of Sciences of the United States of America*, **69**, 2727.
KIVIRIKKO, K. I. & PROCKOP, D. J. (1967) *Proceedings of the National Academy of Sciences of the United States of America*, **57**, 782.
KIVIRIKKO, K. I., SHUDO, K., SAKAKIBARA, S. & PROCKOP, D. J. (1972) *Biochemistry*, **11**, 122.

KRANE, S. M., PINNELL, S. R. & ERBE, R. W. (1972) *Proceedings of the National Academy of Sciences of the United States of America*, **69**, 2899.

LANE, J. M., ROSENBLOOM, J. & PROCKOP, D. J. (1971) *Nature (New Biology)*, **232**, 191.

LAPIÈRE, C. M., LENAERS, A. & KOHN, L. D. (1971) *Proceedings of the National Academy of Sciences of the United States of America*, **68**, 3054.

LAYMAN, D. L., McGOODWIN, E. B. & MARTIN, G. R. (1971) *Proceedings of the National Academy of Sciences of the United States of America*, **68**, 454.

LAZARIDES, E. L. & LUKENS, L. N. (1971) *Nature (New Biology)*, **232**, 37.

LAZARIDES, E. L., LUKENS, L. N. & INFANTE, A. A. (1971) *Journal of Molecular Biology*, **58**, 831.

LENAERS, A., NUSGENS, B., ANSAY, M. & LAPIÈRE, C. M. (1971) *Hoppe-Seylers Zeitschrift für physiologische Chemie*, **352**, 14.

LENAERS, A., ANSAY, M., NUSGENS, B. V. & LAPIÈRE, C. M. (1971) *European Journal of Biochemistry*, **23**, 533.

MILLER, E. J. (1971) *Biochemistry*, **10**, 3030.

MILLER, E. J. & MATUKAS, V. J. (1969) *Proceedings of the National Academy of Sciences of the United States of America*, **64**, 1264.

MILLER, E. J., EPSTEIN, E. H. JR. & PIEZ, K. A. (1971) *Biochemical and Biophysical Research Communications*, **42**, 1024.

MILLER, R. L. & UDENFRIEND, S. (1970) *Archives of Biochemistry and Biophysics*, **139**, 104.

MORGAN, P. H., JACOBS, H. G., SEGREST, J. P. & CUNNINGHAM, L. W. (1970) *Journal of Biological Chemistry*, **245**, 5042.

NIINIKOSKI, J. (1969) *Acta physiologica Scandinavica, Supplement*, **334**, 1.

OBRINK, B. (1973) *European Journal of Biochemistry*, **34**, 129.

O'HARA, P. J., READ, K. K., ROMANE, W. N. & BRIDGES, C. H. (1970) *Laboratory Investigation*, **23**, 307.

PALADE, G. E. (1966) *Journal of the American Medical Association*, **198**, 815.

PIEZ, K. A., BLADEN, H. A., LANE, J. M., MILLER, E. J., BORNSTEIN, P., BUTLER, W. T. & KANG, A. H. (1968) *Brookhaven Symposia in Biology*, **21**, 345.

PINNELL, S. R., KRANE, S. M., KENZORA, J. E. & GLIMCHER, M. J. (1972) *New England Journal of Medicine*, **286**, 1013.

PROCKOP, D. J., DEHM, P., OLSEN, B. R., BERG, R. A., GRANT, M. E., UITTO, J. & KIVIRIKKO, K. I. (1973) In *The Biology of the Fibroblast*, p. 311. Eds. E. Kulonen & J. Pikkarainen. New York: Academic Press.

RAMACHANDRAN, G. N. (1967) In *Treatise on Collagen*, Vol. 1, p. 103. Ed. G. N. Ramachandran. New York: Academic Press.

RAMALEY, P. B. & ROSENBLOOM, J. (1971) *Federation of European Biochemical Societies Letters*, **15**, 59.

REID, K. B. M., LOWE, D. M. & PORTER, R. R. (1972) *Biochemical Journal*, **130**, 749.

RHOADS, R. E. & UDENFRIEND, S. (1968) *Proceedings of the National Academy of Sciences of the United States of America*, **60**, 1473.

RHOADS, R. E. & UDENFRIEND, S. (1970) *Archives of Biochemistry and Biophysics*, **139**, 329.

ROBERTSON, P. B. & MILLER, E. J. (1972) *Biochimica et biophysica acta*, **289**, 247.

ROSENBLOOM, J. & PROCKOP, D. J. (1969) In *Regeneration and Repair: The Scientific Basis for Surgical Practice*, p. 117. Eds. J. E. Dunphy & W. van Winkle Jr. New York: McGraw Hill Book Co.

ROSS, R. & BENDITT, E. P. (1964) *Journal of Cell Biology*, **22**, 365.

SAKAKIBARA, S., INOUYE, K., SHUDO, K., KISHIDA, Y., KOBAYASHI, Y. & PROCKOP, D. J. (1973) *Biochimica et biophysica acta*, **303**, 198.

SCHOFIELD, J. D., FREEMAN, I. L. & JACKSON, D. S. (1972) *Biochemical Journal*, **124**, 467.

SCHOFIELD, J. D. & PROCKOP, D. J. (1973) *Clinical Orthopaedics and Related Research*, **97**, 175.

SEIFTER, S. & HARPER, E. (1971) In *The Enzymes*, Vol. 3, p. 649. Ed. P. D. Boyer. New York: Academic Press.

SMITH, B. E., BYERS, P. H. & MARTIN, G. R. (1972) *Proceedings of the National Academy of Sciences of the United States of America*, **69**, 3260.

SPEAKMAN, P. T. (1971) *Nature (London)*, **229**, 241.

SPIRO, R. G. (1967) *Journal of Biological Chemistry*, **242**, 4813.

SPIRO, R. G. (1969) *Journal of Biological Chemistry*, **244**, 602.

SPIRO, R. G. & SPIRO, M. J. (1971a) *Journal of Biological Chemistry*, **246**, 4899.
SPIRO, R. G. & SPIRO, M. J. (1971b) *Journal of Biological Chemistry*, **246**, 4910.
STARK, M., LENAERS, A., LAPIÈRE, C. M. & KUHN, K. (1971) *Federation of European Biochemical Societies Letters*, **18**, 225.
STOLTZ, M., FURTHMAYR, H. & TIMPL, R. (1973) *Biochimica et biophysica acta*, **310**, 461.
STRAWICH, E. & NIMNI, M. E. (1971) *Biochemistry*, **10**, 3905.
TANZER, M. L. (1973) *Science*, **180**, 561.
TRAUB, W. (1969) *Journal of Molecular Biology*, **43**, 479.
TRAUB, W., YONATH, A. & SEGAL, D. M. (1969) *Nature (London)*, **221**, 914.
TRELSTAD, R. L., KANG, A. H. & GROSS, J. (1972) *Federation Proceedings*, **30**, 1196.
TRELSTAD, R. L., KANG, A. H., IGARASHI, S. & GROSS, J. (1970) *Biochemistry*, **9**, 4993.
TSAI, R. L. & GREEN, H. (1972) *Nature (New Biology)*, **237**, 171.
UITTO, J., JIMENEZ, S. A., DEHM, P. & PROCKOP, P. J. (1972) *Biochimica et biophysica acta*, **278**, 198.
UITTO, J. & PROCKOP, D. J. (1973) *Abstracts of Ninth International Congress of Biochemistry, Stockholm*, p. 425.
VEIS, A. (1972) In *The Comparative Molecular Biology of Extracellular Matrices*, p. 345. Ed. H. Slavkin. New York: Academic Press.
VEIS, A., ANESEY, J. R., GARVIN, J. E. & DIMUZIO, M. T. (1972) *Biochemical and Biophysical Research Communications*, **48**, 1404.
VEIS, A., ANESEY, J. R., YUAN, L. & LEVY, S. J. (1973) *Proceedings of the National Academy of Sciences of the United States of America*, **70**, 1464.
VON DER MARK, K. & BORNSTEIN, P. (1973) *Journal of Biological Chemistry*, **248**, 2285.
VUUST, J. & PIEZ, K. A. (1972) *Journal of Biological Chemistry*, **247**, 856.
WILLIAMSON, A. R. (1969) In *Essays in Biochemistry*, Vol. 5, p. 140. Eds. P. N. Campbell & G. D. Greville. London: Academic Press.
WINTERBURN, P. J. & PHELPS, C. F. (1972) *Nature (London)*, **236**, 147.
WOOLLEY, D. E., GLANVILLE, R. W., LINDBERG, K. A., BAILEY, A. J. & EVANSON, J. M. (1973) *Federation of European Biochemical Societies Letters*, **34**, 267.
YONEMASU, K., STROUD, R. M., NIEDERMEIER, W. & BUTLER, W. T. (1971) *Biochemical and Biophysical Research Communications*, **43**, 1388.

8

Biosynthesis of collagen cross-links:
Relationship of heritable disorders

Allen J. Bailey

In a previous paper Dr Grant (1973) described the biosynthesis of the collagen molecule. The object of this paper is to discuss what happens extracellularly subsequent to the biosynthesis of the collagen molecule; in other words, what holds the molecule together to maintain the integrity of the fibre and, at the same time, gives the collagen fibre its high tensile strength. It is this high tensile strength of the fibre that permits collagen to act as the major mechanical supporting component of the body. Indeed, the role of collagen in the body is almost, but not entirely, mechanical (Harkness, 1961).

The collagen, together with elastin, the other fibrous protein of connective tissue, is embedded in an amorphous ground substance of mucopolysaccharides and salts. These complex connective tissues exist to contain other tissues, e.g. skin and muscle fascia; to connect one tissue to another, e.g. tendons and ligaments; or to act as a support to other tissues, e.g. bone. The variation in physical properties of these tissues possessing such diverse functions is due to the variation in organization and proportion of the various components. The tendons, requiring a high unidirectional tensile strength, contain a high proportion of collagen (80–90 per cent) and the fibres are aligned in parallel. Skin requires more flexibility and, therefore, the collagen fibres are randomly orientated, contain about 40 per cent collagen and a higher proportion of mucopolysaccharide. On the other hand, bone has to be strong and possess a high rigidity. Again, collagen (20 per cent) imparts the strength and the Ca^{++} salts (70 per cent) confer rigidity (for reviews see Bailey, 1968; Ramachandran, 1968).

It is now generally agreed that the high tensile strength of the collagen fibre, required for the ultimate functioning of the above tissues, is due to the presence of covalent cross-links between the collagen molecules making up the fibre (Fig. 1). In the absence of these cross-links, as seen in experimentally induced lathyrism, the apparently normal fibres

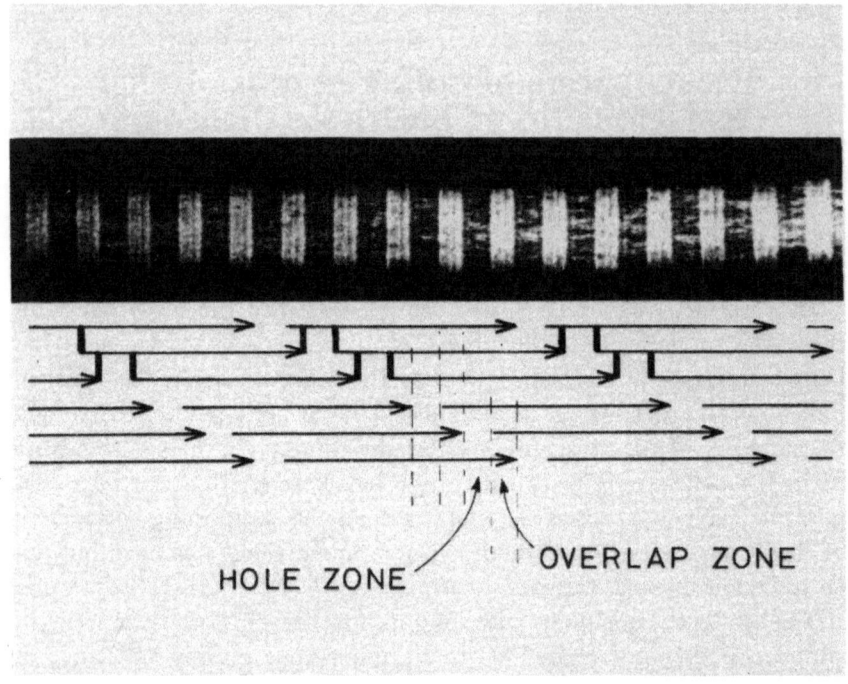

Fig. 1   (a) Electron micrographs of a native collagen fibril negatively stained with phosphotungstic acid; (b) A schematic representation of the alignment of the tropo-collagen molecules in the fibre and the possible location of the intermolecular cross-links stabilizing the fibre.

are extremely fragile and are readily soluble in salt buffers (Levene and Gross, 1959).

The total absence of the stabilizing cross-links, as in lathyritic collagen, is obviously fatal, but these experiments show that cross-link defects on a smaller scale could lead to connective tissue disorders. Clearly, disorders of the connective tissue could result also from defects in any one of the other components. Furthermore, it should be remembered that similarities in phenotypic expression of connective tissue disorders do not necessarily indicate similar aetiologies. However, a number of heritable disorders of connective tissue appear to suggest, at least from the clinical symptoms, that the disorder might be a defect in the cross-linking mechanism. The Ehlers–Danlos syndrome in which skin is hyperextensible, the Marfan syndrome in which the aorta frequently ruptures and osteogenesis imperfecta in which the bones

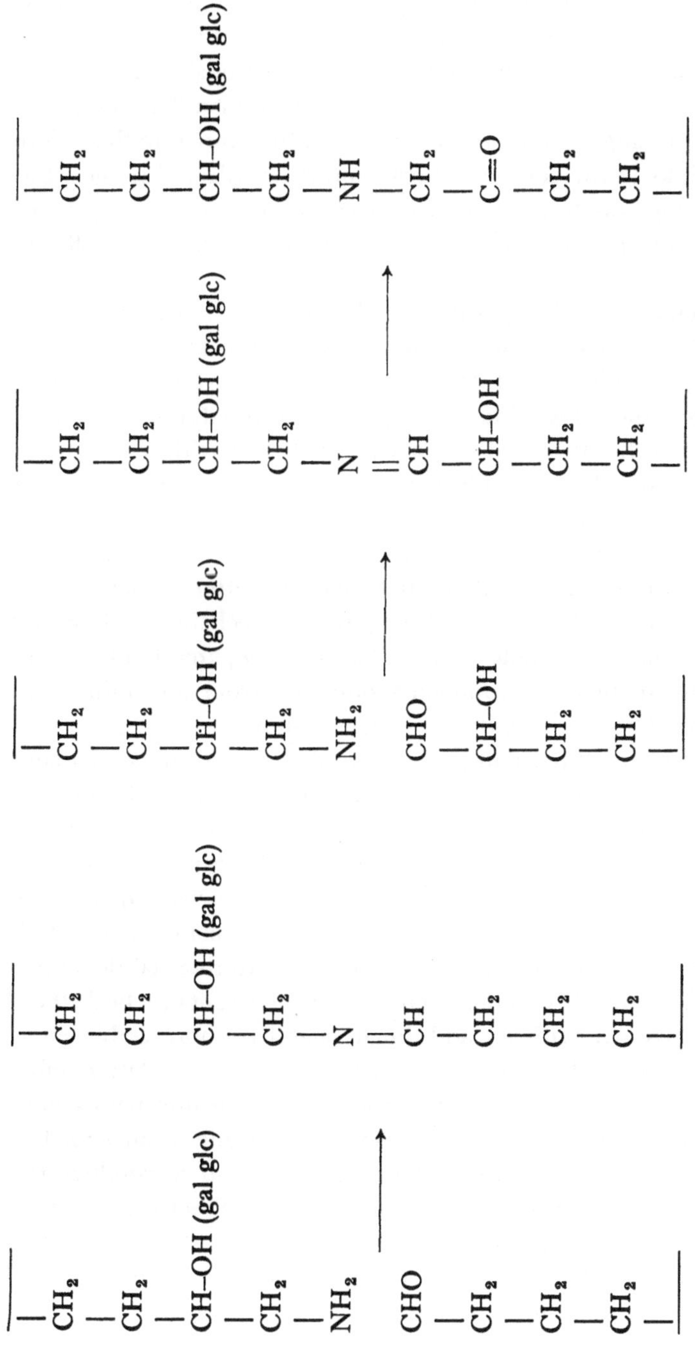

| | CH$_2$ | CH$_2$ | CH–OH (gal glc) | CH$_2$ | NH | CH$_2$ | C=O | CH$_2$ | CH$_2$ | | hydroxylysino–5 keto norleucine |

| | CH$_2$ | CH$_2$ | CH–OH (gal glc) | CH$_2$ | N | =CH | CH–OH | CH$_2$ | CH$_2$ | | dehydro-dihydroxy lysinonorleucine |

↑

| | CH$_2$ | CH$_2$ | CH–OH (gal glc) | CH$_2$ | NH$_2$ | CHO | CH–OH | CH$_2$ | CH$_2$ | | Hydroxyallysine |

↑

| | CH$_2$ | CH$_2$ | CH–OH (gal glc) | CH$_2$ | N | =CH | CH$_2$ | CH$_2$ | CH$_2$ | | Dehydro-hydroxy lysinonorleucine |

↑

| | CH$_2$ | CH$_2$ | CH–OH (gal glc) | CH$_2$ | NH$_2$ | CHO | CH$_2$ | CH$_2$ | CH$_2$ | | Allysine |

SCHEME I *Biosynthesis of the two aldimine cross-links*

are extremely brittle, all strongly suggest that the connective tissue is weaker than normal. Since collagen is the only connective tissue protein possessing a high mechanical strength, it is a reasonable assumption that the cross-links, being the basis of the collagen fibres' strength, are defective. An investigation has been carried out therefore into the nature of the cross-links in the collagen fibres from these affected tissues, but before discussing this work, it is necessary to summarize the present status of the biochemistry of the cross-links stabilizing the collagen fibre.

The first stage in the biosynthesis of the cross-links occurs through the enzyme lysyl oxidase, which oxidatively deaminates specific lysyl and hydroxylysyl residues in the non-helical N- and C-terminal regions of the collagen molecule. The aldehydes so formed then condense spontaneously with the ϵ-NH_2 of a hydroxylysine within the triple helical body of an adjacent molecule, thus forming an intermolecular aldimine bond (for review see Traub and Piez, 1971).

The structure of these cross-links has been obtained by characterization of their reduced forms, isolated from collagen after reduction with tritiated borohydride (Bailey and Peach, 1968; Mechanic, Gallop and Tanzer, 1971; Davis and Bailey, 1971; Tanzer *et al.*, 1973). The structure of all the reducible components obtained from an amino acid chromatogram of reduced tendon collagen is shown in Fig. 2.

Comparison of the types and proportion of the cross-links in tissues which are widely different in their fibre alignment and in the relative proportion of associated glycosaminoglycans revealed significant differences, suggesting a relationship between the type of cross-link and the function of the fibre (Bailey, Peach and Fowler, 1969). Skin collagen was shown to contain two major reducible components, both of which have been shown to be extremely labile to thermal denaturation and mild chemical reagents. Tendon collagen contains both these components, together with an additional relatively more stable component. Bone and cartilage, on the other hand, contain the latter stable component as the only major reducible compound. The unusual stability of this latter aldimine has now been shown to be due to an Amadori rearrangement, i.e. the migration of the double bond to produce the more stable keto form (Robins and Bailey, 1973). Direct confirmation that the non-reduced form does indeed exist as a cross-link *in vivo* has been obtained by isolation of a cross-linked peptide containing this cross-link from non-borohydride reduced collagen (Balian and Bailey,

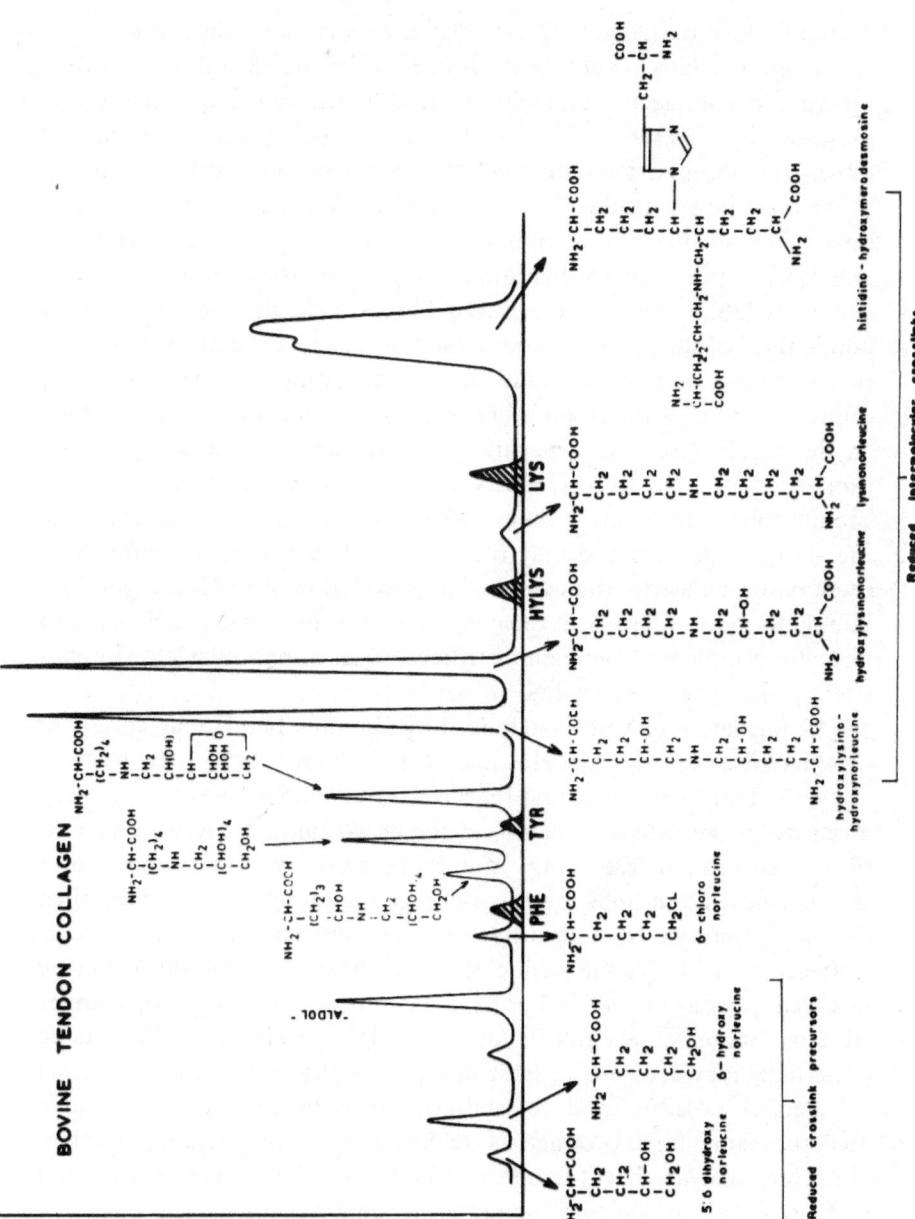

Fig. 2 A typical elution chromatograph of an acid hydrolysate of tendon collagen reduced with tritiated potassium borohydride, depicting the location and structure of all the reduced components.

1975). However, establishing the presence of dehydro-hydroxy-lysinonorleucine (dehydro-OH-LNL) *in vivo* is more difficult owing to its extreme lability. The third reduced aldimine, histidino hydroxy-merodesmosine, seems unlikely to exist in the non-reduced form as proposed by Tanzer *et al.* (1973) and may be an artifact produced during the borohydride reduction procedure (Robins and Bailey, 1973).

We must now consider the physiological role of these aldimine cross-links. The two major reducible components present in skin, dehydro-OH-LNL and dehydro-histidino hydroxymerodesmosine are both extremely labile in the non-reduced fibre. Thus, although as covalent bonds they could readily account for the tensile strength of the fibre, their lability to dilute acids and thermal denaturation means that they cannot account for the insolubility of a high proportion of skin collagen. In the highly insoluble collagens, such as bone and cartilage, a high proportion of dehydro-diOH-LNL is present, which, because of its spontaneous conversion to hydroxylysino-keto-norleucine, is stable to the above conditions and may therefore account for the insolubility of these tissues. Clearly, the extent of hydroxylation of the lysine residues in the N- and C-terminal regions, very low in dermal collagen but virtually complete in bone and cartilage, is an important factor in con-trolling the type of cross-link present.

The formation of a fibre stabilized by aldimine bonds may appear to complete the biosynthesis. However, skin is known to become increas-ingly resistant to chemical and thermal degradation with age, suggesting a change in the extent or nature of the cross-links. Analysis of various tissues, covering a wide range of ages, revealed that the proportion of the reducible cross-links increases during the rapid growth phase, then decreases until at maturity they are virtually absent. This decrease suggests that the labile reducible cross-links are stabilized during maturation to a non-reducible form in some as yet unknown manner (Robins, Shimokomaki and Bailey, 1973). It is possible that these stable cross-links may account, at least in part, for the insolubility of dermal collagen. A possible mode of stabilization is by *in vivo* reduction to give the same final product as achieved by borohydride reduction. However, analyses have demonstrated that *in vivo* reduction does not take place during ageing (Robins, Shimokomaki and Bailey, 1973).

With the limitations that the nature of the permanent stable cross-links have not yet been elucidated, we can apply our present knowledge of cross-linking to the problem of heritable connective tissue disorders mentioned above, in which the clinical symptoms suggest a defect in the stability of the collagen.

Ehlers–Danlos syndrome (E–DS)

The main clinical features of this disorder are the hyperextensibility of the skin and hypermobility of the joints. The skin and the peripheral blood vessels are fragile and split on minor trauma (McKusick, 1972). Determination of the breaking strength of affected skin revealed that it was about one-fifth of control skin (Rollhauser, 1950). Based on the correlation with the tissue fragility experienced in lathyritic skin, these observations strongly suggest a deficiency in the extent of the cross-linking. On the other hand, Graham and Beighton (1969) demonstrated that the Young's Modulus of the E–DS fibre was comparable with that of the fibre from normal skin, and other workers (Harris and Sjoerdsma, 1966) have shown that the solubility of E–DS skin, unlike lathyritic skin collagen, is no higher than normal. Furthermore, Layman, Narayanan and Martin (1972) recently demonstrated that *in vitro* cultures of fibroblasts isolated from E–DS skin, synthesize normal amounts of the amine oxidase, lysyl oxidase, necessary for the formation of the cross-links. At least in cell culture, the enzyme is neither absent nor functionally inert. These latter results suggest that cross-linking is not affected in these subjects.

The E–DS syndrome has been classified on a clinical basis by Beighton (1970) into five types, and Dr Herbert of the Bristol Royal Infirmary and I have now analysed samples of the skin collagen from subjects in each of these five classes. In all cases, the E–DS skins and the age, sex and site matched controls from normal subjects revealed similar patterns of reducible cross-links. However, in the majority of the biopsies the relative proportion of the reducible cross-links appeared to be significantly lower in the E–DS patients relative to normal subjects, although the difference could not be determined in absolute terms of cross-links per molecule. Tissue culture of biopsies and subsequent reduction of the newly synthesized collagen, revealed a high proportion of the cross-link precursors and the intramolecular aldol, confirming the ability of the tissue to synthesize cross-links. In contrast, a report on a single unclassified case of E–DS by Mechanic (1972) indicating that the reducible cross-links are absent in E–DS is not borne out by our own results.

Transmission electron micrographs reveal the fibre to possess the normal periodicity, although the fragility of the fibre is reflected in the large number of fibres with broken ends. Electron micrograph scanning, and also histological examination, indicate that the fibres are thinner and appear to be more randomly organized than normal skin fibres. Thus it may be that, in addition to a possible cross-linking defect, the organization of the fibres is unusual, as originally proposed by Jansen (1958). The lack of organization of the fibres could explain the hyperextensibility of the skin, although perhaps not the fragility.

Very recently, two variants of the disease, designated type VI and VII (McKusick, 1972) on the basis of biochemical differences, have been reported. Both are inherited recessively rather than by a dominant mode as in the other five classes. In the case of type VI ED–S, Pinnell, Krane, Kenzora and Glimcher (1972) first revealed that the collagen was deficient in hydroxylysine, owing to a deficiency in lysyl protocollagen hydroxylase (Krane, Pinnell and Erbe, 1972). Since hydroxylysine is an essential component of all the cross-links so far identified, it was not surprising that analysis of the tissue demonstrated the absence of the normal reducible cross-links (Eyre and Glimcher, 1972). It is surprising, however, that the analogous cross-links involving lysine rather than hydroxylysine were not found. It would seem that perhaps the loss of hydroxylysine is an oversimplification of the problem. A second recessive type, termed dermatosparactic type (type VII) has also been reported recently by Martin and his co-workers (quoted by McKusick, 1972). In this case, the defect demonstrated is the inability of the newly synthesized procollagen to cleave off its additional non-helical region. As far as I am aware no details of this work have been published, but it appears to be a similar defect to that described in cattle by Lapière and his colleagues (Lenaers, Ansay, Nusgens and Lapière, 1971). Unlike E–DS the skin is not hyperelastic in the sense that it returns to normal after stretching, but is lax and it tends to tear on stretching. Analysis of a sample of skin from these cattle, kindly supplied by Professor Lapière, was carried out in order to determine the effects of the extra peptide on the cross-linking. A marked decrease in the proportion of reducible cross-links was observed compared to normal calf skin. This is probably due to the disorganization of the fibre, since removal of the end-peptides with a peptidase extracted from normal skin, and subsequent reprecipitation of the molecules, produced normal uniform fibres and the cross-links also formed normally (Bailey and

Lapière, 1973). Whether this new recessive type of E–DS is a milder form of the disorder observed in cattle remains to be established.

At the present time, of the five major classes in which the disorder is inherited by a dominant mode, no specific defect has been identified. The defects identified in types VI and VII are not present in types I to V, and whether these former two recessive types should be classified as E–DS is debatable.

The Marfan syndrome

The major manifestations of this disease are the long thin extremities, the subjects being tall and loose jointed from birth, joint dislocations occur less frequently and the eyes sometimes have intense blue sclera. The major cardiovascular complication is dilation and dissecting aneurysm of the aorta. The aorta usually appears much thicker, but is weaker than normal. This swelling of the aorta and subsequent aneurysm is very similar to the experimental lathyrism induced by feeding β-aminopropionitrile or by keeping animals on a copper deficient diet. In both cases the lysyl oxidase activity is inhibited, cross-links fail to form in both collagen and elastin and finally the aorta ruptures.

Tissue culture of isolated fibroblasts revealed, as in the case of E–DS, that the lysyl oxidase was present and functional (Layman *et al.*, 1972), suggesting that at least the potential for cross-linking is present. Solubility studies on skin biopsies demonstrated that the skin was slightly more soluble (Laitinen, Uitto, Livanaisen, Hannuksela and Kivirikko, 1968). Tissue or fibroblast cultures (Macek, Kurych, Chvapil and Kadlecova, 1966; Priest, Moinuddin and Priest, 1973) both produced an excess of acid soluble collagen compared with controls. These observations have led to the suggestion by these workers that there is a deficiency of cross-links. However, since such a deficiency would lead to an increase in salt solubility, it is more likely that the increased acid solubility reflects an increased proportion of the collagen cross-linked by aldimine bonds. This suggestion is supported by analysis of diseased tissue for the aldimine bonds, by borohydride reduction. In the limited number of cases analysed a high proportion of aldimine cross-links were found in adult patients, whereas in age matched controls these cross-links were virtually no longer present. This could indicate an impairment in the stabilization of the borohydride reducible cross-links.

Menkes' kinky hair syndrome

Menkes, Alter, Steigleder, Weakly and Sung (1962) described this recessive disorder which, like the Marfan syndrome, results in disruption and fragmentation of the large arteries. In this case, the basic defect has been shown to be a low intestinal absorption of copper (Danks *et al.*, 1972). The absence of the copper leads directly to an inhibition of the cross-linking of both collagen and elastin by the copper dependent lysyl oxidase, analogous to the cross-linking defect in copper deficient swine (Carnes, 1968; Partridge *et al.*, 1964).

Osteogenesis imperfecta

This disorder again represents a generalized defect of the connective tissue, the joints being mobile like E–DS and the Marfan syndrome but the major characteristic in this case is the fragility of the bone (McKusick, 1972). Subjects with this disorder have short arms and legs, the eyes are very often blue and the skin is thin and transparent. Histological examinations have demonstrated the presence of thin agyrophilic fibres, rather than reticulum, leading some workers to suggest an immature type of fibre. As in the case of the other three disorders the biochemical studies have been distressingly few. Analysis of a number of patients with this disease for changes in the nature of the cross-links failed to reveal any significant differences.

Homocystinuria

The presence of homocystine in the urine of subjects is associated with abnormalities of connective tissue. Ectopia lentis of the eye, similar to Marfans syndrome, is always present. Like Marfan's, the media of the aorta appears to be disorganized, but dissecting aneurysms are not observed (McKusick, 1972).

In this disorder the fundamental defect is known, cystathionine synthetase activity is less than 5 per cent of normal in liver and brain. However, the nature of the resultant effect of the homocysteine on connective tissue has not been demonstrated.

We have shown previously that D-penicillamine was capable of cleaving aldimine cross-links by formation of a thiazolidine complex (Bailey, 1968). The structure of homocysteine is very similar to D-penicillamine and, as has been suggested by a number of workers, should be similarly capable of achieving the same effect. Therefore, we carried out some *in vitro* experiments and demonstrated that homocysteine was capable of cleaving the reducible cross-links. The fibre becomes increasingly fragile as the concentration of homocysteine is increased and analysis, after reduction with borohydride, reveals the absence of the reducible cross-links. This is analogous to the effect of D-penicillamine *in vitro* and the feeding of this drug to animals results in a decrease in the tensile strength of the collagen and an increase in the solubility (Nimni, 1968). Homocysteine is obviously capable of achieving the same effect.

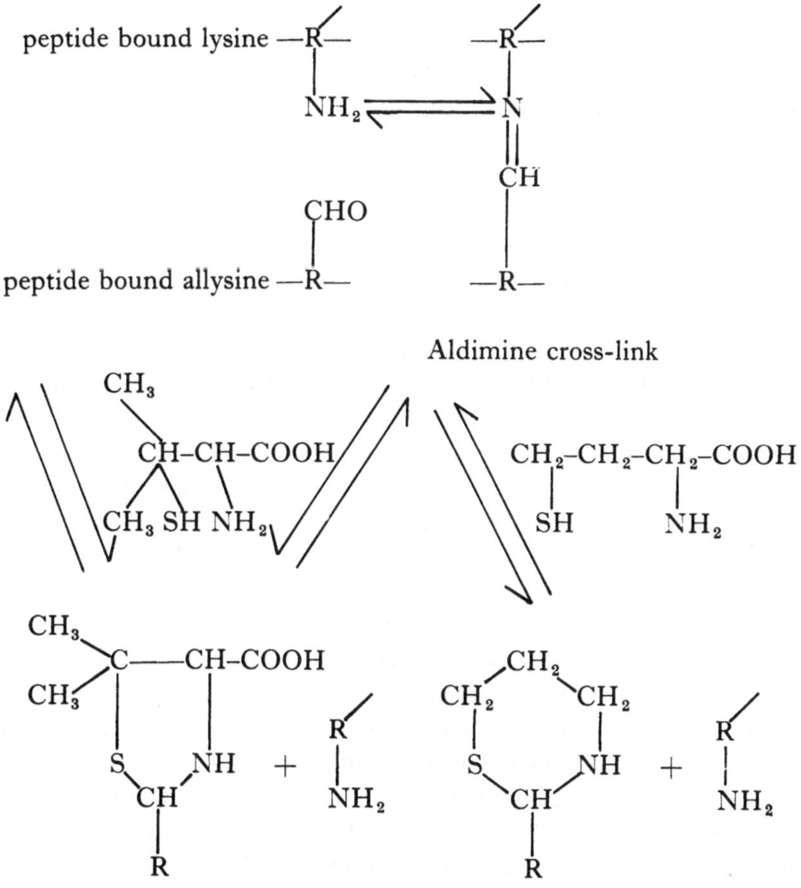

SCHEME 2 *Possible mode of cleavage of aldimine cross-link by homo-cysteine to form a tetrahydro-thiazine complex by analogy with the formation of a thiazolidine complex by D-penicillamine.*

Harris and Sjoerdsma (1966) found a higher solubility of the skin collagen and a higher α-β ratio in patients with this disorder. Therefore, an effect on the cross-links is suggested. In this connection, it is interesting to note that subjects fed D-penicillamine for chelating the excess copper in Wilson's disease have been shown to have a more soluble skin collagen, but no evidence of other connective tissue defects has been reported.

Conclusions

Using our technique for the identification of the cross-links in collagen, we have now studied a large number of cases of these four disorders, but as yet we have been unable to show a definitive effect in any one disease. Clearly the answer to the aetiology of these diseases is not going to be an easy one. Although we started out with some optimism that these disorders were apparently cross-link defects this has not proved to be readily demonstrable. However, it must be remembered that there may be some effect on the as yet unidentified stable cross-links of mature collagenous tissue.

Fig. 3 summarizes the biosynthesis of the collagen fibre. Inserted at a number of points in the scheme are arrows denoting where a defect could occur and result in some disorder of the cross-linking mechanism.

Clearly the biosynthesis of the cross-links is finely controlled and unless all the parameters, primary amino acid sequence, correct enzymes, and fibre alignment, are at an optimum the ultimate fibre strength will not be realized. The importance of the stabilizing cross-links in collagen cannot be over-emphasized.

Although the work to date has revealed only a preliminary insight into the molecular basis for these connective tissue disorders, it is equally obvious that we can reasonably expect that the pathogenesis of some of these disorders will be elucidated in the near future. The subsequent correlation of the fundamental defect and mechanism by which the disorders occur resulting in disease may be even more difficult in some cases, but the solution of these problems will provide an understanding of the normal state of healthy connective tissue in man and lead to both prevention and scientific progress.

Acknowledgements

The author is indebted to Dr Carol Herbert, and Dr S. Robins for constructive discussions.

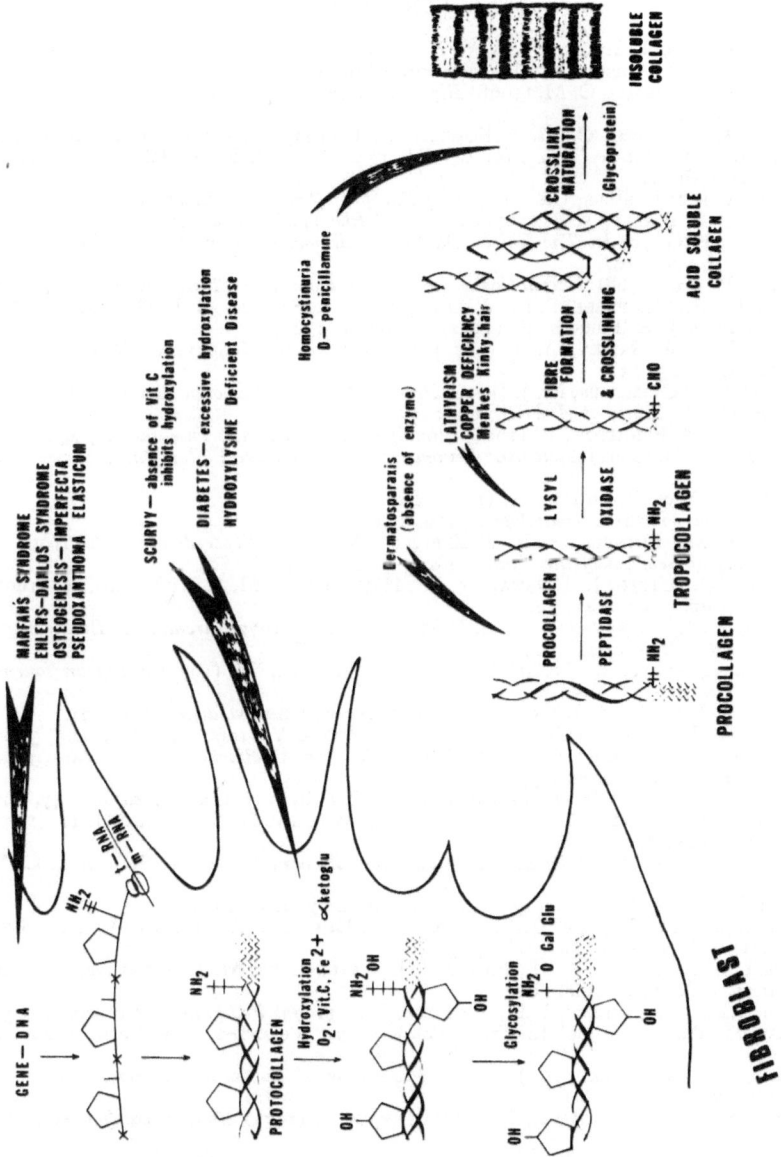

FIG. 3 Schematic representation of the biosynthesis and fibrillogenesis of collagen depicting the possible points in the development of the fibre where a defect could occur leading to a specific disorder.

REFERENCES

BAILEY, A. J. (1968) In *Comprehensive Biochemistry*, Vol. 26B, p. 297. Eds. M. Florkin & E. H. Stotz. Amsterdam: Elsevier Publishing Co.

BAILEY, A. J. & PEACH, C. M. (1968) *Biochemical and Biophysical Research Communications*, **38**, 812.

BAILEY, A. J., PEACH, C. M. & FOWLER, L. J. (1969) In *Chemistry and Molecular Biology of the Intracellular Matrix*, Vol. 1, p. 385. Ed. E. A. Balazs. New York: Academic Press.

BAILEY, A. J. & LAPIÈRE, CH. M. (1973) *European Journal of Biochemistry*, **34**, 91.

BALIAN, G. & BAILEY, A. J. (1975) *Annals of Rheumatic Disease* (In Press).

BEIGHTON, P. (1970) In *The Ehlers–Danlos Syndrome*. London: William Heinemann Medical Books Ltd.

CARNES, W. H. (1968) *International Reviews of Connective Tissue Research*, **4**, 197.

DANKS, D. M., CAMPBELL, P. E., WALKER-SMITH, J., STEVENS, B. J., GILLESPIE, J. M., BLOMFIELD, J. & TURNER, B. (1972) *Lancet*, **1**, 1100.

DAVIS, N. R. & BAILEY, A. J. (1971) *Biochemical and Biophysical Research Communications*, **45**, 1316.

EYRE, D. R. & GLIMCHER, M. J. (1972) *Proceedings of the National Academy of Sciences of the United States of America*, **69**, 2594.

GRAHAM, R. & BEIGHTON, P. (1969) *Annals of the Rheumatic Diseases*, **28**, 248.

HARKNESS, R. D. (1961) *Biological Reviews of the Cambridge Philosophical Society*, **36**, 399.

HARRIS, E. D. & SJOERDSMA, A. (1966) *Lancet*, **ii**, 707.

JANSEN, L. H. (1958) *Dermatologica*, **110**, 108.

KRANE, S. M., PINNELL, S. R. & ERBE, R. W. (1972) *Proceedings of the National Academy of Sciences of the United States of America*, **69**, 2899.

LAITINEN, O., UITTO, J., LIVANAISEN, M., HANNUKSELA, M. & KIVIRIKKO, K. (1968) *Clinica chimica acta*, **21**, 321.

LAYMAN, D. L., NARAYANAN, A. S. & MARTIN, S. R. (1972) *Archives of Biochemistry and Biophysics*, **149**, 97.

LENAERS, A., ANSAY, M., NUSGENS, B. V. & LAPIÈRE, Ch. M. (1971) *European Journal of Biochemistry*, **23**, 535.

LEVENE, C. I. & GROSS, J. (1959) *Journal of Experimental Medicine*, **110**, 771.

MACEK, M., KURYCH, J., CHVAPIL, M. & KADLECOVA, V. (1966) *Humangenetik*, **3**, 87.

MECHANIC, G., GALLOP, P. M. & TANZER, M. (1971) *Biochemical and Biophysical Research Communications*, **45**, 644.

MECHANIC, G. (1972) *Biochemical and Biophysical Research Communications*, **47**, 267.

MENKES, J. H., ALTER, M., STEIGLEDER, S. K., WEAKLY, D. R. & SUNG, J. H. (1962) *Pediatrics*, **29**, 764.

McKUSICK, V. A. (1972) In *Heritable disorders of connective tissue*. St. Louis: C. V. Mosby.

NIMNI, M. E. (1968) *Journal of Biological Chemistry*, **243**, 1457.

PARTRIDGE, S. M., ELSDEN, D. F., THOMAS, J., DORFMAN, A., TELSER, A. & PEI-LEE, H. (1964) *Biochemical Journal*, **93**, 30C.

PINNELL, S. R., KRANE, S. M., KENZORA, J. & GLIMCHER, M. J. (1972) *New England Journal of Medicine*, **286**, 1013.

PRIEST, R. E., MOINUDDIN, J. F., & PRIEST, J. H. (1973) *Federation Proceedings*, 3450.

RAMACHANDRAN, G. (1968) In *Treatise on Collagen*, Vols. 1–2. New York: Academic Press.

ROBINS, S. P. & BAILEY, A. J. (1973) *Federation of European Biochemical Societies Letters*, **33**, 167.

ROBINS, S. P., SHIMOKOMAKI, M. & BAILEY, A. J. (1973) *Biochemical Journal*, **131**, 771.

ROLLHAUSER, H. (1950) *Gegenbaurs morphologische Jahrbuch*, **90**, 249.

TANZER, M. L., HOUSELY, T., BERUBE, L., FAIRWEATHER, R., FRANZBLAU, C. & GALLOP, P. M. (1973) *Journal of Biological Chemistry*, **248**, 393.

TRAUB, W. & PIEZ, K. A. (1971) *Advances in Protein Chemistry*, **25**, 243.

9

Molecular conformations of connective tissue mucopolysaccharides

Edward Atkins

Introduction

The opportunity to glimpse some of the molecular shapes, conformations and structures exhibited by the connective tissue polysaccharides has arisen only within the last two years. This data, obtained in the main from paracrystalline solid-state preparations using X-ray diffraction, should enable valuable inroads to be made concerning our understanding of the molecular architecture, and consequently the molecular behaviour and properties, of these biologically and medically important group of polymeric substances.

For a considerable time the wealth of chemical and biochemical data has favoured linear, unbranched polysaccharide chains with relatively simple covalent sequences: disaccharides in the case of hyaluronate and chondroitin sulphates and possibly tetrasaccharides for heparan sulphate and heparin (for a recent review see Balazs (1970)). On this basis it would be reasonable to expect some ordered arrangements to occur, or to be induced to occur, at a molecular level and a technique such as X-ray diffraction, capable of delineating detailed molecular conformations and interactions, could most usefully be employed. Although attempts were made to induce orientation and crystallization in the hyaluronates and chondroitin sulphates (Bettelheim, 1958, 1964), no substantial information concerning molecular conformations of the connective tissue polysaccharides was obtained until more reliable crystallization techniques, using stress fields and annealing, were developed (Atkins and Mackie, 1972; Atkins and Sheehan, 1972). Within a reasonably short time X-ray photographs of exceptional quality have been obtained for a variety of mammalian polysaccharides, some of which are illustrated in Fig. 1. Such is the richness of data exhibited by these X-ray patterns that trial structures may readily be proposed.

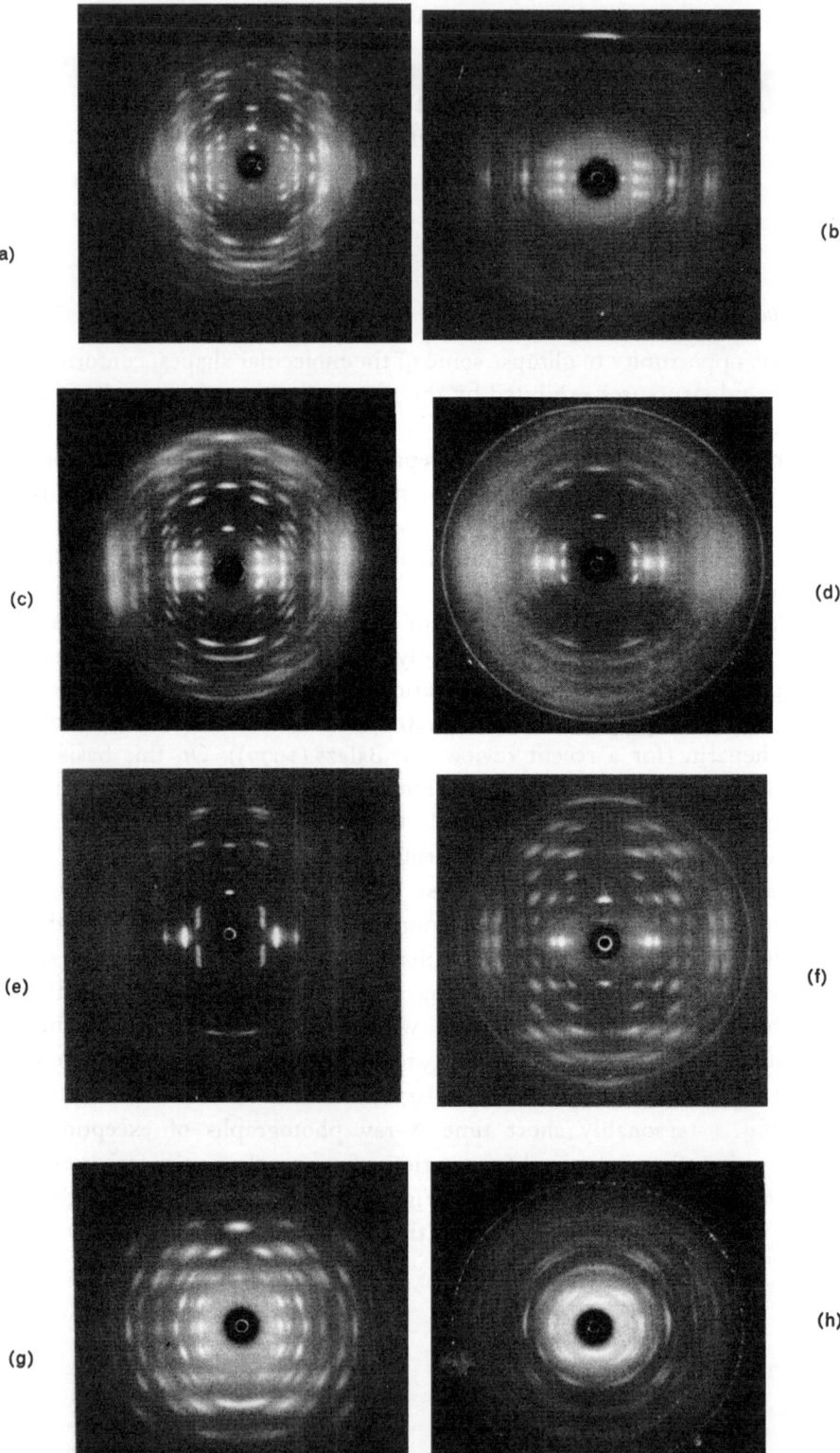

X-ray diffraction

A schematic diagram of the type of X-ray diagram obtained is shown in Fig. 2. The dimensional characteristics of the diffraction pattern (known as a 'fibre' pattern) reveal such parameters as the axial repeats along the chain and lateral periodicities between chains. Examination of the distribution of intensities of the diffraction spots provide an indication of the general features of the structure, such as the type of helix and whether or not a number of chains are intertwined. Additional information from bulk density measurements and model building, using computer procedures as well as space filling molecular models, limits the permissible structures. Ultimately the use of all the intensity data in a high resolution X-ray photograph will define the precise conformation and types of interaction between chains and their environments.

However, in this report it is intended to present a general survey of molecular conformations of individual molecules, rather than details of molecular juxtapositioning in a crystal lattice. Long chain molecules with a relatively simple covalent repeating sequence usually form helices, and the position of meridional reflections with respect to layer lines is

---

FIG. 1   X-ray fibre diffraction patterns obtained from oriented films of the connective tissue polysaccharides.

(a) Potassium hyaluronate: the axially projected disaccharide repeat is quite low at 0·83 nm and the pattern is consistent with the double-stranded molecule proposed by Dea *et al.* (1973). A computer drawn trial structure is shown in Fig. 5.

(b) Sodium hyaluronate: the layer line spacing in this case is 2·85 nm and the meridional reflections occur on the third, sixth and ninth layer lines. The pattern is consistent with a three-fold helical conformation (see Fig. 3(b)) and the disaccharide periodicity of 2·85/3 = 0·95 nm favours single helices.

(c) Chondroitin 4-sulphate, sodium salt form: this pattern clearly indicates a three-fold helical conformation (see Fig. 7(a)) and is rich in structural information.

(d) Sodium salt form of chondroitin 6-sulphate: again the pattern is consistent with a three-fold helical conformation but it is less well developed compared with 1(c). This appears to be a function of the source of the material (Fleming, 1973).

(e) Sodium salt of dermatan sulphate: the pattern has a very large layer-line spacing of 7·44 nm (Atkins and Laurent, 1973) and may be interpreted as a helix with eight disaccharide units repeating in three complete turns (Atkins and Isaac, 1973). See computer drawn projections in Fig. 11.

(f) By altering the chemical and thermodynamic environment of the sample the pattern in 1(c) may be converted into this two-fold conformation. The projected axial rise per disaccharide is 0·97 ± 0·01 nm and therefore firmly rules out the 1C chair for the L-iduronic acid moiety in these preparations.

(g) Calcium salt of heparan sulphate.

(h) Heparin, sodium salt form: the chain periodicity is 1·59 nm. The generally accepted all α, 1→4 linked system is ruled out and other possible models are shown in Fig. 12.

a helpful indicator of the number of covalent repeats per turn of helix (see Fig. 2).

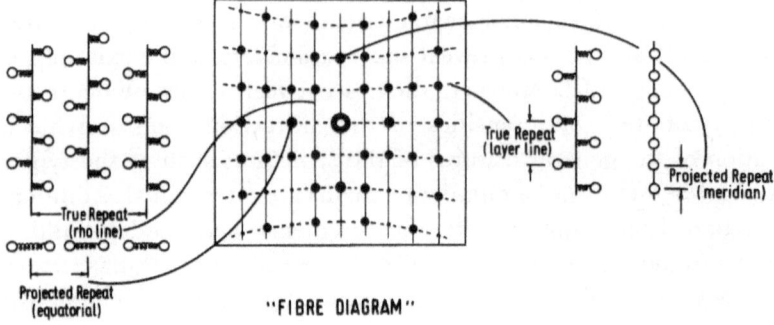

"FIBRE DIAGRAM"

FIG. 2   Schematic illustration of a Fibre Diagram. The spacing of the dashed layer lines represents the true repeat. Those reflections which occur on the central vertical line, called the meridian, represent the repeat projected on to the molecular axis. Thus the relative positions of meridional reflections on the layer lines can very often indicate the type of helix. In the example shown the two-fold helical conformation has meridional reflections occurring on layer lines which are multiples of two. Similar data concerning the packing of molecules may also be derived from consideration of the vertical rho lines.

Molecular conformations

The mammalian polysaccharide hyaluronates, chondroitin sulphates and dermatan sulphate are based on a disaccharide covalent repeating sequence with alternating 1→3 and 1→4 glycosidic linkages while the evidence concerning heparan sulphate and heparin favours a more complicated tetrasaccharide covalent repeat (for recent reviews see Bettelheim, 1970; Jeanloz, 1970). The details of such covalent repeating sequences including schematic diagrams are given in Table I.

Hyaluronates. One of the first X-ray patterns to be obtained was from a sample of sodium hyaluronate (Fig. 3(a)). It may be noted that the meridional reflections occur on the third, sixth and ninth layer lines indicating a three-fold helical conformation. On analysis these reflections represent orders of the covalent disaccharide repeat distance as projected on to the helix axis (Atkins and Sheehan, 1971, 1972). The measured spacing of 0·95 nm, only a little less than the fully extended hyaluronate chain, favours single three-fold helices as depicted by the computer generated trial structure shown in Fig. 3(b). By changing the experimental conditions such as pH, ionic strength, relative humidity, etc. other distinct conformations have been observed. For example,

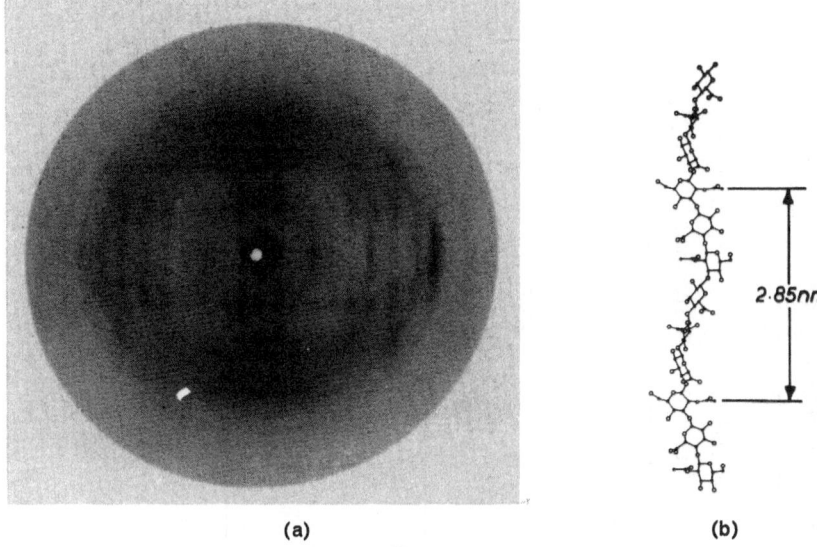

(a)   (b)

FIG. 3

(a) X-ray diffraction pattern of sodium hyaluronate. Note the meridional reflections occur on the third, sixth and ninth layer lines suggesting a three-fold helical conformation.

(b) Computer drawn projections (perpendicular and parallel to the chain axis) of a trial conformation consistent with the general features of the X-ray data. The lower projection is drawn to a larger scale to enable more detail to be seen.

lowering the pH to 2·5 allows the three-fold salt form to relax to a two-fold free acid form with a slight increase in the projected axial disaccharide repeat from 0·95 nm to 0·98 nm (Atkins, Phelps and Sheehan, 1972). Thus the turn angle between successive disaccharides has rotated 60°, from 120° to 180°, with little change in the axially projected disaccharide periodicity. This suggests that a major part of the rotation occurs about the 1eq→4eq glycosidic linkage which controls the proximity of the acetamido and carboxyl groups (see diagrams in Table 1). The two-fold conformation may be thought of as a mean conformation and rotation about the glycosidic linkage bonds could give possible helical conformations of either chirality (depending on the directions of rotation) up to a maximum of just over four disaccharides per turn (Rees, 1969).

The X-ray pattern shown in Fig. 4(a) shows such four-fold character with the first meridional reflection occurring on the fourth layer line with a spacing of 0·93 nm (Atkins and Sheehan, 1973). A computer drawn trial conformation is illustrated in Fig. 4(b). The X-ray pattern

TABLE I   *Details of the connective tissue polysaccharides under consideration*

Polysaccharides	Chemical and structural repeating sequence	Probably chair conformation	Glycosidic linkages	Typical occurrence
Hyaluronic acid	Heteropolyuronides–disaccharide repeat N-acetylglucosamine D-glucuronic acid	both C1	1e*→4e alternating with 1e→3e	Vitreous humour of the eye, human umbilical cord, synovial fluid
Chondroitin 6-sulphate (chondroitin sulphate C or D)	N-acetylgalactosamine 6-sulphate D-glucuronic acid	both C1	1e→4e alternating with 1e→3e	Intercellular matrix in cartilage
Chondroitin 4-sulphate (chondroitin sulphate A)	N-acetylgalactosamine 4-sulphate D-glucuronic acid	both C1	1e→4e alternating with 1e→3e	Intercellular matrix in cartilage

Dermatan sulphate (chondroitin sulphate B)	N-acetylgalactosamine L-iduronic acid	both CI	1e→4e alternating with 1e→3e	Intercellular matrix in skin
Heparin†	*Heteropolyuronides–tetrasaccharide repeat* (c) 1ax 4eq 0 1eq 0 4eq 1ax 4ax 1ax 4eq 4eq *n* sulphated N-acetyl-glucoamine / D-glucuronic acid / sulphated N-acetyl-glucoamine / sulphated L-iduronic acid	CI and IC	1a→4e, 1e→4e, 1a→4a, 1a→4e depending on the uronic acid composition	Liver tissue
Heparan sulphate	Similar to heparin but usually with only one sulphated group per tetrasaccharide repeat	CI and IC	similar to heparin	Human aorta

* The symbol 'e' represnts equatorially directed linkage bonds and 'a' axially directed linkage bonds.
† The structure drawn is one of a number of possibilities which are compatible with the tetrasaccharide repeat of 1.58 nm (see Nieduszynski and Atkins (1973)).

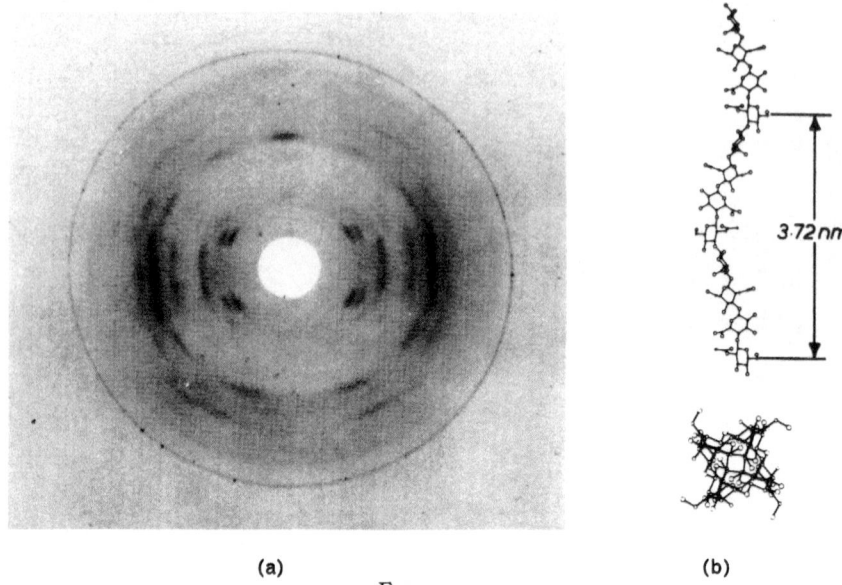

(a)   (b)

Fig. 4

(a) X-ray diffraction pattern of potassium hyaluronate. The pattern is consistent with
a four-fold helical conformation as shown in (b). Again the lower projection (repre-
senting a view down the chain axis) is at a somewhat larger scale.

shown in Fig. 1(a) has certain features similar to Fig. 4(a) but an
important difference is that the axial rise per disaccharide is considerably
reduced, to 0·83 nm. This substantial lowering in the axial periodicity
allows room for another helix to intertwine to form a double-stranded
molecule (Dea *et al.*, 1973). A trial computer generated model is
shown in Fig. 5. The ability for two hyaluronate chains to associate in
double helix formation is thought to be of considerable importance in
gelation (Rees, 1972) and may well explain some of the remarkable
properties of the hyaluronates.

To summarize, a range of molecular conformations have been
observed from two-fold through to four-fold and from single strand to
double strand, all as a function of environment. Thus, not only is
crystallization of the hyaluronates possible but further molecular
variation and conformational versatility may also be controlled.

Chondroitin 4-sulphate. Examination of Table I shows that chondroitin 4-sulphate differs from hyaluronate by replacement of the
N-acetylglucosamine moiety by N-acetylglactosamine together with
sulphation of the axial hydroxyl in the 4-position. The material is

extremely sensitive to humidity and Fig. 6 illustrates a sequence of X-ray diffraction photographs taken with the sample maintained at various degrees of relative humidity during exposure. The conformation of the sodium salt form is three-fold (Fig. 7(a)), with similar dimensions to the corresponding sodium hyaluronate. Note that the axially positioned sulphate groups lie at the periphery of the molecule, at a radius comparable with the equatorially positioned hydroxymethyl in the 6-positions (Fig. 7(a)). On conversion to the free acid form a relaxation to a two-fold conformation is observed (Isaac and Atkins, 1973).

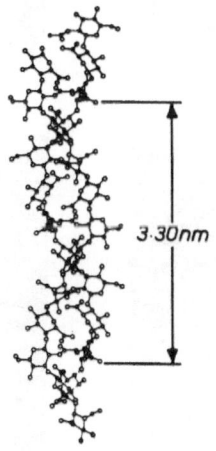

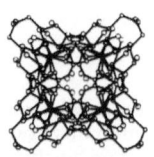

FIG. 5　A trial computer generated model of the double-stranded conformation similar to that proposed by Dea *et al.* (1973). The corresponding X-ray pattern is shown in Fig. 1(a).

Chondroitin 6-sulphate. The sulphate group in chondroitin 6-sulphate is equatorially positioned (see diagram in Table I) and extends some 0·2 nm further from the helix axis than in the case of chondroitin 4-sulphate. Both three-fold and two-fold conformations have been observed similar to, but not identical with, chondroitin 4-sulphate (Atkins, Gaussen, Isaac, Nandanwar and Sheehan, 1972). An X-ray

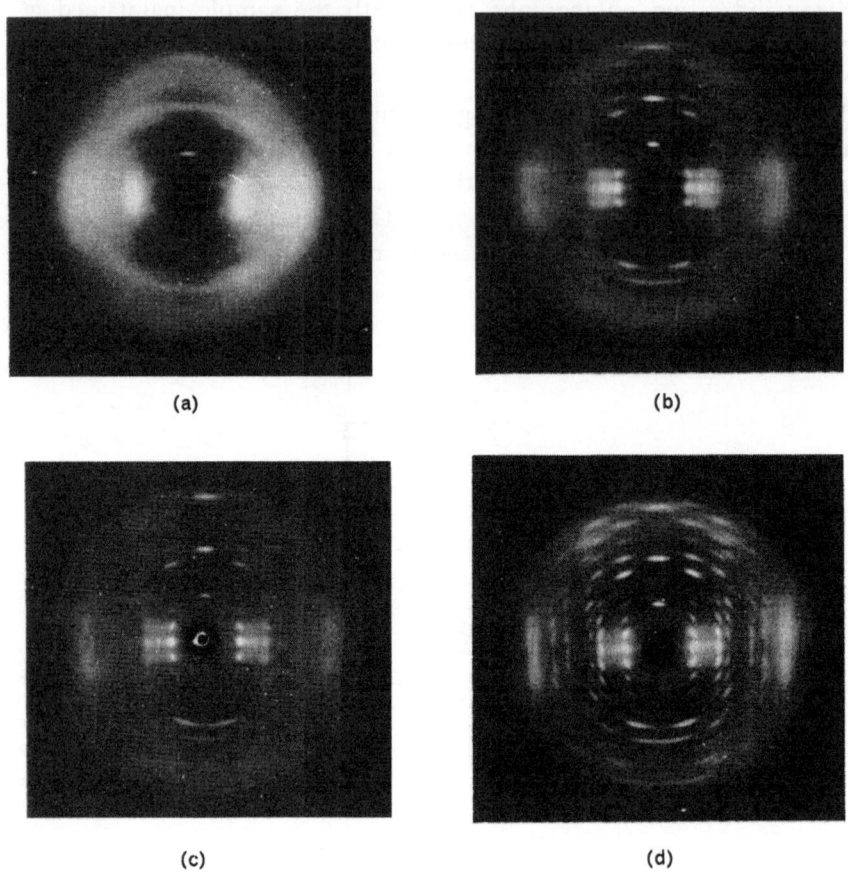

FIG. 6   X-ray diffraction patterns obtained from the sodium salt of chondroitin 4-sulphate as a function of relative humidity. (a) at room humidity ∼60 per cent (b) at 86 per cent; (c) at 90 per cent and finally (d) at 93 per cent. The process is reversible.

diffraction pattern of the three-fold sodium salt form is shown in Fig. 1(d) and the corresponding computer generated trial molecular model is illustrated in Fig. 7(b). In addition, Arnott, Guss, Hukinsa and Mathews (1973) have reported yet another distinct X-ray pattern which they interpret as an eight-fold helix (eight units in one turn) with a turn angle of 45° between successive disaccharide. Such a model is shown in Fig. (8a) and it implies considerable distortion, involving a

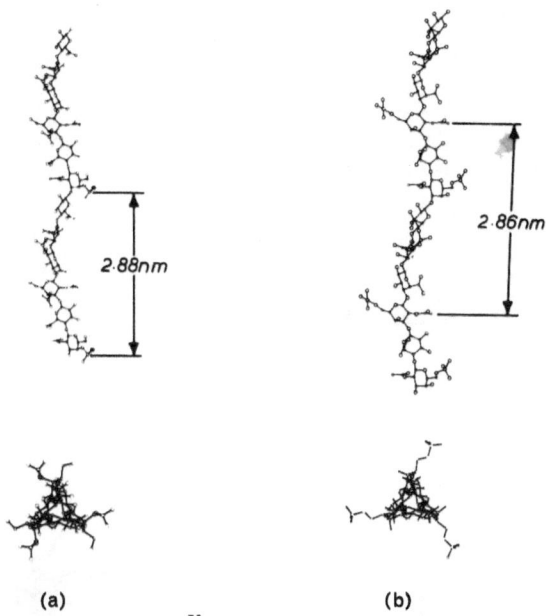

FIG. 7

(a) Chondroitin 4-sulphate: projections of a trial three-fold helical conformation consistent with the X-ray data shown in Fig. 6(d). Note the positions of the axially positioned sulphate groups.

(b) Chondroitin 6-sulphate: projections of the corresponding three-fold helix showing how the equatorially positioned sulphate groups in the 6-positions extend out beyond the periphery of the molecule.

rotation of $135°$ from the mean two-fold conformation. Such a conformation was ruled out on stereochemical criteria by Rees (1969), and an alternative model involving eight disaccharides in three turns (see Fig. 8(b)) has been suggested by Fleming (1973). It will be worthwhile referring to this particular conformation when discussing dermatan sulphate in the next section.

Dermatan sulphate. Of those connective tissue polyuronides based on the hyaluronic acid covalent repeat, the molecular shape of dermatan sulphate has probably aroused most discussion. The covalent repeat is characteristically distinguished by replacement of the usual D-glycuronic acid by its $C(5)$ epimer L-iduronic acid. A schematic representation of the shape and disposition of side groups for both uronic acids in the C1 chair form are shown in Fig. 9(a). Such a chair conformation for D-gluronic acid appears quite satisfactory with all the side groups favourably positioned equatorially. On the other hand, the $C(5)$ epimer

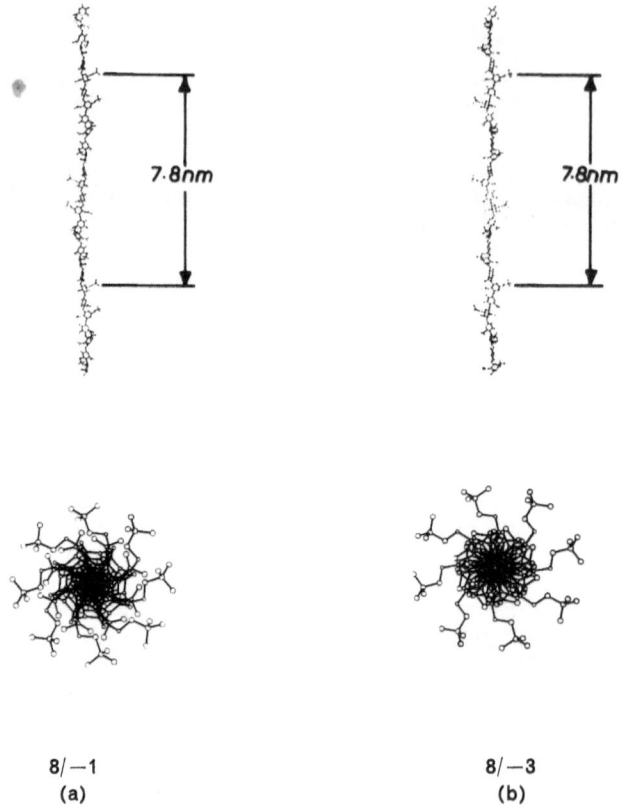

8/—1   8/—3
(a)   (b)

FIG. 8   Possible models to explain the eight-fold type helix.
(a) A trial model similar to the type proposed by Arnott *et al.* (1973) where each
successive disaccharide rotates through 45° giving an 8/–1 (negative sign denotes a
left-handed structure) helical conformation.
(b) An alternative model, similar to the one discussed for dermatan sulphate, where
each successive disaccharide rotates through 135° to give an 8/–3 helix with eight
disaccharides in three turns.

L-iduronic acid has the large carboxyl group axially positioned (Fig.
9(a)) and serious consideration must be given to the alternate 1C chair
form for this particular uronic acid moiety.

   Certainly, there is an analogous situation in the brown seaweed
polysaccharide alginates where the C(5) epimers, D-mannuronic acid
and L-guluronic acid, exist in different chair conformations which
radically alter the molecular shape of the polysaccharide (Atkins, Mackie
and Smolko, 1970, Atkins, Mackie, Nieduszynski, Parker and Smolko,
1973).

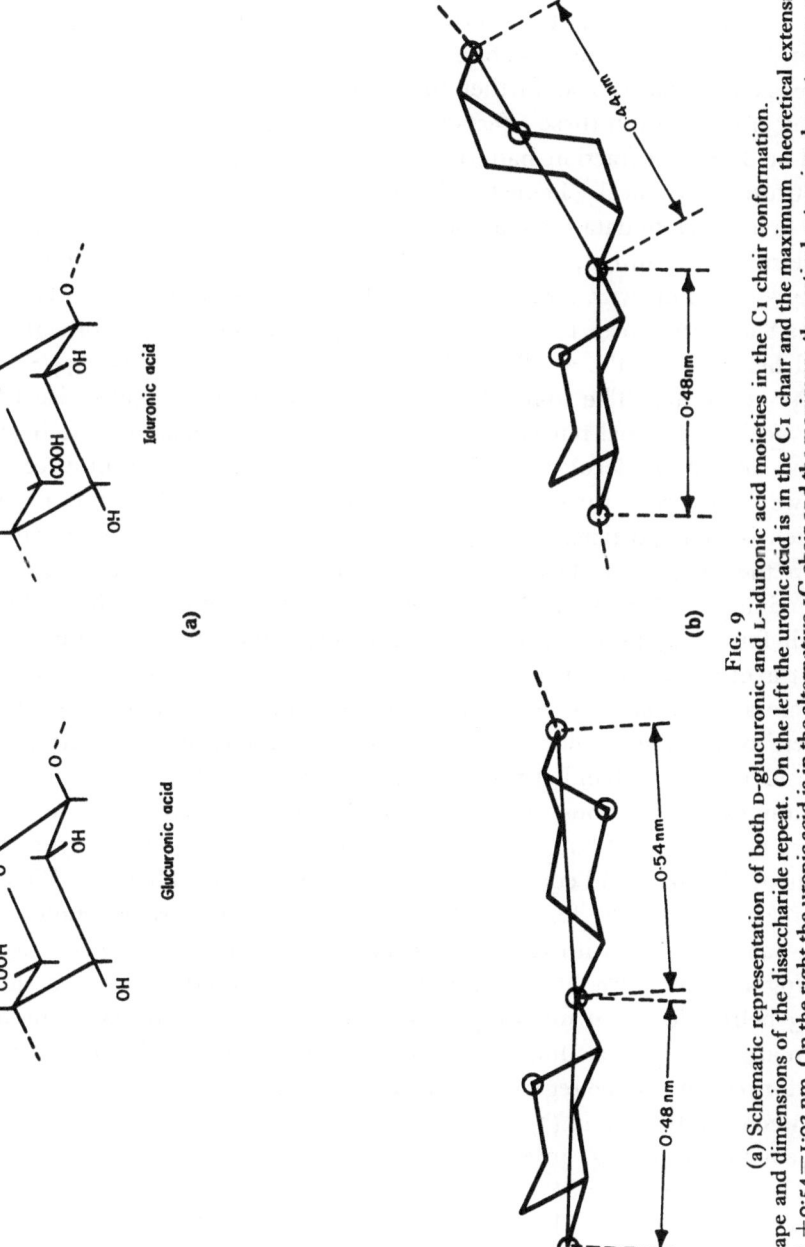

FIG. 9

(a) Schematic representation of both D-glucuronic and L-iduronic acid moieties in the C1 chair conformation.

(b) Shape and dimensions of the disaccharide repeat. On the left the uronic acid is in the C1 chair and the maximum theoretical extension is 0·48 ±0·54=1·02 nm. On the right the uronic acid is in the alternative 1C chair and the maximum theoretical extension drops to 0·92 nm.

Returning to dermatan sulphate, the effect of converting the L-iduronic acid moiety to the alternate 1C chair would be to substantially alter the shape of the backbone by introducing diaxially positioned glycosidic linkages, and further to reduce the disaccharide repeat by about 0·1 nm. Both these effects are illustrated in Fig. 9(b).

The X-ray diffraction pattern shown in Fig. 1(e), obtained at the Institute of Medical Chemistry. Uppsala in August 1972, represented the first concrete data for solid-state preparations of dermatan sulphate (Atkins and Laurent, 1973). The layer-line spacings are orders of 7·44 ±0·08 nm, with strong meridional reflections occurring on layer lines 8 and 16. These results may be interpreted as some type of eight-fold helix, where the axially projected disaccharide repeat is 7·44/8 = 0·93 ±0·01 nm. The four-fold pseudo character, which gives rise to the weak meridional reflections on layer lines 4 and 12, appears to be a result of intermolecular packing forces in the tetragonal unit cell. However it is the projected axial repeat of the disaccharide at this stage which is of importance. The measured spacing of 0·93 nm is greater than the maximum allowed repeat (see Fig. 9(b)) for a disaccharide containing L-iduronic acid the alternate 1C chair and, therefore, this chair form may be ruled out, at least in these solid-state preparations.

It is of some interest to consider this eight-fold helix in more detail. There are *a priori* four fundamentally different conformations to consider, two for each chirality. To avoid confusion let us arbitrarily consider only left-handed helices. (There is some evidence from model building considerations that left-handed helices are stereochemically more favourable, although the same arguments concerning the type of eight-fold helix could equally well apply to right-handed helices.) First, there is the straight forward 8/−1 helix (the negative sign denotes a left-handed helix) with eight disaccharide units in one complete turn giving a turn angle of 45° (see Fig. 10(b)). Secondly, there is the 8/−3 helix with eight units repeating in three complete turns giving a turn angle of 135°, as illustrated schematically in Fig. 10(c). This latter conformation may be regarded as a 2·66/−1 helix and lies nearly halfway between the three-fold (3/−1) helix and the two-fold (2/1) helix, shown schematically in Fig. 10(a) and (d).

The merits of both 8/−1 and 8/−3 conformations have been discussed in some detail recently by Atkins and Isaac (1973). These authors have shown that by perturbing the chemical and thermodynamic environment of the sample the eight-fold helix will transform to both three-fold

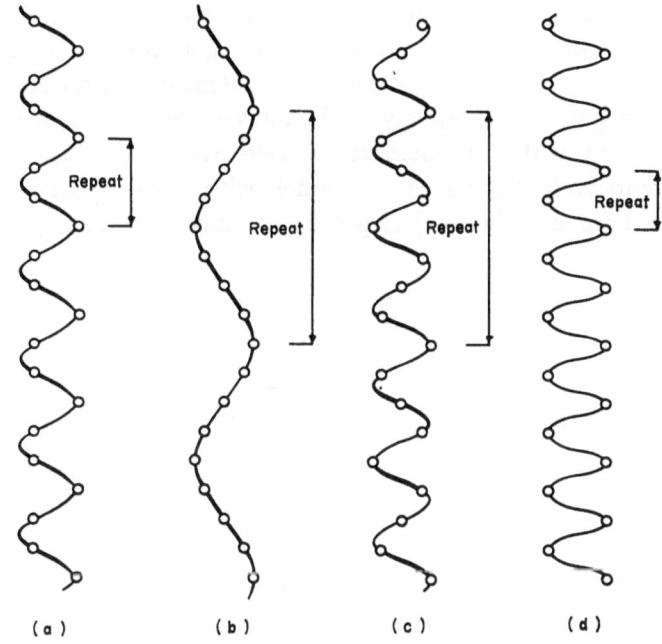

(a)   (b)   (c)   (d)

FIG. 10 Schematic diagrams of helical conformations relevant to some of the
proposed structures.
(a) Three-fold (3/–1) helix, left-handed.
(b) Eight-fold (8/–1) helix, left-handed.
(c) 8/–3 helix with the same repeat as (b) but may be considered as a 2·66/–1 helix
lying partway between (a) and (d).
(d) Two-fold helix.

and two-fold conformations, which strongly suggests that the eight-fold
conformation is more consistent with the 8/–3 computer generated
model shown in Fig. 11.

Heparan sulphate and heparin. The detailed covalent repeat of heparan
sulphate and heparin has not been established with the same degree of
certainty as those of the other galactosaminoglycuronans, but has been
thought to involve D-glucuronic acid and D-glucosamine units joined
by α-(1→4) linkages (Wolfram, Weisblat, Karabinor, McNeedy and
McLean, 1943). More recently, Cifonelli and Dorfman (1962) have
indicated the presence of L-iduronic acid; furthermore, for the case of
heparin in particular, Perlin, Ng Yink Kin and Battacharjee (1972)
have suggested that L-iduronic acid is the major uronic acid and Lindahl
and Axelsson (1971) have indicated that L-iduronic acid is the major
sulphated uronic acid present.

The diffraction data for heparan sulphate gives a layer-line spacing of 1·86 nm, with a meridional streak on the first layer-line (Atkins and Laurent, 1973). The maximum theoretical extension of a tetrasaccharide repeat having all α-D-(1→4)-glycosidic links is 1·80 nm and is therefore not consistent with the measured periodicity. Atkins and Laurent (1973) tentatively suggested a model with α-(1→4)(1ax→4eq)-D-glucosaminidic and β-(1→4)(1eq→4eq)-D-glucuronic linkages respectively.

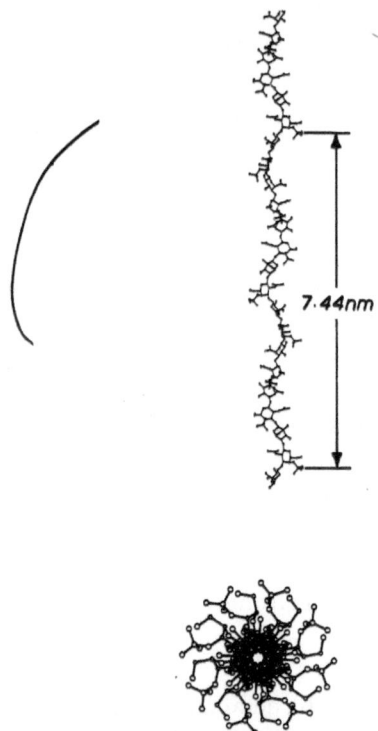

7·44nm

FIG. 11   Computer drawn projections of a trial conformation of the 8/−3 dermatan helix. Note the backbone oscillates three times in the repeat of 7·44 nm.

The X-ray photograph obtained from heparin is shown in Fig. 1(h). Nieduszynski and Atkins (1973) have shown that the data again rules out the generally accepted α-(1→4) (1 ax→4 eq)-linkage system and suggest three possible alternative covalent shapes depending on the uronic acid composition (see Fig. 12). Certainly the evidence favours the L-iduronic acid, when sulphated, to exist in the alternative 1C chair

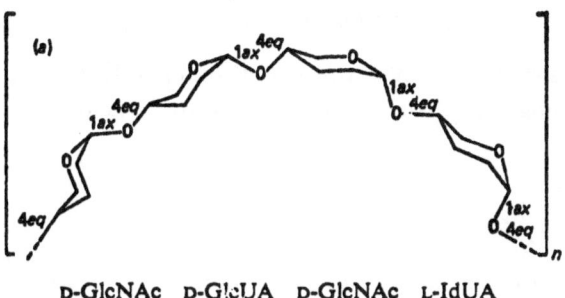

D-GlcNAc D-GlcUA D-GlcNAc L-IdUA

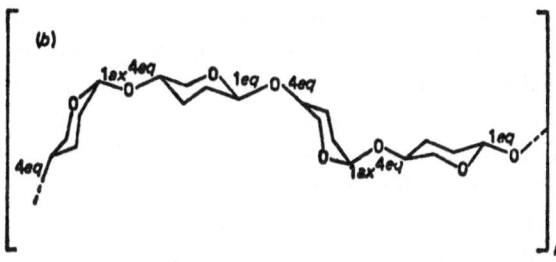

D-GlcNAc UA (C1) D-GlcNAc UA (C1)

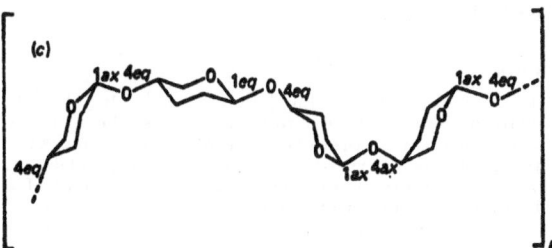

D-GlcNAc UA (C1) D-GlcNAc UA (1C)

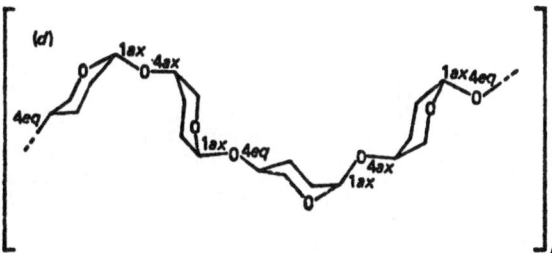

D-GlcNAc UA (1C) D-GlcNAc UA (1C)

FIG. 12 Molecular conformations of heparin.
(a) Generally accepted conformation.
(b) (c) and (d) are three possible tetrasaccharide repeats depending on the proportion
of D-glucuronic/L-iduronic acid.

form. Fransson (1975) has presented independent evidence which favours a change in chair shape for L-iduronic acid as a function of sulphation.

Conclusion

We have witnessed an avalanche of molecular information relevant to the connective tissue polysaccharides which will naturally take time to be completely digested and fully understood, yet we have probably only scratched the surface. Much work will be needed to be done in refining the trial molecular structures outlined in this report. However, instinctively one feels that this is an exciting period, since not only has crystallization of those macromolecules been achieved, but a whole variety of molecular conformations are evident as a function of the chemical and thermodynamical environment. The ability to monitor detailed molecular conformation as a function of such parameters will greatly facilitate our general understanding of their properties and molecular behaviour.

Acknowledgements

I am indebted to my colleagues, Dr Ian Nieduszynski, Dr John Sheehan and Mr David Isaac, for sharing some of the exciting discoveries, the so many valuable discussions and for allowing me to reproduce some of their results. My thanks also to Dr Charles Phelps, Professor Torvard Laurent, Dr Ulf Lindahl, Dr Per-Henrik Iverius and Dr Lars-Ake Fransson for their invaluable biochemical advice and the supply of material which made much of this work possible. In addition, I am grateful to Professors F. C. Frank, FRS, and A. Keller, FRS, for their constant support and encouragement.

The work was financed by the Arthritis and Rheumatism Research Council and the Science Research Council.

REFERENCES

ARNOTT, S., GUSS, J. M., HUKINS, D. W. L. & MATHEWS, M. B. (1973) *Science*, **180, 743**.
ATKINS, E. D. T. & ISSAC, D. H. (1973) *Journal of Molecular Biology*, **80**, 773
ATKINS, E. D. T. & LAURENT, T. C. (1973) *Biochemical Journal*, **133**, 605.
ATKINS, E. D. T. & MACKIE, W. (1972) *Biopolymers*, **11**, 1685.
ATKINS, E. D. T. & SHEEHAN, J. K. (1971) *Biochemical Journal*, **125**, 92.
ATKINS, E. D. T. & SHEEHAN, J. K. (1972) *Nature (New Biology)*, **235, 253**.
ATKINS, E. D. T., PHELPS, C. F. & SHEEHAN, J. K. (1972) *Biochemical Journal*, **128, 1255.**
ATKINS, E. D. T. & SHEEHAN, J. K. (1973) *Science*, **179**, 562.
ATKINS, E. D. T., GAUSSEN, R., ISAAC, D. H., NANDANWAR, V. & SHEEHAN, J. K. (1972) *Journal of Polymer Science; Part B: Polymer Letters*, **10**, 863.
ATKINS, E. D. T., MACKIE, W. & SMOLKO, E. E. (1970) *Nature (London)*, **225**, 626.
ATKINS, E. D. T., MACKIE, W., NIEDUSZYNSKI, I. A., PARKER, K. D. & SMOLKO, E. E. (1973) *Biopolymers*, **12**, 1865.
BALAZS, E. A. (1970) In *Chemistry and Molecular Biology of the Intercellular Matrix*, Vol. II. Ed. E. A. Balazs. London and New York: Academic Press.
BETTELHEIM, F. A. (1958) *Nature (London)*, **182**, 1301.

BETTELHEIM, F. A. (1964) *Biochimica et biophysica acta*, **83**, 350.
BETTELHEIM, F. A. (1970) In *Biological Polyelectrolytes*, p. 131. Ed. A. Veis. New York: Marcel Dekker.
CIFONELLI, J. A. & DORFMAN, A. (1962) *Biochemical and Biophysical Research Communications*, **7**, 41.
DEA, I. C. M., MOORHOUSE, R., REES, D. A., ARNOTT, S., GUSS, J. M. & BALAZS, E. A. (1973) *Science*, **179**, 560.
FLEMING, M. (1973) M.Sc. Thesis, University of Bristol.
FRANSSON, L-Å (1975) *Proceedings of the Society for the Study of Inborn Errors of Metabolism*, **11**, *Inborn Errors of Skin, Hair and Connective Tissue*, Eds. J. B. Holton & J. T. Ireland. Lancaster: Medical and Technical Publishing Co.
ISAAC, D. H. & ATKINS, E. D. T. (1973) *Nature (New Biology)*, **244**, 252.
JEANLOZ, R. W. (1970) In *The Carbohydrates*, p. 589. Eds. W. W. Pigmann & D. Horton. New York: Academic Press.
LINDAHL, U. & AXELSSON, O. (1971) *Journal of Biological Chemistry*, **246**, 74.
NIEDUSZYNSKI, I. A. & ATKINS, E. D. T. (1973) *Biochemical Journal*, **135**, 729.
PERLIN, A. A., NG YINK KIN, N. M. K. & BATTACHARJEE, S. S. (1972) *Canadian Journal of Chemistry*, **50**, 2437.
REES, D. A. (1969) *Journal of the Chemical Society, Section B: Physical Organic Chemistry*, p. 217.
REES, D. A. (1972) *Biochemical Journal*, **126**, 257.
WOLFRAM, M. L., WEISBLAT, D. I., KARABINOR, J. A., McNEEDY, W. H. & McLEAN, J. (1943) *Journal of the American Chemical Society*, **65**, 2077.

10

Mucopolysaccharides in ageing

David A. Hall

If age changes in mucopolysaccharides are to be discussed, it is of interest first to ascertain whether a suitable definition of ageing exists; particularly one which suggests that ageing phenomena themselves may be due to inborn errors of the body's overall metabolism.

Theories of ageing may be divided broadly into two groups (Bjorksten, 1969). There are those which ascribe age changes to the accumulation of the results of random insults to our physiology throughout life, and those which rely for their explanation of the changes which can be observed on genetically determined factors. As with most disciplines, there are adherents to both these groups of theories, some being very outspoken in their condemnation of the views of colleagues in the other camp. As always, there are probably elements of truth in both approaches. It may not be exciting to sit with a foot in either camp, but in this instance one is possibly more than justified in doing so. If life is considered as a parabola, similar to that described by a stone which is thrown through the air, some of the parameters which determine its path can be correlated with factors involved in the ageing process (Fig. 1). Thus the distance travelled before the stone returns to the ground is comparable to life span. In the dynamic situation, this distance is partly dependent on adverse atmospheric conditions: contrary winds, atmospheric pressure, etc. which restrict the flight of the stone. Similarly, throughout life, disease, and the accumulation of random errors and mutations, can alter the slope of the falling segment of the curve and affect the rate of ageing. However, the optimum distance travelled by the stone is more dependent on the force with which it is propelled and the angle of its trajectory, than by any incidental changes in conditions which may exist during flight. It is, however, also controlled to a considerable extent during flight by the forces of gravity. The first two of these factors which affect the launch of the stone can be compared with inborn determinants of life span, and gravity with those physiological changes which affect all members of any one species.

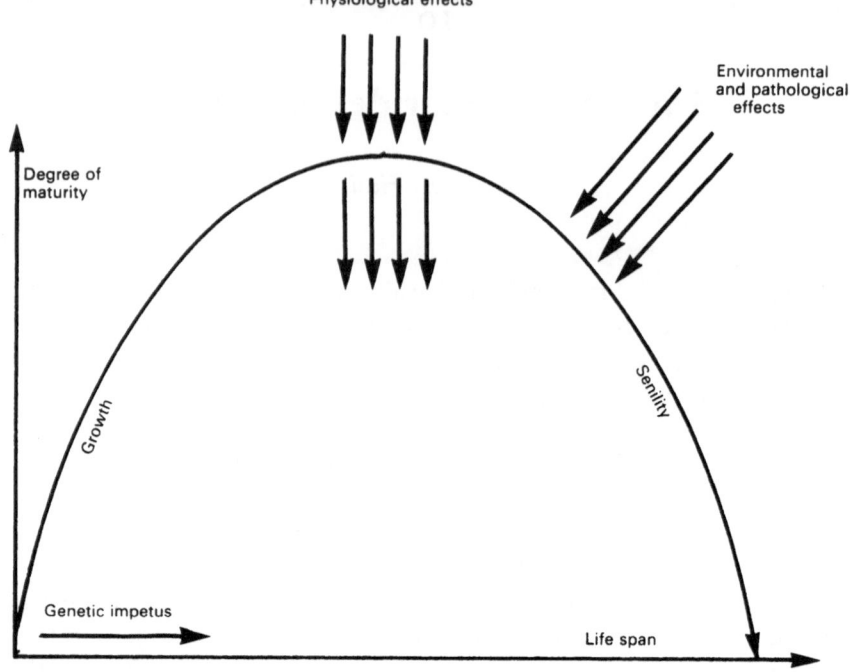

FIG. 1

All of these particular effects are genetically determined, and therefore fall within the province of this discussion. Since each effect can be ascribed to the activity of a single gene, or group of genes, the ageing phenomena which are induced may vary from individual to individual, but whether this variation can be ascribed to a deviation from some hypothetical norm remains to be seen.

Age changes in mucopolysaccharides are dependent on alterations in the metabolic processes of the cells which produce them and, theoretically, it is at the cellular level that alterations in mucopolysaccharide, or any other extracellular component of a tissue, should be studied. However, although there have been many improvements in glycosaminoglycan analysis during the past ten years, and much more is known about the enzymes which synthesize them, the stage where complete metabolic studies can be carried out for all mucopolysaccharides has still not been reached. It is necessary to rely in many instances on descriptive studies of the glycosaminoglycan contents of tissues, and on differential analyses of polysaccharide types. The age determined metabolic pathways, which synthesize these polysaccharides, have been studied in only a limited number of cases. In this communication, observations will be restricted to changes in cartilage, where the mucopolysaccharide compounds occur in greatest concentrations and where, in load bearing cartilage at least, any age-induced changes may have a marked role to play in the senile decrepitude of the subject.

Glycosaminoglycans are of varying types depending on the proportions of glucosamine, galactosamine, glucuronic and iduronic acids, and on the position and degree of sulphation. In general, vertebrates possess cartilage which contains two specific forms of glycosaminoglycan, namely chrondroitin sulphate and keratan sulphate. The proteoglycans, of which these glycosaminoglycans form a part, are not necessarily homogenous. Any one protein chain may be substituted along its length by different glycosaminoglycans. During foetal life the human costal cartilage is rich in chondroitin-6-sulphate (CS6) and chondroitin-4-sulphate (CS4) but, also, contains a portion of unsulphated polysaccharide (Mathews and Glagov, 1966). The content of these unsulphated disaccharide units falls to zero by the time the foetus has reached full term and it is never present thereafter. After birth, the level of CS4 rises slightly during infancy and then falls over the next forty years. The CS6 fraction also rises during early infancy, but then falls to only about 80 per cent of highest level. During early development and childhood, the CS4 is replaced by keratan sulphate (KS), which is completely absent before birth. The rate of removal with age of polysaccharide sulphated in the 6 position, from the proteoglycan, appears to vary according to the tissue in which it is present, the change over from rise to fall occurring at 1 to 2 years in the case of costal cartilage (Mathews 1973), and between 60 and 70 in the knee joint cartilage (Greiling and Bauman, 1973).

In the intervertebral disc the nuclear concentration of the glycosaminoglycans, CS4, CS6 and KS, which is initially higher than that in the annulus, also changes its composition with age. The total content of CS6 and CS4 in the nucleus decreases with age (Buddecke and Seigoleits, 1964) and the ratio of (CS4+CS6)/KS decreases from 1:1 to 1:4, whilst the CS4/CS6 ratio changes from 2:1 to a situation in which CS6 represents the major chondroitin sulphate components.

The alterations can affect a number of different properties of the disc. In our laboratory we have chosen the effect of age on water sorptive properties for study (Hall and Reed, 1973). The water content of a glycosaminoglycan rich tissue is dependent on a variety of factors:

1. The number of free hydroxyl groups.
2. The number and position of the sulphate groups.
3. The degree of binding to protein.

Thus Bethelheim and Ehrlich (1963) have shown that the degree of uptake of water by Ca salts of glycosaminoglycans can be arranged in the following order: $CS_6 > Heparin > Dermatan\ sulphate > CS_4$, whilst the effect of the sulphate group in CS_6 is far less than in CS_4.

Since the amounts of the polysaccharides with the higher sorbtive properties in the nucleus decrease with age, it would be expected that the water content would decrease with age. Conversely, the observations of Galante (1967) on the annulus, which indicate that there is a replacement of chondroitin sulphate by keratan sulphate between 10 and 70 years of age, could indicate an increase in water content.

Most workers over the past forty years (Armstrong, 1965) have continued to report the observations of Püschel (1930) on water content of intervertebral disc, in which he stated that both regions of the disc lose water with age.

Our observations (Reed, 1971; Hall and Reed, 1973) indicate that, whereas in agreement with Püschel the water content of the nucleus decreases continuously with age (13 mg water/g dry tissue/year), at ages above 30 the moisture content of the annulus increases by 8·5 mg water/g dry tissue/year. The slight loss that occurs in the annulus at ages below 30 may not be significant, since relatively few samples were examined within this age range.

The synthesis of the various glycosaminoglycans from glucose has been shown to be dependent on the oxidation and amination of nucleotide sugars and their subsequent sulphation by the action of sulphotransferase, in the presence of 3-phosphoadenyl sulphate (Roden, 1970).

The specificity of this enzyme appears to be controlled by the adjacent sugar molecule. Thus, in the heterogeneous dermatan sulphate of the umbilical cord 6-sulphation occurs adjacent to glucuronic acid residues, whereas 4-sulphation is spatially associated with iduronic acid. This type of specificity could not determine the change from CS_4 to CS_6 with advancing age since the chondroitin disaccharide unit is common to both, but it would appear likely that these changes in glycosaminoglycan content are enzymically determined, and thus come under genetic control.

It is possible, therefore, that as far as age changes are concerned the variations in glycosaminoglycans result from chronological alterations in gene repressor action.

REFERENCES

ARMSTRONG, J. R. (1965) In *Lumbar Disc Lesion*, 3rd Edition. Edinburgh: E. & S. Livingstone Ltd.

BETHELHEIM, F. A. & EHRLICH, S. H. (1963) *Journal of Physical Chemistry*, **67**, 1948.

BJORKSTEN, J. (1969) In *Aging Life Processes*. Ed. S. Baderman. Springfield: C. C. Thomas.

BUDDECKE, E. & SEIGOLEITS, M. (1964) *Hoppe–Seylers Zeitschrift für physiologische Chemie*, **337**, 105.

GALANTE, J. O. (1967) *Acta orthopaedica Scandinavica*, Supplement 100.

GREILING, H. & BAUMAN, G. (1973) In *Connective Tissue and Ageing*, p. 160. Ed. H. G. Vogel. Amsterdam: Excerpta Medica.

HALL, D. A. & REED, F. B. (1973) *Age and Ageing* (in press).

MATHEWS, M. B. (1973) In *Connective Tissue and Ageing*, p. 151. Ed. H. G. Vogel. Amsterdam: Excerpta Medica.

MATHEWS, M. B. & GLAGOV, S. (1966) *Journal of Clinical Investigation*, **45**, 1103.

PÜSCHEL, J. (1930) *Beiträge zur pathologischen Anatomie und zur allgemeinen Pathologie*, **84**, 123.

REED, F. B. (1971) Ph.D. Thesis, University of Leeds.

RODEN, L. (1970) In *Chemistry and Molecular Biology of the Intercellular Matrix*, p. 797. Ed. E. A. Balazs. London: Academic Press.

DISCUSSION
(of papers by Drs M. E. Grant, E. Atkins, A. J. Bailey and David Hall)

Teller (Ulm). In Dr Grant's lecture he described two types of collagen disorder, the hydroxylysine deficiency and dermatosparaxis. Where does the Ehlers–Danlos syndrome fit into these?

Grant (Manchester). The patients which were studied in Boston by Pinnell and co-workers, presented with some of the clinical features of the Ehlers–Danlos syndrome. It is becoming clear that there may be as many as seven different subtypes of this syndrome, one of which is now defined by a deficiency in protocollagen lysyl hydroxylase in certain tissues.

The dermatosparactic condition arising from a defect in the conversion of procollagen to collagen has been detected in both cattle and sheep. The possibility that a similar condition might occur in man cannot be excluded and there are some preliminary indications that in one form of Ehlers–Danlos syndrome there may be a partial defect in procollagen peptidase activity.*

Bailey (Bristol). There is little I can add to what Dr Grant has just said. Certainly both the hydroxylysine deficient (ED–S type 6) and dermatosparactic (ED–S type 7) result in defective cross linking which could, at least in part, account for the fragility of the fibres. However, no similar defect could be shown in our analyses of Ehlers–Danlos types 1–5. Indeed since the latter are characterized by autosomal dominant inheritance it is unlikely that the basic defect is an enzyme deficiency as in the autosomal recessive types 6 and 7. Whether types 6 or 7 should still be classified as Ehlers–Danlos is debatable.

Harris (Sheffield). The description of dermatosparaxis sounds similar to epidermolysis bullosa (foetalis lethalis type). Have any studies been done on the collagen of patients with this disease?

Dorfman (Chicago). I think I might comment that electronmicroscopy has been done on epidermolysis bullosa and there is a defect at the basal layer. I don't think it looks like the pathology of the dermis— it's actually at the epidermal junction as I recall.

Muir (London). How far does a deficiency in hydroxylase affect

* See, Lichtenstein, J. R., Martin, G. R., Kohn, L. D., Byers, P. M. and McKusick, V. A. (1973) *Science*, **182**, 298.

basement membranes since hydroxylation is more important for basement membrane collagen?

Grant. I don't think anyone has had an opportunity to look at the
basement membrane collagen from patients with the lysyl hydroxylation
deficiency.

Muir. Do they have any signs suggesting abnormal glomerular
filtration?

Grant. I am afraid I can't answer that question but as far as I can recall,
in the patients studied, the amino acid analyses of their urines were
normal. I should point out, however, that considerable variation in the
degree of hydroxylysine deficit has been seen in different collagen-
containing tissues studied by the Boston group. Whereas dermal collagen contains only 5 per cent of the normal levels of hydroxylysine,
bone collagen was found to contain 50 per cent of control levels. Thus,
it is conceivable that other collagens may contain their normal complement of hydroxylysine and basement membrane collagen could possibly
be unaffected.

Marshall (London). Do you have any information concerning the
amino acid sequence around the hydroxylysine residue which acts as
the acceptor for allysine (or hydroxyallysine) in the formation of
the cross-links? Is it always in the sequence -Gly-X-Hylys-Y-Arg-
which appears to be that requisite for glycosylation of collagen, or
does it occur also in other sequences? If it is present always in the former
then it might be deduced that the carbohydrate of collagen has at least
one specific function, namely to assist in some undefined way in the
cross-linking as has been suggested, and there might be a subsequent
partial removal of the sugars in the collagen of the adult after formation
of the cross-link.

Bailey. The hydroxylysine residues which act as the acceptor for the
allysine cross-link precursor are, assuming the quarter-stagger and
overlap hypothesis is correct, at positions 103 and 943 along the α-chain.
The hydroxylysine residue at 103 is glycosylated in rat, guinea pig
and human skin and occurs in the sequence gly met-hylys-gly-his-arg-.
The sequence around 943 is similar but the hydroxylysine is not glycosylated in all tissue. Furthermore, the extent of glycosylation of the
cross-link varies considerably with the tissue, hence it is at present
difficult to see a relation between glycosylation and cross-linking.

Steinman (Zurich). What is the function of 3-OH proline?

Bailey. I do not know.

Muir. Could Dr Atkins give us any idea of the energies involved in the formation of the double helix in hyaluronic acid?

Atkins. We do not know the exact linkage mechanism that occurs in the double helix of hyaluronic acid. In fact both hyaluronic acid and sodium hyaluronate form double helices and we only know, at this stage, that the carboxyl groups are buried in the interior.

Dorfman. I would like to call attention to some work in reference to Dr Hall's paper—not specifically his presentation but rather to the Symposium in general. I suspect that the one clear cut error of ageing that we know is progeria, and just recently the successful growth of fibroblast cultures from patients with progeria has been reported.* This has proved very difficult, but it has now been found, apparently, that they have a defect in their repair mechanism following γ radiation. There have been previous reports, of course, of work with U.V. radiation in genetic disease, but this is the first metabolic lead on ageing, in terms of an inborn error of metabolism, that I know of.

Teller. Studies on urinary excretion patterns during the course of life, as performed by us, have shown a relative increase in the excretion of dermatan sulphate and a concomitant decrease of heparan sulphate. I wonder whether Dr Hall also studied these glycosaminoglycans with regards to ageing of cartilage.

Hall (Leeds). The answer to that is no, but the amounts of dermatan sulphate which are present in the cartilage are small compared to those in the skin. I think the changes to which you refer are mainly due to the metabolism of the skin glycosaminoglycans.

The amounts of any tissue component which appear in the urine over long periods of time are often difficult to measure and the sort of excretion pattern observed daily in the urine of a child, where massive remodelling is taking place, is very much more specific than those which occur over longer periods of time in the urine of an adult.

This sort of effect can be shown, for instance, in the hydroproline content of urine. If one assumes that a certain amount of collagen is lost from the tissues over a period of ten years or more, calculations of the number of microgrammes of hydroxyproline lost per day shows it to be well within the normal limits, and I think the same may well occur in the case of the polysaccharides.

* Epstein, J., Williams, J. R. and Little, J. B. (1973) *Proceedings of the National Academy of Science of the United States of America*, **70**, 977.

11

Genetic aspects of mucopolysaccharidoses with special reference to heterozygous carriers

Walter M. Teller

Introduction

Mucopolysaccharidoses (MPS), disorders of connective tissue with abnormal storage of acid mucopolysaccharides (glycosaminoglycans), are relatively rare hereditary diseases. According to Lowry and Renwick (1971) they occur as seldom as 1:1,000,000 (MPS I), 1:150,000 (MPS II) and 1:300,000 (MPS IV). It is generally accepted that within a MPS-afflicted family only the same type of mucopolysaccharidosis occurs. This has been apparent ever since the first cases were reported at the beginning of this century. Comprehensive reviews including discussions of genetic aspects have been published (Halperin and Curtis, 1942; Ullrich, 1943; Spranger, 1972; McKusick, 1972; Neufeld and Barton, 1973).

Following a survey of our current knowledge of genetics of MPS, in this report particular attention will be given to the detection of heterozygous carriers of different MPS.

Genetics of the mucopolysaccharidoses

In Table I the modes of inheritance of the 'classical' types of MPS (including a recently described form) are compiled. It also contains our present knowledge of the enzyme deficiencies involved. Except for MPS II, all MPS are transmitted as an autosomal recessive disorder. Boys are affected as often as girls. MPS II (Hunter) reveals the x-linked recessive mode of inheritance. The first reported cases were two brothers published by Hunter (1917).

The reproductive capacity of MPS is rather low although one family was reported by McKusick (1972) in which the grandfather and his two grandsons were affected with MSP II. Altogether the ratio MPS I: MPS II: MPS III appears to be 2:1:3. Therefore the heterozygous

TABLE I   *Survey of mucopolysaccharidoses, their modes of inheritance and the enzymes found to be deficient*

Type	Mode of inheritance	Enzyme deficiency
I Hurler	Autos.	α-L-iduronidase
II Hunter	X-link. rec.	Iduronate sulphatase
III A Sanfilippo	Autos. Rec.	Heparan sulphate sulphatase
III B Sanfilippo	Autos. Rec.	N-acetyl-α-D-glucos-aminidase
IV Morquio	Autos. Rec.	?
V Scheie	Autos. Rec.	α-L-iduronidase
VI Maroteux–Lamy	Autos. Rec.	N-acetylgalactose-amine 4-sulphatase
β-glucuronidase deficiency	Autos. Rec.	β-Glucuronidase

carriers of MPS I and III seem to have a slight reproductive advantage compared to their MPS II counterparts.

There is considerable variability of clinical manifestations within the MPS. This may be genetically influenced. MPS II can present itself in a severe form causing death before the age of about 15 years and a mild form surviving into the 30th to 50th year of life. Also, MPS VI (Maroteaux-Lamy) may occur in a mild and a severe form (Spranger *et al.*, 1970). The Morquio syndrome (MPS IV) is considered to exist in more than one allelic variant. According to different adult heights attained, Spranger (1972) proposed a pseudo-Morquio I and II and a Dale-variant. The latter is taller ($>$115 cm) than the 'true' Morquio (height $<$115 cm). MPS V (Scheie) which most authors including our-selves still classify as a separate entity may very well be a mild form of MPS I (Hurler) (McKusick, 1972). This became apparent when Bach, Friedman, Weissmann and Neufeld, 1972, found the same enzyme, α–L–iduronidase, to be lacking in both entities. There was no mutual correction in cultures of fibroblasts (Wiesmann and Neufeld, 1970). The Hurler corrective factor obtained from non-Hurler cultures normalized the incorporation of ^{35}S in both Hurler and Scheie cell cultures (Barton and Neufeld, 1971). Patients with MPS who clinically fitted neither the picture of MPS I nor of MPS V were considered by McKusick *et al.* (1972) as intermediates with a possible genetic compound (MPS I/MPS V), analogous to the compound of hemoglobin S/C disease.

Detection of heterozygous carriers

Heritable diseases as involving and of such poor prognosis as some of the MPS stimulate the effort for detecting clinically inconspicuous heterozygotes in order to give them pertinent genetic counselling. Wiedemann (1951) and Rampini and Adank (1964) found abnormal granulations of peripheral neutrophilic leucocytes of heterozygous carriers. Also the bone marrow of these subjects contained unusually granulated cells. Mittwoch (1962) observed an increased nuclear segmentation of the neutrophils of heterozygous carriers of MPS (also formerly called gargoylism). As a whole this approach to the detection of heterozygotes proved to be rather unreliable and has largely been abandoned.

In 1961 Teller, Rosevear and Burke found qualitatively abnormal excretion of acid mucopolysaccharides in the urine of parents of patients with MPS I. The total excretion of acid mucopolysaccharides was normal; also clinically the parents were healthy and free from any of the symptoms of MPS. Although several authors were unable to confirm these findings (for review see Spranger, 1972) subsequent studies using more refined methods largely confirmed the early results (Teller and Kruger, 1967; Teller, Busch and Bode, 1969; Robertson, 1968; Jozsa and Szabo, 1972). In MPS III (Sanfilippo) the qualitative analysis of urinary mucopolysaccharides seems to be most reliable (Robertson, 1968), while in one family with Hunter disease (MPS II) our own studies gave an erroneous result in a father who should have been a normal excretor (Table II).

Figure 1 shows the column chromatographic pattern of urinary acid mucopolysaccharides in a girl with MPS III, her parents and a normal control child. Measuring hyaluronidase activity in urine, Jozsa and Szabo (1972) obtained pathological results in a total of 71·4 per cent of parents whose children had all types of MPS (Table III).

In cell cultures abnormal mucopolysaccharide storage has been found in leucocytes (Foley, Danes and Bearn, 1969) and fibroblasts of heterozygous carriers of MPS (Danes and Bearn, 1966, 1967).

TABLE II *Urinary excretion of acid mucopolysaccharides in patients with mucopolysaccharidoses and their kin*
(*Teller et al.*, 1969)

	Total carbazole (mg GA/24 h)	No. of subjects with pathol. values	% HS-fr.	Column chromatography† % CSA/C-fr.	CSB-fr.	KS fr.	No. of subjects with pathol. patterns
Type I (Hurler)							
Patients* (n=5)	11·2-**61.2**	4	34 -**56**	21·8-53·8	7·2-**21·0**	trace	5
Fathers (n=2)	8·6	0	38 -**44·5**	28·4-45·5	16·5-**27**	trace	2
Mothers (n=3)	3·6- 7·1	0	**41·2-52·8**	30·5-36·0	15·5-**28·2**	trace	3
Siblings* (n=3)	9·8	0	12·5-34	53·5-76·6	10·8-19·0	trace	0
Type II (Hunter)							
Patients* (n=4)	**39·0-42·6**	4	33·3-39·9	28·1-35·5	**31·2-33·5**	trace	4
Fathers (n=3)	5·2-12·2	0	4·4-50·3	21·4-79·5	16·1-**31·5**	trace	1
Mothers (n=3)	12·2-12·8	0	32·6-50·0	16·1-33·0	17·0-**51·4**	trace	3
Siblings* (n=2)		0	10·2-39·5	59·3-78·0	10·2-11·8	trace	0
Type III (Sanfilippo)							
Patients* (n=6)	**40·0-59·0**	6	**70·0-85·5**	8·2-**25·0**	**4·5- 6·7**	trace	6
Fathers (n=3)	6·5-16·0	(1)	35·0-**56·4**	**28·8-50·5**	14·5-16·0	trace	3
Mothers (n=4)	4·6- 9·5	0	**40·5-89·0**	**11·0-43·2**	**12·8-16·8**	trace	4
Siblings* (n=4)	7·4-14·8	0	13·0-34·2	52·5-63·0	9·8-**34·5**	trace	(1)
Control subjects (Teller & Krüger, 1967)							
Adults (n=9)	4 -12		28·2±5·4	54·0±4·3	19·1±4·8	trace	
Children (age 3-8) (n=7)	3 -14		31·8±7·0	57·5±6·5	10·9±2·7	trace	

*age less than 14 yrs.
GA = glucuronic acid; fr. = fraction.
HS = heparan sulphate (heparitin sulphate).
CSA/C = chondroitin-4-sulphate/chondroitin-6-sulphate (chondroitin sulphate A/C).
CSB = dermatan sulphate (chondroitin sulphate B).
KS = keratan sulphate (keratosulphate).

† values expressed in per cent total carbazole material eluted from the column.

Abnormal value are given in heavy print; questionable results are given in brackets.

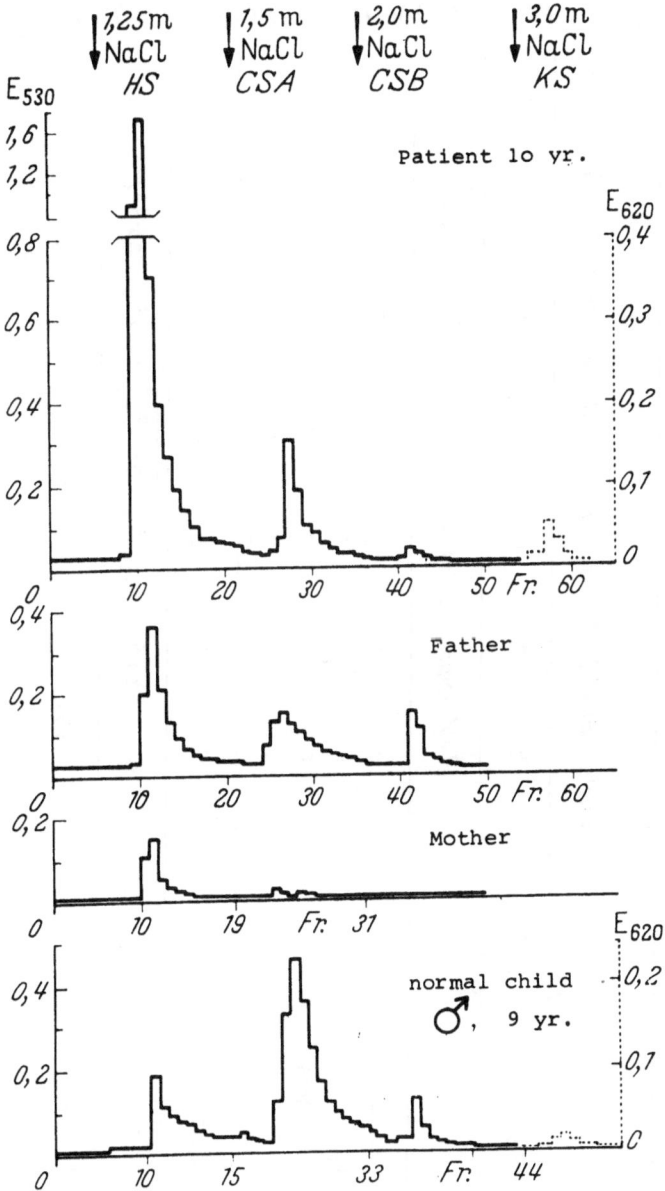

FIG. 1 Column chromatographic fractionation (method of Teller and Ziemann, 1966) of urinary acid mucopolysaccharides in the urine of a patient with MPS III, her father, mother, and a normal control child (Teller, Bechtelsheimer and Totovic, 1967).

TABLE III *Hyaluronidase activity in the urine of parents of children suffering from different forms of mucopolysaccharidoses (Józsa and Szabó, 1972)*

Type of MPS	Total No. of parents	Parents with normal MPS excretion				Parents excreting pathologic fractions			
		Total	CS	A	N	Total	CS	A	N
			Hyaluronidase activity				Hyaluronidase activity		
Hurler–Hunter (types I–II)	18	6	0	1	5	12	7	4	1
Sanfilippo (type III)	15	2	0	1	1	13	11	1	1
Types IV, V, VI and others	13	7	0	1	6	6	3	3	0
Hurler variant	17	3	0	0	3	14	7	5	2
Total	63	18	0	3	15	45	28	13	4
		28·6%	0%	16·6%	83·4%	71·4%	62·2%	28·8%	9%
			16·6%				91%		

Normal (N)=250–400 U; somewhat reduced (A)=200 U; markedly reduced (CS)=below 200 U.

Matalon and Dorfman (1969) determined chemically the mucopoly-saccharide material stored in cultured fibroblasts of MPS heterozygotes and found abnormally high amounts of dermatan sulphate.

All procedures employing cell cultures are rather cumbersome and fallible. They can hardly be considered suitable for routine use. Also, about 20 different disease entities have been described so far, all of which reveal abnormally high metachromasia of fibroblast cultures. Therefore Milunsky and Littlefield (1969) raised a word of caution about interpreting the results obtained in tissue cultures.

TABLE IV *Mean values and standard deviations of N-acetyl-α-D-glucosaminidase activity in the serum of homozygous and heterozygous carriers of the Sanfilippo B gene and of normal individuals (v. Figura et al., 1973)*

		Test I	Test II	Test III
		mumoles/min./ml		
Humozygotes ..	x̄†	0·01	0·06	0·14
Parents	x̄	0·12	0·21	0·31
	s	0·01	0·03	0·07
Presumed heterozygotes ..	x̄	0·13	0·23	0·35
	s	0·01	0·06	0·09
Normals (1/2–76 years)* ..	x̄	0·44	0·70	0·88
	s	0·17	0·22	0·26
		n=30	n=130	n=159

* No age dependency of *N*-acetyl-α-D-glucosaminidase activity was found for normal individuals.

† Symboles used are x̄: mean value and s: standard deviation.

Following the detection of single enzyme deficiencies being responsible for MPS (for reviews see Neufeld and Barton, 1973, and McKusick, 1972; also Table I), the determination of activities of the enzyme involved became the most logical approach to diagnosis of a certain MPS. It also proved to be a feasible means of detecting heterozygous carriers. v. Figura, Lögering, Mersmann and Kresse (1973) determined N-acetyl-α-D-glucosaminidase in serum to patients with MPS III B (Sanfilippo B) and their kin by three different methods (Table IV). In homozygotes the values were low, in parents and presumed heterozygotes they were intermediate to normal controls. Sly, Quinton, McAllister and Rimoin (1973), who described a new type of MPS with β-glucuronidase deficiency, found intermediate activities of these enzymes in white cell lysates of the proband's parents and some of his relatives. The subjects with low levels may be presumed to be heterozygous carriers (Fig. 2).

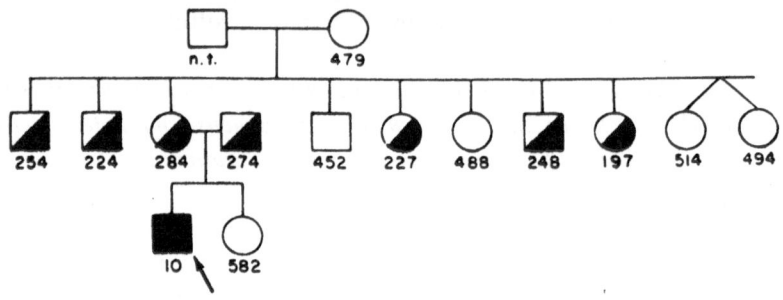

FIG. 2   Pedigree of family with β-glucuronidase deficiency. Numbers indicate β-glucuronidase activities (m μ mol/mg/3 h) in white cell lysates (Sly *et al.*, 1973) ↑ = proband. n.t. = not tested.

In fibroblast cultures of the same patient and his parents, Hall, Cantz and Neufeld (1973) determined low and intermediate activities, respectively, of β-glucuronidase compared to normal controls. Tables Va and Vb summarize our present knowledge of the various means of detecting heterozygous carriers of different MPS.

Prenatal diagnosis and genetic counselling

Like several heritable metabolic and chromosomal diseases, MPS can be diagnosed antenatally. Besides metachromasia of cultured fibroblasts, the direct determination of stored mucopolysaccharides in cultured cells has been employed (Matalon, Dorfman, Nadler and Jacobsen, 1970). These approaches have proved not to be entirely satisfactory. Therefore new impulses may be expected to arise from direct determination of mucopolysaccharide content of amnoitic fluid (Duncan, Logan, Ferguson–Smith and Hall, 1973) or, possibly, of the enzyme deficient in a given MPS. Since in MPS all therapeutic attempts, including plasma infusions, have failed to be effective (Crocker, 1972) it is ethically warranted to suggest termination of the pregnancy, once the

TABLE V *Survey of mucopolysaccharidoses and various means of detecting their heterozygous carriers*

TABLE Va URINE

Heterozygous carriers

Type	Urine	Authors
I Hurler	Dermatan sulphate ↑	Teller *et al.* (1961)
II Hunter	Heparatan sulphate ↑	Teller *et al.* (1969)
IIIA Sanfilippo A	Hyaluronidase ↑	Józsa and Szabó (1972)
	Heparan sulphate ↑	Teller, Betchtel-sheimer and Totovic (1967)
		Teller, Busch and Bode (1969)
		Robertson (1968)
IIIB Sanfilippo B	Heparan sulphate ↑	Józsa and Szabó (1972)
IV Morquio		
V Scheie		
VI Maroteau–Lamy		
β-Glucuronidase deficiency		

foetus is found to be affected. An easy and reliable procedure for the detection of heterozygous carriers in families with MPS should be used as a basis for a judicious and pertinent genetic counselling in heterozygous individuals who intend to get married.

Summary

Except for Hunter disease which is x-linked recessive, all mucopolysaccharidoses are transmitted by an autosomal recessive mode of inheritance.

Various means were employed to detect heterozygous carriers: abnormal granulations of leucocytes, abnormal urinary mucopolysaccharide excretion pattern, metachromasia of cultured fibroblasts

TABLE Vb   SERUM AND FIBROBLASTS

Type	Serum	Authors	Heterozygous carriers	
			Fibroblasts	Authors
I Hurler			Metachromasia ↑	Danes and Bearn (1966)
II Hunter			Metachromasia ↑	Danes and Bearn (1967)
			(Leucocytes: Metachromasia) ↑	Foley et al. (1969)
IIIA Sanfilippo A				
IIIB Sanfilippo B	n-Acetyl-D-Glucosaminidase 26–35%	v. Figura et al. (1973)		
β-Glucuronidase deficiency			β-Glucuronidase ↓ (Intermediate)	Hall et al. (1973)
			(Leucocytes: Intermediate)	Sly et al. (1973)

and leucocytes, mucopolysaccharide contents of cultured cells, and, finally, the determination of the activities of the enzyme which is lacking in a given mucopolysaccharidosis. At the present time the latter procedure seems to be the most promising and reliable approach to diagnosis of the disease and to detection of its heterozygotes. It may also prove useful in the antenatal diagnosis. In mucopolysaccharidoses a judicious genetic counselling seems to be appropriate and feasible, especially since no effective therapy is available as yet.

Acknowledgement

I wish to thank Mrs Rupp for secretarial help and typing of the manuscript.

REFERENCES

BACH, G., FRIEDMAN, R., WEISSMANN, B. & NEUFELD, E. F. (1972) The defect in the Hurler and Scheie syndromes: deficiency of α-L-iduronidase. *Proceedings of the National Academy of Sciences of the U.S.A.*, **69**, 2048.

BARTON, R. W. & NEUFELD, E. F. (1971) The Hurler corrective factor: purification and some properties. *Journal of Biological Chemistry*, **246**, 7773.

CROCKER, A. C. (1972) Commentary: Plasma infusion therapy for Hurler's syndrome. *Pediatrics*, **50**, 683.

DANES, B. S. & BEARN, A. G. (1966) Hurler's syndrome. A genetic study in cell culture. *Journal of Experimental Medicine*, **123**, 1.

DANES, B. S. & BEARN, A. G. (1967) Cellular metachromasia: a genetic marker for studying the mucopolysaccharidoses. *Lancet*, **i**, 241.

DUNCAN, D. M., LOGAN, R. W., FERGUSON–SMITH, M. A. & HALL, F. (1973) The measurement of acid mucopolysaccharides (glycosaminoglycans) in amniotic fluid and urine. *Clinica Chimica Acta*, **45**, 73.

v. FIGURA, K., LÖGERING, M., MERSMAN, G. & KRESSE, H. (1973) Sanfilippo B disease: serum assays for detection of homozygotes and heterozygotes in three families. *Journal of Pediatrics* (in press).

FOLEY, K. M., DANES, B. S. & BEARN, A. G. (1969) White blood cell cultures in genetic studies of the human mucopolysaccharidoses. *Science*, **164**, 424.

HALL, C. W., CANTZ, M. & NEUFELD, E. F. (1973) A β-glucuronidase deficiency mucopolysaccharidosis: Studies in cultured fibroblasts. *Archives of Biochemistry and Biophysics*, **155**, 32.

HALPERIN, S. L. & CURTIS, G. M. (1942) The genetics of gargoylism. *American Journal of Mental Deficiency*, **46**, 298.

HUNTER, C. (1917) *Proceedings of the Royal Society of Medicine*, **10**, pt. 1, 104.

JOZSA, L. & SZABO, L. (1972) Determination of the heterozygous state from the urine of the parents of children suffering from mucopolysaccharidosis. *Acta Paediatricia, Academy of Science (Hungary)*, **13**, 39.

LOWRY, R. B. & RENWICK, D. H. G. (1971) Relative frequency of the Hurler and Hunter syndromes. *New England Journal of Medicine*, **284**, 221.

MATALON, R. & DORFMAN, A. (1969) Acid mucopolysaccharides in cultured fibroblasts. *Lancet*, **ii**, 838.

MATALON, R., DORFMAN, A., NADLER, H. L. & JACOBSEN, C. B. (1970) A chemical method for the antenatal diagnosis of mucopolysaccharidoses. *Lancet*, **i**, 83.

McKUSICK, V. A. (1972) In *Heritable Disorders of Connective Tissue*, Fourth edition, p. 521. Saint Louis: C. V. Mosby.

McKUSICK, V. A., HOWELL, R. R., HUSSELS, I. E., NEUFELD, E. F. & STEVENSON, R. E. (1972) Allelism, non-allelism, and genetic compounds among the mucopolysaccharidoses. *Lancet*, **i**, 993.

MILUNSKY, A. & LITTLEFIELD, J. W. (1969) Diagnostic limitations of metachromasia. *New England Journal of Medicine*, **281**, 1128.

MITTWOCH, U. (1962) Nuclear segmentation of the neutrophils in heterozygous carriers of gargoylism. *Nature (London)*, **193**, 1209.

NEUFELD, E. F. & BARTON, R. W. (1973) Genetic disorders of mucopolysaccharide metabolism. In *Biology of Brain Dysfunction*, Vol. I, p. 1. Ed. G. E. Gaull. New York, London: Plenum Press.

RAMPINI, S. & ADANK, W. (1964) Hamatologische Befunde bei Patienten mit Gargoylismus und heterozygoten Genträgern. *Helvetic Paediatrica Acta*, **19**, 101.

ROBERTSON, W. V. B. (1968) Patterns of mucopolysaccharide excretion during development and in disease. *XIIth International Congress of Pediatrics*, Mexico City, III, 38.

SLY, W. S., QUINTON, B. A., McALISTER, W. H. & RIMOIN, D. L. (1973) Beta glucuronidase deficiency: report of clinical, radiological and biochemical features of a new mucopolysaccharidosis. *Journal of Pediatrics*, **82**, 249.

SPRANGER, J., KOCH, F., McKUSICK, V. A., NATZSCHKA, J., WIEDEMANN, H. R. & ZELLWEGER, H. (1970) Mucopolysaccharidosis VI (Maroteaux–Lamy's disease). *Helvetica Paediatrica Acta*, **25**, 337.

SPRANGER, J. (1972) The systemic mucopolysaccharidoses. *Ergebnisse Inneren Medizin Kinderheilk*. N.F., **32**, 165.

TELLER, W., ROSEVEAR, J. W. & BURKE, E. C. (1961) Identification of heterozygous carriers of gargoylism. *Proceedings of Society of Experimental Biology (N.Y.)*, **108**, 276.

TELLER, W. & ZIEMANN, A. (1966) Die saulenchromatographische Fraktionierung der sauren Mucopolysaccharide im Harn. *Klinische Wochenschrift*, **44**, 1141.

TELLER, W. & KRUGER, CH. (1967) Age-dependent changes of acid mucopolysaccharide excretion patterns in human urine. *Experientia*, **23**, 908.

TELLER, W., BECHTELSHEIMER, R. & TOTOVIC, V. (1967) Die Heparitusulfate-Mucopolysaccharidose (Sanfilippo); Klinische, biochemische, genetische und morphologische Untersuchungen. *Klinische Wochenschrift*, **45**, 497.

TELLER, W., BUSCH, C. & BODE, H. H. (1969) Re-evaluation of heterozygous carriers of mucopolysaccharidoses. *Hormone Metabolism Research*, **1**, 78.

ULLRICH, O. (1943) Die Pfaundler-Hurler'sche Krankheit. *Ergebnisse der Inneren Medizin Kinderheilk*, **63**, 929.

WIEDEMANN, H. R. (1951) Beitrage zur Pfaundler-Hurler'schen Krankheilk. *Zeitschrift fur Kinderheilk*, **70**, 81.

WIESMANN, U. & NEUFELD, E. F. (1970) Scheie and Hurler syndromes: apparent identity of the biochemical defect. *Science*, **169**, 72.

DISCUSSION
(of paper by Professor Teller)

Spranger (Keil). Do you find an abnormal excretion pattern of mucopolysaccharides in the parents? I would be interested to know how you explain this because if you culture fibroblasts from heterozygotes they do not show the storage defect. Although the parents obviously have an intermediate enzyme activity, the amount of enzyme is sufficient to prevent storage occurring *in vitro* and to ensure they are clinically normal. How then do you explain the abnormal urinary excretion patterns?

I would also like to ask whether you know any means of counselling the mother of a patient with Hunter disease? There the question is quite important if she is to have a second child, so maybe you would like to tell us something about cloning studies, or about the mother's fibroblasts, or about Dr Nadler's findings that mothers' fibroblasts do show some abnormal mucopolysaccharide accumulation, which has some problems with the Lyon hypothesis.

Teller. I really cannot answer this question completely, the only thing I know is that the heterozygote carriers do show abnormal storage in their fibroblasts so, despite the fact that they can correct their disease state *in vivo*, in culture their fibroblasts do show some storage. *In vivo* these people are healthy, but, from the data of Danes and others, the fibroblasts of the heterozygous carriers are different from the homozygous normals. Also, if one considers the enzymes, for instance in Sanfilippo disease, one can speculate that the metabolism is working at a certain level, just competing with normal requirements, and keeping the patient healthy apparently. But the enzyme is abnormal, so we may find on a qualitative analysis of urine a shifting of the different fractions in the direction of the disease.

The other question is about the difficulty of detecting Hunter heterozygotes because of the fact that if you culture fibroblasts from a Hunter heterozygote you might find the cells are all normal. Because of the Lyon hypothesis you get normal cells and diseased cells but only if you see them side by side in the same culture can you be sure that this is a Hunter mother. But the original material may not have been diseased if you just hit the area where normal cells are lying, then you just pick up the normal cell line on tissue culture.

I should say that the detection of heterozygotes in the Hunter disease should be made by enzyme interpretation. We saw this morning that the dermatan sulphatase is deficient and one can set up an easy assay to determine the enzyme, in serum for instance. One can then follow up a similar line to that which others have used in Sanfilippo. Unless we have this test, the only way would be to do several cultures of different sides of the suspected child and then see whether they have metachromasia.

Sinclair (London). I was very impressed with Professor Spranger's analysis of urine but I have a family in which it was very difficult to sort out the family relationships. Was the father the natural father of the patient. When we measured the urinary acid mucopolysaccharides against the urinary creatinine concentration everything fell into place, fitting in with the blood groups as well. I wonder whether it is worth going back on your stored specimens which you mentioned, and trying to correlate the excretion of the various metabolites against the concentration of creatinine in the urine. It might be an interesting parameter to consider.

The Second Milner Lecture

12

Genetic defects of the degradation of glycosaminoglycans: the mucopolysaccharidoses

Albert Dorfman
with *Reuben Matalon, Jerry N. Thompson, J. Anthony Cifonelli, Glyn Dawson, Allen C. Stoolmiller and Stanford T. Lamberg*

Introduction

Elsewhere in this volume the clinical characteristics and genetics of the mucopolysaccharidoses are discussed. Extensive reviews of historical aspects, clinical features and pathology have been published (Dorfman and Matalon, 1972; Spranger, 1972; McKusick, 1972). Modern understanding of the metabolic basis of these diseases started with the demonstration by Brante (1952) that livers of patients with Hurlers disease contain increased quantities of substances composed of hexosamine, uronic acid and sulphate. More definitive evidence of involvement of glycosaminoglycans became available when Dorfman and Lorincz (1957) discovered that dermatan sulphate and heparan sulphate were excreted in large amounts in the urine of a patient with the Hurler syndrome. Although it was clear on genetic grounds that Hunter's and Hurler's syndromes represented different mutations, the distinction of individual mucopolysaccharidoses on chemical grounds was established after Harris (1961) and Sanfilippo, Podosin, Langer and Good (1963) observed that the excessive urinary excretion of only heparan sulphate was characteristic of a distinctive clinical entity. The classification of the mucopolysaccharidoses by McKusick *et al.* (1965) served to clarify the concept that the mucopolysaccharidoses consisted of a group of clinically distinct diseases.

More recent understanding of the etiology of this group of diseases was advanced by the discovery by Danes and Bearn (1965) that fibroblasts cultured from the skin of Hurler and Hunter patients contain large numbers of metachromatic granules. Independently Matalon and Dorfman (1966) found that such cultured fibroblasts accumulate large amounts of dermatan sulphate.

Van Hoof and Hers (1964), on the basis of electron microscopic studies, first suggested that Hurler's syndrome represents a lysosomal disease due to faulty degradation of glycosaminoglycans. On the basis of kinetic studies, Frantantoni, Hall and Neufeld (1968a) concluded that accumulation of glycosaminoglycans results from impaired degradation. These investigators (1968b) observed that growth of Hunter or Hurler fibroblasts in the presence of normal fibroblasts results in the disappearance of metachromasia and the correction of the metabolic defect as measured by the uptake or disappearance of $^{35}SO_4$-containing macromolecules. Correction was also demonstrated by the culture of fibroblasts derived from Hurler and Hunter patients in the presence of growth medium previously exposed to normal cells. Subsequent studies showed that fibroblasts derived from each of the syndromes were deficient in specific factors produced by fibroblasts of normal individuals or patients with any of the other syndromes. Addition of the appropriate factor to fibroblast cultures resulted in correction of the specific metabolic defect. In the case of Scheie's and Hurler's syndromes mutual correction was not observed (Wiesmann and Neufeld, 1970). Since Neufeld and Cantz (1971) discovered that fibroblasts of certain patients with the Sanfilippo's disease cross-correct each other, they concluded that there existed two biochemically distinct syndromes, each presumably lacking a different factor required for mucopolysaccharide degradation.

Corrective factors were found in various tissues and in urine, and Barton and Neufeld (1971) have extensively purified the Hurler factor. Sanfilippo A factor has been purified by Kresse and Neufeld (1972), and the Hunter factor has been partially purified by Cantz, Chramack and Neufeld (1970).

Degradation of Glycosaminoglycans

The presence of glycosidases in mammalian tissues has been long known. Recent appreciation of their localization in lysosomes and their role in the pathogenesis of glycosphingolipidoses and mucopolysaccharidoses has stimulated a more detailed study of their properties. In general, such glycosidases had been previously considered specific with respect to the aglycone and the anomeric linkage of the glycoside bond. However, exceptions to this concept are already known to exist, e.g. β-N-acetylhexosaminidase hydrolyzes glycosides of both N-acetylglucosamine and N-acetylgalactosamine. In contrast, α-N-acetylgluco-saminidase is specific for the glucosamine configuration (Leaback, 1970). Different isozymes of a given glycosidase may have different specificities.

TABLE I *Glycoside linkages of acidic glycosaminoglycans*

	β-Xyl	β-Gal	β-Glc NAc	α-Glc NAc	α-Glc NSO_4	β-Gal NAc	βGlcNAc $AspNH_2$	βGlc UA	α-IdUA
Hyaluronic acid			X					X	
Chondroitin 4/6-SO_4	X	X				X		X	
Dermatan sulphate	X	X				X		X	X
Heparan sulphate	X	X		X	X			X	X
Heparin	X	X		X	X			X	X
Keratan sulphate		X	X				X		
Keratan sulphate		X	X			X	?		

Our approach to the study of the etiology of the mucopolysaccharidoses has been on the basis of the structural features of the glycosaminoglycans. Table I indicates the established glycoside linkages of the known glycosaminoglycans. Those listed seem reasonably well-established although certain structural features of the keratan sulphates remain to be elucidated. Table II indicates the known sulphate linkages.

TABLE II *Sulphate linkages in glycosaminoglycans*

	GlcNAc-6-SO_4	GalNAc-6-SO_4	GalNAc-.4-SO_4	Gal-6-SO_4	IdUA-2-2-SO_4	GlcN-SO_4
Chondroitin-4-SO_4			X			
Chondroitin-6-SO_4		X				
Dermatan sulphate		X	X		X	
Heparan sulphate	X				X	X
Heparin	X				X	X
Keratan sulphate I	X			X		
Keratan sulphate II	X			X		

Some chondroitin sulphates may contain both 4- and 6-sulphate groups.

In considering genetic diseases it must be remembered that glycoproteins, glycosphingolipids and glycosaminoglycans share specific glycoside linkages. It is, therefore, to be anticipated that absence of a specific hydrolase should lead to accumulation of macromolecules or portions derived therefrom which are degraded by that hydrolase. If the same hydrolase is involved in degradation of more than one macromolecule, storate of multiple substances is to be expected. This has already been demonstrated in the case of GM_1-gangliosidosis which is characterized by the storage of GM_1-ganglioside and a 'keratan sulphate-like' material (Suzuki, 1968). Similarly, the accumulation of globoside in addition to GM_2-ganglioside has been demonstrated in Sandhoff-Jatzkewitz disease (Sandhoff, Andreae and Jatzkewitz, 1968).

The situation is complicated by lack of detailed knowledge concerning the mutliple forms of various hydrolases and their specificity. Assay with artificial substrates, although frequently helpful, has been misleading in many cases.

In the case of metabolism of acid glycosaminoglycans many questions remain unanswered. The specificity of sulphatases for specific linkages and the sequence of action of glycosidases and sulphatases is not clear. The studies of Tudball and Davidson (1968) indicated that partial degradation of chondroitin sulphate precedes sulphatase action.

The studies of Knecht, Cifonelli and Dorfman (1967) showed that the glycosaminoglycans excreted in urine and deposited in tissues of patients with the Hurler syndrome are partially degraded. In the case of dermatan sulphate such degradation could be accounted for by the action of hyaluronidase. The finding of N-acetylgalactosamine-SO_4 non-reducing terminal groups in dermatan sulphate fragments isolated from the urine of a Hurler patient by Fransson, Sjöberg, Matalon and Dorfman (1974) indicates the possibility that hyaluronidase degraded fragments are acted on by β-glucuronidase.

The fragments of heparan sulphate that were isolated by Knecht, Cifonelli and Dorfman could have arisen by the action of an endoglycosidase though no such enzyme acting on heparin or heparan sulphate has yet been discovered. The finding by Matalon and Dorfman (1968b) that the molecular weight of dermatan sulphate isolated from Hurler fibroblasts is high is consistent with the finding that skin fibroblasts are devoid of hyaluronidase activity and degrade dermatan sulphate by the sequential action of exoglycosidases. Assays of fibroblast extracts for hyaluronidase by the sensitive viscosity reduction method failed to reveal hyaluronidase activity (Matalon, R. and Dorfman, A., unpublished results). When labelled chrondroitin sulphate was subjected to digestion by extracts of normal fibroblasts, no oligosaccharides could be detected by gel chromatography, but the presence of small amount of material which behaved as a monosaccharide was observed. These findings led to the conclusion that degradation of dermatan sulphate may proceed by two different pathways. In hyaluronidase-containing tissues such as liver, degradation occurs by the action of hyaluronidase followed by the serial degradation by exoglycosidases. In fibroblasts, degradation is confined to the action of exoglycosidases.

Defects in degradation in mucopolysaccharidoses

Examination of the linkages in Tables I and II indicates that dermatan sulphate and heparan sulphate, the glycosaminoglycans deposited and excreted in Hurler, Hunter and Scheie's disease, share α-L-iduronosyl and idurono-sulphate linkages. When our studies were inaugurated no specific α-L-iduronidase was known. Search for such an enzyme was initially hampered by the lack of an adequate substrate. In an attempt to demonstrate α-L-iduronidase, desulphated dermatan sulphate was incubated with testicular hyaluronidase, β-glucuronidase and tissue extracts (Matalon, Cifonelli and Dorfman, 1971). Hyaluronidase and β-glucuronidase were used to bare a maximal number of non-reducing terminal iduronic acid residues. L-Idurone was released from this substrate by extracts of normal human fibroblasts, leukocytes and liver as well as by preparations obtained from normal urine. However, only very small amounts of L-idurone were released by extracts of fibroblasts cultured from Hurler patients. An improved substrate became available when the disaccharide, α-L-iduronosyl-anhydromannose, was prepared by the action of nitrous acid on desulphated heparan sulphate (Cifonelli, Matalon and Dorfman, 1971). With this substrate, α-L-iduronidase activity was demonstrated in extracts of normal fibroblasts, liver, leukocytes and urine but was found to be deficient in preparations derived from Hurler patients. Enzyme preparations derived from Hunter and Sanfilippo patients showed α-L-iduronidase activities comparable to those of preparations from normal individuals.

Subsequently Weissmann and Santiago (1972) demonstrated the presence of α-L-iduronidase in rat liver utilizing a synthetic substrate, α-phenyl-L-iduronide. When this substrate was made available by Dr Bernard Weissmann of the University of Illinois, more quantitative studies became possible. The absence of α-L-iduronidase in extracts of Hurler fibroblast was once again demonstrated (Matalon and Dorfman, 1972). The data in Table III summarizes these results. The low iduronidase activity in 'I-cell' disease is similar to the diminished activity of a number of lysosomal enzymes in fibroblasts derived from such patients. Mixing experiments indicated that the lack of iduronidase activity in Hurler's fibroblasts was not due to the presence of inhibitors.

TABLE III   α-L-*iduronidase activity of liver and cultured fibroblast extracts*

	Extract	Phenol μM/mg prot./24 h
Fibroblasts*	Normal	0·260
	Hurler	0·020
	Scheie	<0·002
	Hunter	0·310
	Sanfilippo A	0·180
	'I-cell'	0.080
Liver†	Normal	0·042
	Hurler	<0·002
	Sanfilippo A	0·067
	'I-cell'	0·033

* Assays performed with 300 μg of phenyliduronide per assay.

† Assays performed with 60 μg of phenyliduronide per assay.

Bach, Friedman, Weissmann and Neufeld, (1972) have also shown diminished α-L-iduronidase activity in Hurler and Scheie fibroblasts. Purified Hurler factor isolated from normal urine was found to exhibit α-L-iduronidase activity.

Hurler's and Scheie's syndromes thus appear to be due to diminished or absent α-L-iduronidase. Presumably these two genetic diseases result from allelic mutations.

The other linkage shared by dermatan sulphate and heparan sulphate (but not by other acid glycosaminoglycans except heparin) is iduronosulphate. Since Hunter's disease is genetically distinct from Hurler disease and extracts of Hunter's fibroblasts demonstrate normal levels of α-L-iduronidase, it seemed possible that absence of iduronosulphate sulphatase might be responsible for this syndrome. This suggestion has now been verified as indicated by the end group studies of Fransson *et al.* (1974) presented elsewhere in this volume and the studies of Coppa, Singh, Nichols and Di Ferrante (1973) and Bach, Eisenberg, Cantz and Neufeld (1973).

Sanfilippo A and Sanfilippo B syndromes are characterized by excretion of heparan sulphate. Reference to Table I indicates that at least two linkages, sulphamide and α-N-acetylglucosaminide, occur in heparan sulphate and heparin but are absent in other connective tissue glycosaminoglycans.

TABLE IV *Sulphamidase activity of fibroblast extracts*

Extract	$^{35}SO_4$ cpm/mg	Per cent cts applied (Corr.)
Normal (JT)	768	0·8
Normal (RA)	2202	3·0
Hurler (DR)	528	0·8
Hunter (DR)	2060	1·8
Sanfilippo A (SM)	0	0
Sanfilippo A (AB)	39	<0·1
Sanfilippo A (CB)	0	0
Sanfilippo B (PL)	1670	2·1
Sanfilippo B (KP)	999	1·3
Sanfilippo B (AS)	728	1·1

Substrate: $^{35}SO_3$-N-heparin

On the basis of some properties of the heparan sulphate stored in fibroblasts and the release of sulphate on incubation with Sanfilippo A factor, Kresse *et al.* (1972) concluded that the absence of a specific heparan sulphate sulphatase is probably responsible for Sanfilippo A disease. This conclusion has been verified in this laboratory by the use of a commercially available heparin specifically labelled in the N-sulphate position (Amersham-Searle) (Matalon and Dorfman, 1973). The data in Table IV demonstrate a lack of release of $^{35}SO_4$ when this substrate is incubated with extracts of fibroblasts derived from San-filippo A patients. In contrast extracts of all other strains of fibroblasts appear to hydrolyze the sulphamide linkage. The existence of a specific sulphamidase has previously been demonstrated by Dietrich (1970) and Friedman and Arsenis (1972).

O'Brien (1972) and von Figura and Kresse (1972) have recently demonstrated that α-N-acetylglucosaminidase is absent from extracts of fibroblasts of patients with Sanfilippo B disease. The data in Table IV confirm these findings. Some of the fibroblasts studied were from the same patients as those studied by O'Brien.

An additional defect of glycosaminoglycan metabolism involving the absence of β-glucuronidase has been recently discovered by Hall, Cantz and Neufeld (1973). Stumpf and Austin (1972), in a preliminary report, have observed a diminution of arylsulphatase B in tissues of a patient with Maroteaux–Lamy disease.

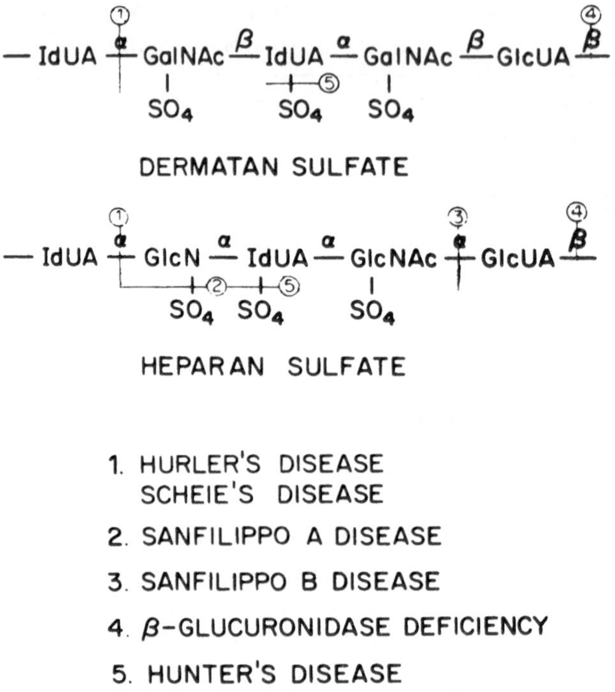
— IdUA α GalNAc β IdUA α GalNAc β GlcUA β
SO4 SO4 SO4
DERMATAN SULFATE
— IdUA α GlcN α IdUA α GlcNAc α GlcUA β
SO4 SO4 SO4
HEPARAN SULFATE
1. HURLER'S DISEASE
SCHEIE'S DISEASE
2. SANFILIPPO A DISEASE
3. SANFILIPPO B DISEASE
4. β-GLUCURONIDASE DEFICIENCY
5. HUNTER'S DISEASE

FIG. 1 Summary of enzymic defects of mucopolysaccharidoses.

Available information now permits the delineation of the enzymic defects responsible for six different mucopolysaccharidoses. The defects, together with their relationship to the stored polysaccharides, are summarized in Fig. 1.

Interrelationships of storage diseases

The similarity of linkages in acidic glycosaminoglycans, glycoproteins and glycosphingolipids suggests the possibility of accumulation of incompletely degraded products from more than one class of carbohydrate-containing macromolecule as a result of the absence of a specific hydrolase. It is now well-established that Tay-Sachs disease is characterized by an absence of β-N-acetylhexosaminidase A (Okada and O'Brien, 1969), while Sandhoff-Jatzkewitz disease is characterized by an absence of both N-acetylhexosaminidase A and B (Sandhoff *et al.*, 1968). The chemical interrelationship of the two isozymes is not yet clear.

Structural considerations suggest that hexosaminidases are concerned with the degradation of the glycosaminoglycans; yet neither Tay-Sachs disease nor Sandhoff–Jatzkewitz disease show clinical or chemical characteristics of mucopolysaccharidoses. Strecker and Montreuil (1971) found an increased amount of an oligosaccharide fraction composed primarily of N-acetylglucosamine and mannose but no increased levels of uronic acid-containing glycosaminoglycans in the urine of a patient with Sandhoff-Jatzkewitz syndrome.

In order to investigate this anomaly further, a labelled oligosaccharide was prepared biosynthetically by the following reaction:

$$\text{UDP-}[^{14}\text{C}]\text{GalNAc} + (\text{GlcUA-GalNAc})_3 \rightarrow$$
$$| $$
$$\text{SO}_4$$
$$[^{14}\text{C}]\text{GalNAc-}(\text{GlcUA-GalNAc})_3$$
$$|$$
$$\text{SO}_4$$

The transferase was prepared from 13-day-old chick epiphyses by the method of Telser, Robinson and Dorfman (1966), and the product was isolated by chromatography on a Sephadex G-25 column (Thompson, Stoolmiller, Matalon and Dorfman, 1973).

When the substrate was incubated with extracts of normal cultured skin fibroblasts, it was readily hydrolyzed as indicated in Fig. 2. The free $[^{14}\text{C}]$-N-acetylgalactosamine is separated from unreacted heptasaccharide by gel filtration of Sephadex G-25. Unlike the cleavage brought about by extracts of normal fibroblasts, neither extracts of fibroblasts derived from a Tay-Sachs patient nor those derived from a Sandhoff-Jatzkewitz patient cleaved this substrate. In contrast, assay of such extracts with 4-methylumbelliferyl-β-D-N-acetylglucosaminide as substrate, demonstrated the expected activity due to β-N-acetyl-hexosaminidase B in the Tay-Sachs extracts.

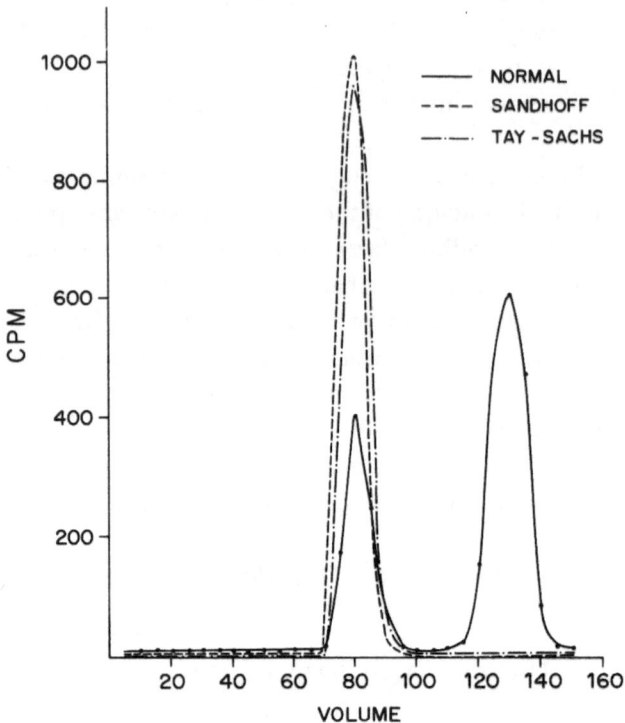

FIG. 2   Degradation of heptasaccharide substrate by fibroblast extracts.

The results of an experiment comparing the activity of a series of fibroblast extracts on the radioactive heptasaccharide showed a marked diminution of activity in fibroblasts of an 'I-cell' patient which is in accord with the previous finding of diminished lysosomal enzyme activities in this disease. In keeping with the inactivity of Tay–Sachs extracts was the almost complete absence of activity of heat-treated extracts of normal fibroblasts.

These studies indicate that hexosaminidase A is required for the degradation of the heptasaccharide. From the fact that Strecker *et al.* (1971) found a marked difference in the urinary oligosaccharide pattern of Tay–Sachs and Sandhoff–Jatzkewitz diseases, one might deduce that N-acetylhexosaminidase B plays a role in degradation of glycoproteins.

The results presented seem to clearly implicate β-N-acetylhexosaminidase A in the degradation of glycosaminoglycans but fail to explain the lack of storage of glycosaminoglycans in the GM_2-gangliosidosis. As indicated in Table I, β-N-acetylhexosaminide linkages occur in hyaluronic acid, chondroitin $4/6$-SO_4 dermatan sulphates and keratan sulphates. In the case of chondroitin $4/6$-SO_4 and hyaluronic acid, the β-N-acetylhexosaminide bonds may be cleaved by the endoglycosidase, hyaluronidase. Such cleavage results in production of oligosaccharides, primarily tetra-hexa and octasaccharides. Complete degradation nevertheless requires the participation of β-N-acetylhexasaminidases. It is possible that oligosaccharides accumulate in Tay–Sachs and Sandhoff–Jatzkewitz diseases which have so far escaped detection. Although hyaluronidase has not been detected in cultured skin fibroblasts, it is plentiful in liver and spleen. Another possible explanation of the lack of accumulation of glycosaminoglycans in the GM_2-gangliosidoses may be the existence of an alternate pathway involving an enzyme that removes a GalNAc-SO_4 group. No such enzyme has so far been demonstrated.

The pathway of degradation of dermatan sulphate is complicated by the fact that GalNAc residues may be bound to either L-iduronic acid or D-glucuronic acid. Fransson and Rodén (1967a, b) demonstrated that testicular hyaluronidase degrades dermatan sulphate at GalNAc-GlcUA linkages but not at GalNAc-IdUA linkages. Whether a specific β-N-acetylhexosaminidase exists for degradation of the GalNAc-IdUA linkage is unknown. Likewise the role of β-N-acetylhexosaminidases in keratan sulphate degradation is unknown.

Purification of β-N-acetylhexosaminidase

The apparent specificity of β-N-acetylhexosaminidase A for the heptasaccharide derived from chondroitin sulphate suggested a new approach to separation of the isozymes of this enzyme. For this purpose an affinity column with the structure shown in Fig. 3 was made by treating chondroitin sulphate proteoglycan with trypsin and chromotrypsin, alcoholic MeOH, testicular hyaluronidase and β-glucuronidase. Such treatment results in the formation of partially degraded disulphated chondroitin sulphate which contains non-reducing terminal β-N-acetylgalactosaminide groups and amino acids at the reducing end of the molecules. Such chains can be linked to cyanogen bromide-activated Sepharose.

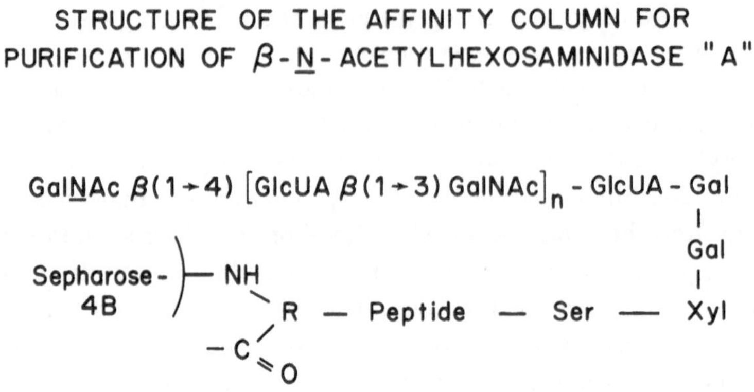

STRUCTURE OF THE AFFINITY COLUMN FOR
PURIFICATION OF β-$\underline{N}$-ACETYLHEXOSAMINIDASE "A"

$$Gal\underline{N}Ac\ \beta(1\rightarrow4)\ \left[GlcUA\ \beta(1\rightarrow3)\ GalNAc\right]_n - GlcUA - Gal$$

Sepharose-4B — NH — R — Peptide — Ser — Xyl — Gal

$-C\overset{\nearrow}{\underset{\searrow}{}}O$

FIG. 3   Structure of affinity matrix for purification of β-N-acetylhexosaminidase A.

Preliminary evidence suggests that such matrices selectively absorb β-N-acetylhexosaminidase A from crude fibroblast or liver extracts (Dawson, Propper and Dorfman, 1973).

Marfan's syndrome

In the course of our earlier studies of mucopolysaccharidoses, meta-chromasia was observed in fibroblasts cultured from patients with Marfan's syndrome (Matalon and Dorfman, 1968a). Unlike the accu-mulated glycosaminoglycans in other mucopolysaccharidoses, the prin-cipal increase is in the hyaluronic acid fraction. In contrast to various mucopolysaccharidoses and glycosphingolipidoses, all of which are recessive diseases, Marfan's syndrome is an autosomal dominant disease. Up to now the biochemical bases of dominant diseases have remained unknown. We have found that Marfan's fibroblasts incorporate [^{14}C]acetate and [^{14}C]glucosamine into hyaluronic acid at a rate of 4–6 times that of normal fibroblasts (Lamberg and Dorfman, 1973). Increased hyaluronic acid was evident not only within the cells but also in the medium. Kinetic studies favour an increase in the rate of synthesis of hyaluronic acid rather than decreased degradation. Until the details of the biochemical mechanisms of these effects are elucidated, it remains impossible to be certain whether this effect on hyaluronic acid metabolism is primary. In any case it opens up a new view of possible genetic disturbances of glycosaminoglycan metabolism.

Summary

The studies reviewed in this paper indicate that there are a number of human genetic diseases which are based on defective degradation of glycosaminoglycans. Elucidation of these defects has resulted in increased understanding of the pathways of glycosaminoglycan degradation. Nevertheless many questions regarding pathways of degradation remain unanswered. There is already evidence of at least one specific sulphatase and a sulphamidase, but the possible specificity of the enzymes responsible for the removal of other sulphate groups have been inadequately explored. The relationship of arylsulphatase A, B, C to glycosaminoglycan metabolism is not clear, although such a relationship is suggested by the finding of acid glycosaminoglycan excretion in a variant of metabolic leukodystrophy characterized by markedly diminished levels of aryl sulphatase A, B, and C (Austin, 1973).

Much remains to be learned of the chemistry of lysosomal enzymes with particular reference to whether the various isozymes represent different products or the results of post translational modification. Considerable evidence indicates that most if not all lysosomal enzymes are glycoproteins. It has been suggested that the carbohydrate portions of the molecule are necessary for interaction with specific cell receptors which facilitate pinocytosis (Hickman and Neufeld, 1972). The possible role of carbohydrate side chains in determining enzyme specificity is not clear. Unravelling of these intriguing interrelationships will undoubtedly permit more rational predictions of the relationship of the stored material and the enzymic defect in any given disease.

The possibility has been raised of another type of mucopolysaccharide disease involving regulation of biosynthesis. Striking increases in synthesis of hyaluronic acid have been observed in Marfan's disease, but the mechanism of this change is as yet unknown.

REFERENCES

AUSTIN, J. H. (1973) *Archives of Neurology and Psychiatry* (Chicago), **28**, 258.
BACH, G., EISENBERG, F., CANTZ, M. & NEUFELD, E. F. (1973) *Proceedings of the National Academy of Sciences of the U.S.A.*, **70**, 2134.
BACH, G., FRIEDMAN, R., WEISSMANN, B. & NEUFELD, E. F. (1972) *Proceedings of the National Academy of Sciences of the U.S.A.*, **69**, 2048.
BARTON, R. W. & NEUFELD, E. F. (1971) *Journal of Biological Chemistry*, **246**, 7773.
BRANTE, G. (1952) *Scandinavian Journal of Clinical Laboratory Investigation*, **4**, 43.
CANTZ, A. M., CHRAMACK, A. & NEUFELD, E. F. (1970) *Biochemical and Biophysical Research Communications*, **39**, 936.

CIFONELLI, J. A., MATALON, R. & DORFMAN, A. (1971) *Federation Proceedings. Federation of American Societies for Experimental Biology*, **30**, 127.

COPPA, G. C., SINGH, J., NICHOLS, B. & DiFERRANTE, N. (1973) *Analytical Letters*, **6**, 225.

DANES, B. S. & BEARN, A. G. (1965) *Science*, **149**, 987.

DAWSON, G., PROPPER, R. L. & DORFMAN, A. (1973) *Biochemical and Biophysical Research Communications* (in Press).

DIETRICH, C. P. (1970) *Canadian Journal of Biochemistry*, **48**, 725.

DORFMAN, A. & LORINCZ, A. E. (1957) *Proceedings of the National Academy of Science of the U.S.A.*, **43**, 443.

DORFMAN, A. & MATALON, R. (1972) *In the Metabolic Basis of Inherited Disease*, p. 1218. Eds. J. B. Stanbury, J. B. Wyngaarden & D. S. Frederickson. New York: McGraw-Hill.

FRANSSON, L.-A. & RODEN, L. (1967a) *Journal of Biological Chemistry*, **242**, 4161.

FRANSSON, L.-A. & RODEN, L. (1967b) *Journal of Biological Chemistry*, **242**, 4170.

FRANSSON, L.-A., SJÖBERG, I., MATALON, R. & DORFMAN, A. (1975) In *S.S.I.E.M. Symposium No. 11, Inborn Errors of Skin, Hair and Connective Tissues.* Eds. J. B. Holton & J. T. Ireland. Lancaster: Medical and Technical Publishing Co.

FRANTANTONI, J. C., HALL, C. W. & NEUFELD, E. F. (1968a) *Proceedings of the National Academy of Science of the U.S.A.*, **60**, 699.

FRANTANTONI, J. C., HALL, C. W. & NEUFELD, E. F. (1968b) *Science*, **162**, 570.

FRIEDMAN, Y. & ARSENIS, C. (1972) *Biochemical and Biophysical Research Communications*, **48**, 1133.

HALL, C. W., CANTZ, M. & NEUFELD, E. F. (1973) *Archives of Biochemistry and Biophysics*, **155**, 32.

HARRIS, R. C. (1961) *American Journal of Diseases of Childhood*, **102**, 741.

HICKMAN, S. & NEUFELD, E. F. (1972) *Biochemical and Biophysical Research Communications*, **49**, 992.

KNECHT, J., CIFONELLI, J. A. & DORFMAN, A. (1967) *Journal of Biological Chemistry*, **242**, 4652.

KRESSE, H. & NEUFELD, E. F. (1972) *Journal of Biological Chemistry*, **247**, 2164.

LAMBERG, S. I. & DORFMAN, A. (1973) *Journal of Clinical Investigation* (in Press).

LEABACK, D. H. (1970) In *Metabolic Conjugation and Metabolic Hydrolysis*, Vol. *II*. Ed. W. H. Fishman. New York: Academic Press.

MATALON, R., CIFONELLI, J. A. & DORFMAN, A. (1971) *Biochemical and Biophysical Research Communications*, **42**, 340.

MATALON, R. & DORFMAN, A. (1966) *Proceedings of the National Academy of Science of the U.S.A.*, **56**, 1310.

MATALON, R. & DORFMAN, A. (1968a) *Biochemical and Biophysical Research Communications*, **32**, 150.

MATALON, R. & DORFMAN A. (1968b) *Proceedings of the National Academy of Sciences of the U.S.A.*, **60**, 179.

MATALON, R. & DORFMAN, A. (1972) *Biochemical and Biophysical Research Communications*, **47**, 959.

MATALON, R. & DORFMAN, A. (1973) *Pediatric Research*, **7**, 156.

McKUSICK, V. A. (1972) In *Heritable Disorders of Connective Tissue.* St. Louis: C. V. Mosby Company.

McKUSICK, V. A., KAPLAN, D., WISE, D., HANLEY, W. B., SUDDARTH, S. B., SEVICK, M. E. & MAUMENEE, A. E. (1965) *Medicine*, **44**, 445.

NEUFELD, E. F. & CANTZ, M. J. (1971) *Annals of the New York Academy of Sciences*, **179**, 580.

O'BRIEN, J. S. (1972) *Proceedings of the National Academy of Science of the U.S.A.*, **69**, 1720.

OKADA, S. & O'BRIEN, J. S. (1969) *Science*, **165**, 698.

SANDHOFF, K., ANDREAE, U. & JATZKEWITZ, H. (1968) *Life of Science*, **7**, 283.

SANFILIPPO, S. J., PODOSIN, R., LANGER, L. O. Jr. & GOOD, R. A. (1963) *Journal of Pediatrics*, **63**, 837.

SPRANGER, J. (1972) *Ergebnisse der inneren Medizin und Kinderheilkunde*, **32**, 165.

STRECKER, G. & MONTREUIL, J. (1971) *Clinica chimica acta*, **33**, 395.

STUMPF, D. & AUSTIN, J. H. (1972) *Proceedings of the American Neurology Association*, (Chicago), 6.

SUZUKI, K. (1968) *Science*, **159**, 1471.

TELSER, A., ROBINSON, H. C. & DORFMAN, A. (1966) *Archives of Biochemistry and Physics*, **116**, 458.
THOMPSON, J. N., STOOLMILLER, A. C., MATALON, R. & DORFMAN, A. (1973) *Science*, **181**, 866.
TUDBALL, N. & DAVIDSON, E. A. (1968) *Biochemica et biophysica octa*, **171**, 113.
VAN HOOF, F. & HERS, H. G. (1964) *Comptes Rendus de l'Academie des Sciences* [D] (Paris), **259**, 1281.
VON FIGURA, K. & KRESSE, H. (1972) *Biochemical and Biophysical Research Communications*, **48**, 262.
WEISSMANN, B. & SANTIAGO, (1972) *Biochemical and Biophysical Research Communications*, **46**, 1430.
WIESMANN, U. & NEUFELD, E. F. (1970) *Science*, **169**, 72.

13

Chemistry of dermatan sulphate accumulated intracellularly in Hunter's disease

Lars-Åke Fransson and Ingrid Sjöberg
(with *Albert Dorfman and Reuben Matalon*)

Introduction

The Hurler and Hunter syndromes are hereditary glycosaminoglycan storage diseases (mucopolysaccharidoses I and II) which are characterized by deposition in tissues and excretion in the urine of dermatan sulphate and heparan sulphate (Dorfman, 1966). However, the two diseases differ with respect to their modes of inheritance. Whereas the Hurler syndrome is transmitted in an autosomal recessive fashion, the Hunter syndrome is sex-linked.

The metabolic error of both syndromes is perpetuated in fibroblast cultures (Danes and Bearn, 1966; Matalon and Dorfman, 1966). Through the work of Neufeld and co-workers (Fratantoni, Hall and Neufeld, 1968), it has been established that fibroblasts from patients afflicted with these diseases synthesize and secrete glycosaminoglycan at a normal rate. However, the rate of intracellular degradation is slow. For adequate degradation the fibroblasts require a specific corrective factor which can be supplied by normal fibroblasts or by fibroblasts of a different genotype (Fratantoni, Hall and Neufeld, 1969).

By degrading chemically desulphated dermatan sulphate with hyaluronidase, β-glucuronidase and β-acetylhexosaminidase, Matalon, Cifonelli and Dorfman (1971) were able to prepare a substrate from which free L-iduronic acid was released upon incubation with extracts of normal human liver and fibroblasts. The finding of diminished L-iduronidase activity in Hurler fibroblasts raised the possibility that lack of this enzyme constituted the defect in Hurler's disease. By using phenyl α-L-iduronide as substrate, Matalon and Dorfman (1972) were able to confirm that α-L-iduronidase was deficient in Hurler fibroblasts. Accordingly, Hurler corrective factor purified from normal human urine was found to be associated with α-L-iduronidase activity (Bach, Friedman, Weissman and Neufeld, 1972). Hunter corrective factor has also been purified from normal human urine (Cantz, Chrambach, Bach and Neufeld, 1972). This proteinaceous factor assisted cultured Hunter fibroblasts in degrading glycosaminoglycans. However, no specific hydrolase activity has yet been ascribed to this factor.

It has become increasingly evident that intralysosomal degradation of glycosaminoglycan is a multi-step process catalyzed by several acid hydrolases. Step-wise erosion of dermatan sulphate from the non-reducing end can be accomplished by the alternate action of hexo-saminidase and α-L-iduronidase as shown in Fig. 1. Whereas the re-moval of L-iduronosyl units is catalyzed by α-L-iduronidase, it is not yet clear how the *N*-acetyl-galactosamine residues are split-off. A combination of sulphatase and β-acetylhexosaminidase (Weissmann, Hadjiioannou and Tornheim, 1964) could execute this removal as in step 1. However, it is conceivable that the entire sulpho-*N*-acetyl-galactosamine residue is removed by a specific hexosaminidase. Finally, some of the L-iduronosly units in dermatan sulphate are substituted with sulphate in the 2- or 3- position (Malmström and Fransson, 1971). Therefore, an additional sulphatase may be postulated (sulphatase b in step 3).

A deficiency of one of the enzymes involved in degradation of der-matan sulphate (Fig. 1) would cause an intracellular accumulation of this polysaccharide. The accumulated polysaccharide pool would contain the substrate for the defective or missing enzyme. Therefore analysis of the non-reducing terminal sugar residue of accumulated dermatan sulphate might be expected to give a clue as to the nature of the deficient enzyme. Such analyses of normal and Hunter dermatan sulphate are described in the present communication. It will be shown that the latter polysaccharide contains significant amounts of non-reducing terminal O-sulpho-L-iduronic acid suggesting that the Hunter syn-drome may be classified as an O-sulpho-L-iduronosyl sulphatase deficiency disease.

Materials

Enzymes. Crystalline papain was isolated from a crude preparation essentially as described by Kimmel and Smith (1954). Nucleases (DNAse and RNAse from bovine pancreas) and a bacterial protease (subtilisin) were purchased from Sigma Chemical. Chondroitinase-ABC from Proteus vulgaris (Yamagata, Saito, Habuchi and Suzuki,

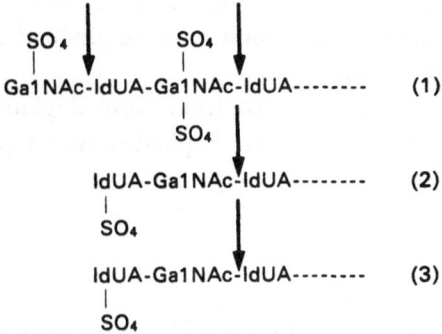

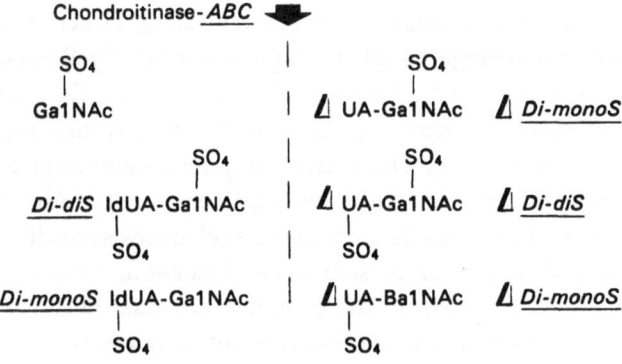

FIG. 1   Step-wise erosion of dermatan sulphate from the non-reducing end catalysed by exoglycosidases and sulphatases.

1968) was a product of Seikaguka Fine Biochemicals, Tokyo, Japan, and purchased from Miles Laboratories, Elkhart, Indiana, U.S.A.

Carbohydrates. Oversulphated chondroitin sulphate (type CS-D) from shark cartilage was obtained from the Seikagaku Kogyo Co., Tokyo, Japan. N-acetyl galactosamine[1] was purchased from Calbiochem. Chondroitin 4-sulphate, N-acetyl chondrosine (Di-OS), 4- or 6-sulphate N-acetylgalactosamine, 4- or 6-sulphated 4,5-unsaturated disaccharides, and 4- or 6-sulphated saturated disaccharides were the same preparations as described previously (Fransson and Havsmark, 1970). Unsulphated, 4,5-unsaturated disaccharide and disulphated, 4,5-unsaturated disaccharide were obtained after chondroitinase-ABC digestion of chemically desulphated chondroitin sulphate (Kantor and Schubert, 1957) and oversulphated chondroitin sulphate (Malmström and Fransson, 1971), respectively.

Miscellaneous. Amnifluor was obtained from New England Nuclear and Instagel from Packard Instruments. Sephadex was a product of Pharmacia Fine Biochemicals.

Methods

Analytical methods. Analysis for uronic acid was carried out by the carbazole method (Dische, 1947). Reducing power was estimated by the method of Park and Johnson (1949). Radioactivity was measured in a TriCarb liquid scintillation spectrometer using either omnifluor in toluene (4 g/l) or Instagel (4 ml of sample and 5 ml of gel) as scintillators.

Chromatographic and electrophoretic techniques. Di- and mono-saccharides obtained after digestion with chondroitinase-ABC were resolved by ion exchange chromatography on a column (1·2 × 40 cm) of AG 1-X 8 (Cl- form) eluted with a linear LiCl gradient (0–3 M). This procedure separates di- and monosaccharides according to charge density as well as degree of saturation (Fransson, Roden and Spach, 1968). Fractions eluted from the column were assayed for radioactivity with Instagel. The various radioactive components were desalted on Sephadex G-10, lyophilized, dissolved in 70 per cent (v/v) ethanol and stored at −18°C.

High voltage paper electrophoresis was carried out as described previously (Fransson *et al.*, 1970). The buffers used were A, 0·1 M pyridine acetate, pH 5·0 and B, 1·6 M pyridine acetate, pH 3·0. Compounds separated by preparative paper electrophoresis were eluted from the paper with distilled water and lyophilized. Descending paper chromatography was performed on Whatman No. 3MM paper in isobutyric acid–0·5 M ammonia (5:3) for 48 h. Papers were cut and strips were assayed for radioactivity in Ominfluor/toluene.

Periodate oxidation. Oxidations were performed in 0·1 ml of 0·05 M acetate buffer, pH 4·5 containing NaIO$_4$ (0·04 M) at 37°C for 1 h.

After terminating the reaction by addition of 0·2 ml of 3 per cent (w/v) mannitol the solution was concentrated on a rotary evaporator and spotted on paper.

Partial acid hydrolysis. Radioactive di- and mono-saccharides were dissolved in 0·5 ml or 0·04 M HC1 and heated at 100°C for 1 h. After evaporation, the samples were spotted on paper.

Isolation and degradation of dermatan sulphate from Hunter fibroblasts. Hunter fibroblasts were allowed to accumulate $^{35}SO_4$=—labelled glycosaminoglycan for five days in tissue culture (Matalon and Dorfman, 1966). The cells were extracted twice with 9 vols of acetone, dried, and suspended in 20 ml of 1·0 M NaCl—0·15 M Na_4 EDTA—0·01 M cysteine hydrochloride-0·05 M phosphate buffer, pH 6·9. After digestion with 2·25 mg of twice crystallized papain at 65° overnight the mixture was dialyzed against 3 × 1 litres of distilled water. The retentate was lyophilized and dissolved in 20 ml of 0·05 M $CaCl_2$ —0·05 M Tris-acetate, pH 7·5 and digested with 1 mg of subtilisin at 37°C overnight. The solution was subsequently concentrated on a rotary evaporator and subjected to gel chromatography on a column (1·1 × 200 cm) of Sephadex G-50, superfine, eluted with 0·2 M pyridine acetate, pH 5·0 at a rate of 12 ml/h. The excluded material was recovered, lyophilized and dissolved in 5 ml of 0·05 M $MgSO_4$—0·05 M phosphate buffer, pH 7·3. Nuclease digestion was then performed with RNAse and DNAse (0·5 mg each) at 37°C overnight. Glycosaminoglycans and oligonucleotides were separated by gel chromatography on Sephadex G-50 as described above. The excluded material was recovered, concentrated and dissolved in 1 ml of 0·5 M Tris, pH 8·0. Dermatan sulphate was degraded with chondroitinase-ABC (0·5 units) at 37°C for 24 h. The dermatan sulphate split products were separated from undegraded polysaccharide (primarily heparan sulphate) by gel chromatography on Sephadex G-25. All of the included radioactive material was recovered and subjected to ion exchange chromatography as described above.

Radioactive dermatan sulphate was also isolated from normal fibroblasts and degraded by chondroitinase-ABC in an identical manner.

Abbreviations

GalNAc-S and GalNAc=N-acetyl galactosamine with or without sulphate.

GalNAc-4S and GalNAc-6S=4- and 6-sulphated N-acetylgalactos-amine, respectively.

Di-OS, Di-monoS, and Di-diS=Unsulphated, monosulphated and disulphated saturated disaccharides, respectively.

ΔDi-OS, ΔDi-monoS and ΔDi-diS=The same series of disaccharides with 4,5- unsaturated uronic acid moieties.

Di-4S and ΔDi-4S, 4-sulphated (mono-sulphated)=Saturated and unsaturated disaccharides, respectively.

Di-6S and ΔDi-6S=The analogous 6-sulphated (monosulphated) disaccharides.

Results

Chondroitinase-ABC cleaves hexosaminidic bonds to L-iduronic as well as D-glucuronic acid residues with concomitant formation of 4,5-unsaturated uronosyl moities (Yamagata *et al.*, 1968). Treatment of dermatan sulphate with this enzyme produces a large quantity of unsaturated disaccharides originating from the internal repeating periods (Fig. 2). However, the non-reducing terminal portion is released unchanged. When GalNAc-S constitutes the terminal moiety this monosaccharide is released in free form (chain 1 in Fig. 2), whereas terminal uronosyl moieties are recovered in the form of saturated disaccharides (chains 2 and 3 in Fig. 2). As shown in Fig. 3 these mono- and disaccharides may be resolved by ion exchange chromatography on AG1-X8 (upper graph). Although a reference sample of Di-diS was not available its position in the chromatogram may be deduced from the positions of ΔDi-OS, ΔDi-monoS and ΔDi-diS in relation to those of their saturated counterparts Di-OS and Di-monoS. The principal non-reducing sugar moiety of normal dermatan sulphate was GalNAc-S (middle graph), whereas dermatan sulphate from Hunter fibroblasts yielded, in addition, two non-reducing terminal disaccharide peaks (1 and 5 in lower graph). The latter disaccharides were eluted in the positions of Di-monoS and Di-diS, respectively.

The various mono- and disaccharide components (1–6) obtained from Hunter dermatan sulphate were also characterized by paper electrophoresis (Fig. 4). It is seen that peaks 1, 3 and 4 had the mobili-ties of Di-monoS, peaks 5 and 6 had the mobilities of Di-DiS, and peak 2 migrated as a GalNAc-S. Whereas peaks 1 and 3 correspond to saturated and unsaturated disaccharides, respectively (Di-monoS and

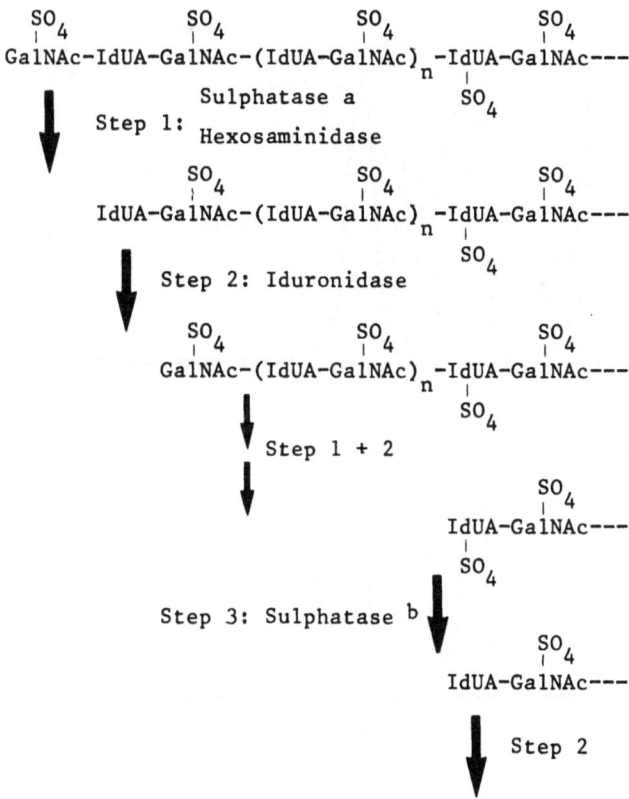

FIG. 2 Scheme for the degradation of dermatan sulphate by chondroitinase-ABC. This enzyme cleaves the hexosaminidic bonds indicated by thin arrows. The three terminal sequences depicted at the top (1, 2 and 3) yield different terminal units (lower left) in addition to a large excess of unsaturated disaccharides (lower right).

ΔDi-monoS), the nature of peak 4 remains unclear. (It is possible that peak 4 consists of the unsaturated disaccharide UA-GalNAc. Work is

$$\underset{SO_4}{\overset{|}{}}$$

in progress to clarify this point.)

In order to determine the structure of the various disaccharides periodate oxidations and partial acid hydrolysis were performed. Unsubstituted, non-reducing terminal uronosyl residues carry two periodate-sensitive glycol groupings. Oxidation of these glycols causes an extensive degradation of the uronosyl residue. However, substitution

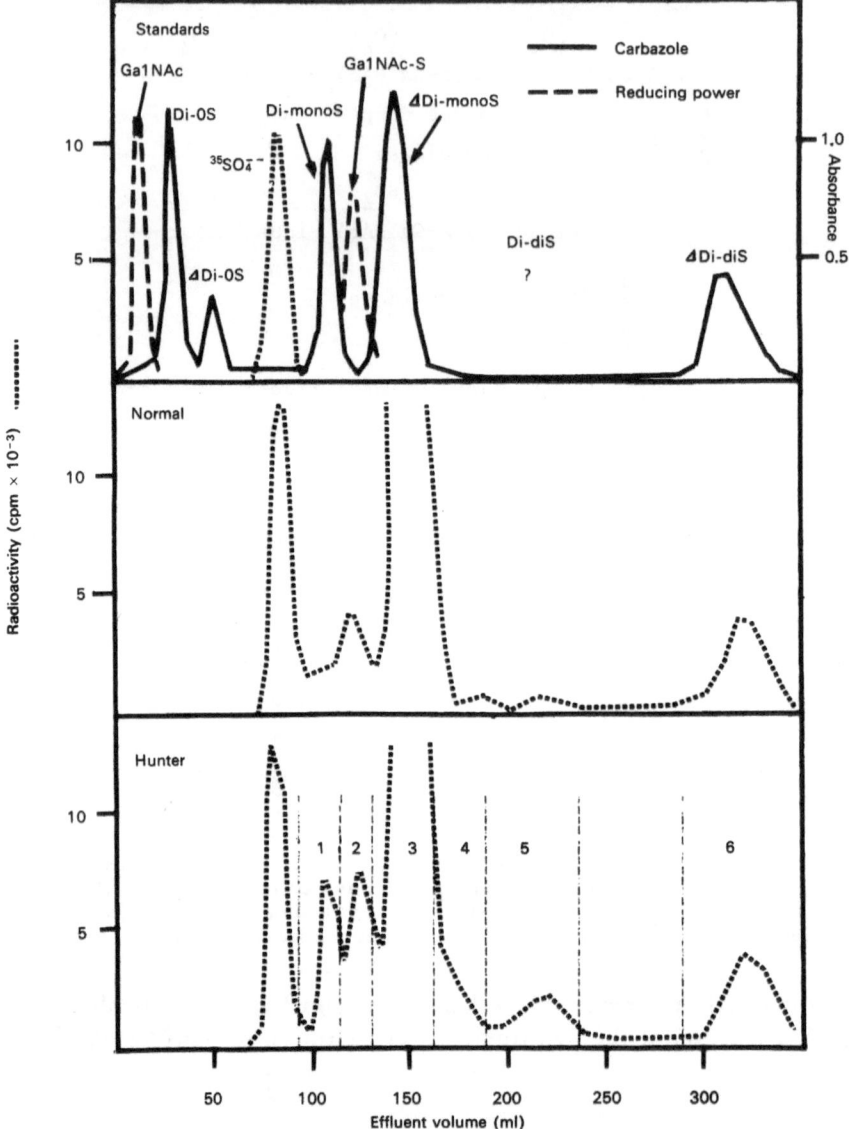

FIG. 3   Ion exchange chromatography of various mono- and disaccharides. A chromatogram of standard compounds is shown in the upper graph. Chromatograms of chondroitinase-ABC digests of radioactively labelled dermatan sulphate from normal and Hunter cells are shown in the middle and lower graphs, respectively. The samples were partially desulphated on standing in concentrated solutions, presumably due to radiolysis. The amount of free sulphate was approximately 10 per cent of the total radioactivity. The fractions from Hunter dermatan sulphate were pooled as indicated (1–6 in lower graph).

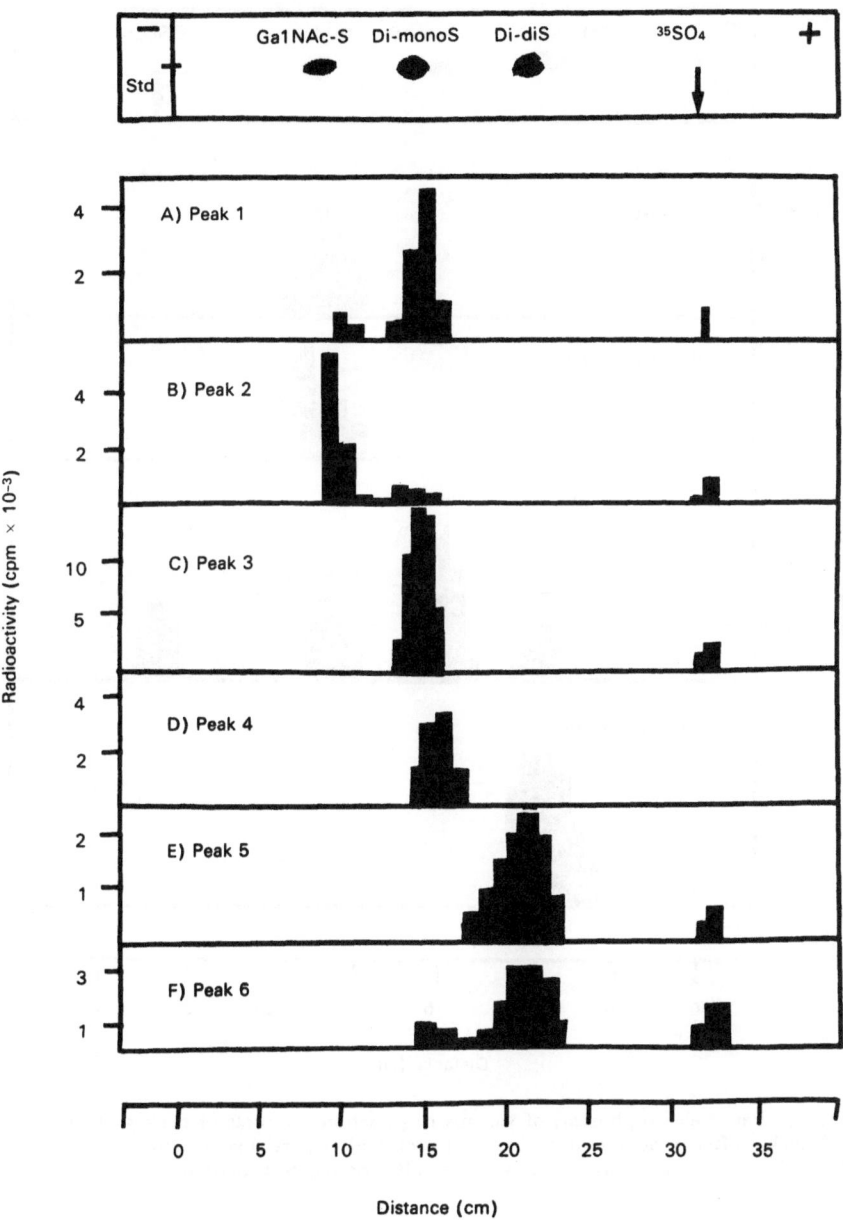

FIG. 4 Paper electrophoresis of various mono- and disaccharides at pH 5·0. In the top electrophoretogram the mobilities of various standards are depicted. It should be noted that saturated and unsaturated disaccharides have the same mobility in this system (peaks 1 and 3; peaks 5 and 6).

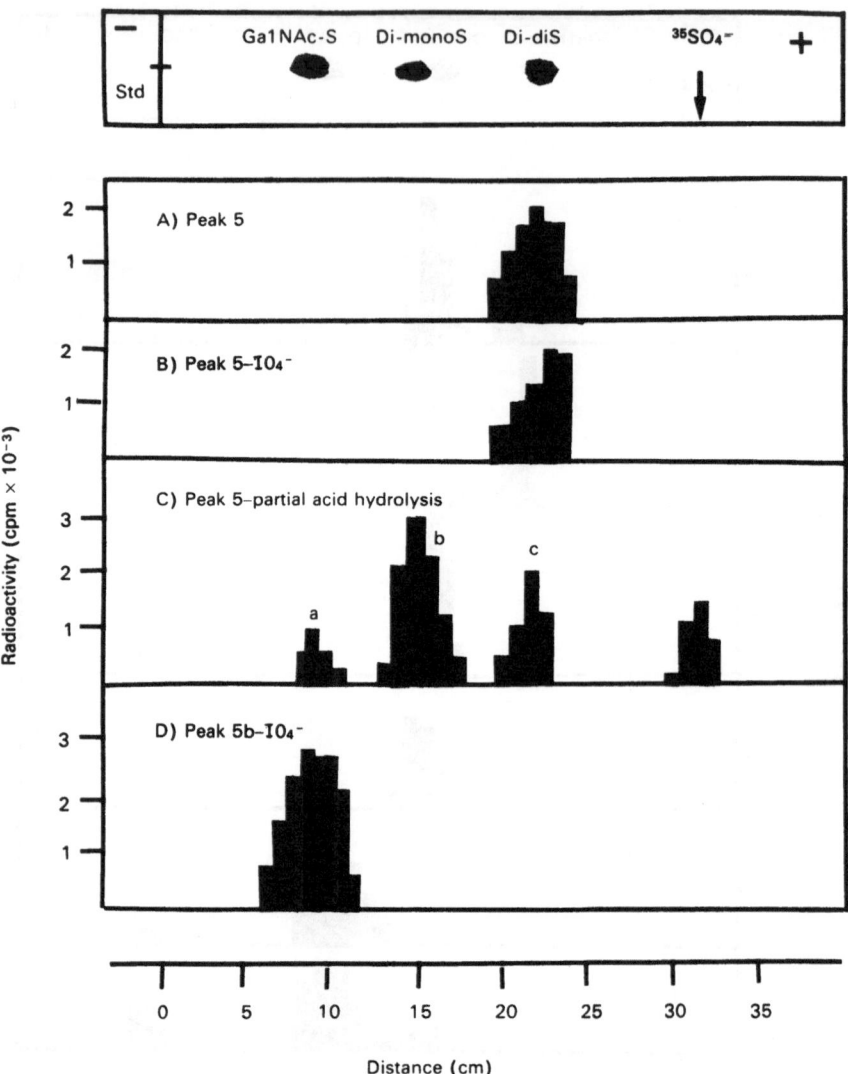

FIG. 5   Paper electrophoresis of various degradation products of peak 5 at pH 5·0; (B) peak 5 after periodate oxidation; (C) peak 5 after partial acid hydrolysis and (D) the hydrolysis product 5b after periodate oxidation.

with sulphate, at C-2 or C-3 will partly or completely prevent destruction of this residue. When peak 5 (Di-diS) was oxidized with periodate little effect was observed (Figs. 5 A and B). The mobility appeared to increase slightly which would suggest a limited attack by periodate, possibly between C-3 and C-4. The Di-diS was also subjected to partial acid hydrolysis (Fig. 5C) which afforded four components, free sulphate, undegraded Di-diS, Di-monoS and GalNAc-S. The Di-monoS component (peak 5b) was also subjected to periodate oxidation. Since this treatment quantitatively transformed the Di-monoS to GalNAc-S (Fig. 5D) it may be inferred that the sulphate group on the uronosyl residue had been released during hydrolysis. These data indicate that Di-diS carried one sulphate on the hexosamine moiety and one sulphate on the uronosyl moiety.

The Di-monoS component (peak 5b) obtained by partial acid hydrolysis of Di-diS was further characterized by paper electrophoresis at pH 3·0 (Fig. 6A). The material appeared heterogeneous; a minor portion had the mobility of a chondroitin sulphate disaccharide while the major portion had a lower mobility. The Di-monoS component (peak 1) obtained directly by chondroitinase-ABC digestion of Hunter dermatan sulphate was also subjected to electrophoresis at pH 3·0 (Fig. 6B). It is seen that this component was resolved into three peaks the middle of which (peak 1b) had the mobility of a chondroitin sulphate disaccharide. Since L-iduronic acid has a higher pk_a value than D-glucuronic acid (Mathews, 1961) the slow moving components (the major portion of 5b and the entire peak 1a) should represent L-iduronic acid-containing Di-monoS.

A preliminary experiment indicated that peak 1 was partially resistant to periodate. It was therefore of interest to investigate whether Di-monoS which carried sulphated uronosyl moieties were present in peak 1. Consequently, the various components obtained by electrophoresis at pH 3·0 (Fig. 6) were subjected to partial acid hydrolysis. It is seen from Fig. 7 that peaks 1a and 1b both yielded GalNAc-S in addition to free sulphate and undegraded Di-monoS, whereas 1c yielded only free sulphate. It is concluded that peak 1c was a Di-monoS with the sulphate on the uronosyl moiety.

In order to gain further information about the position of the sulphate substituents, the various components were subjected to paper chromatography. As shown in Fig. 8 the Di-monoS component (peak 1)

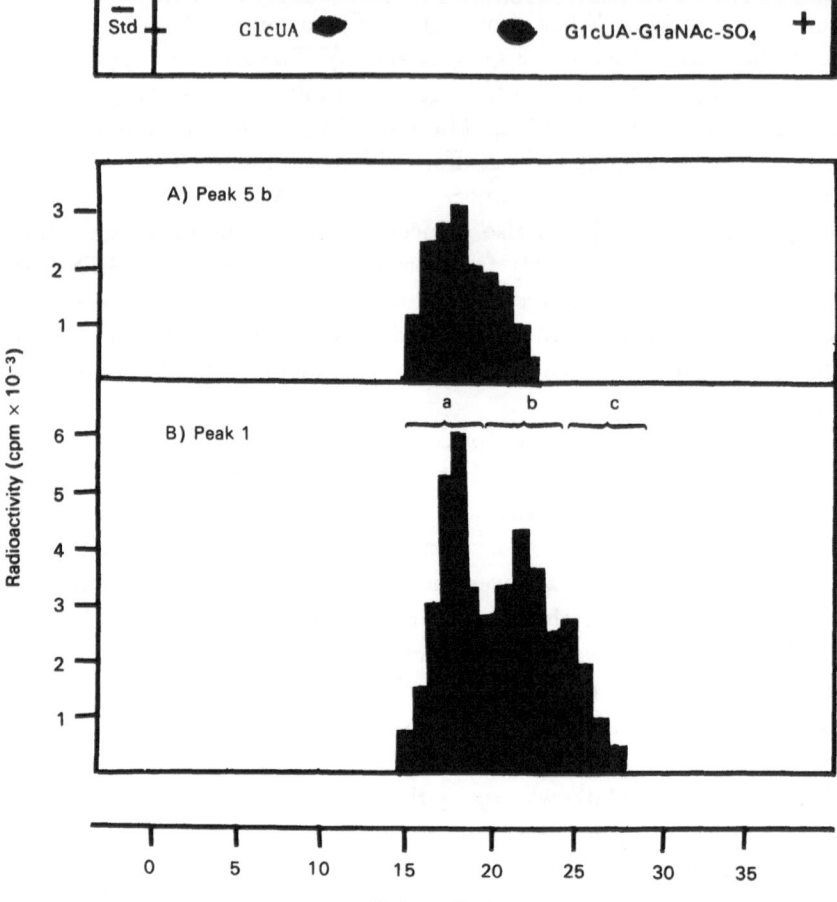

FIG. 6   Paper electrophoresis of the Di-monoS fractions 5b (A) and 1 (B) at pH 3·0.
It should be noted that, in this system, iduronic acid-containing disaccharides have a
lower mobility than glucuronic acid-containing ones. The subfractions of peak 1 were
pooled as indicated by brackets.

appeared extremely heterogeneous, while peak 2 (GalNAc-S) contained
more GalNAc-6S than GalNAc-4S, and peak 3 corresponded to
ΔDi-4S. The mobility of peak 4 was clearly different from that of
Di-monoS, although it was eluted close to this material in the ion
exchange procedure. (Since Di-monoS (peak 3) was the dominating
component in the column chromatogram (Fig. 3) it was not clearly
separated from the preceding GalNAc-S (peak 2). Therefore the slow-

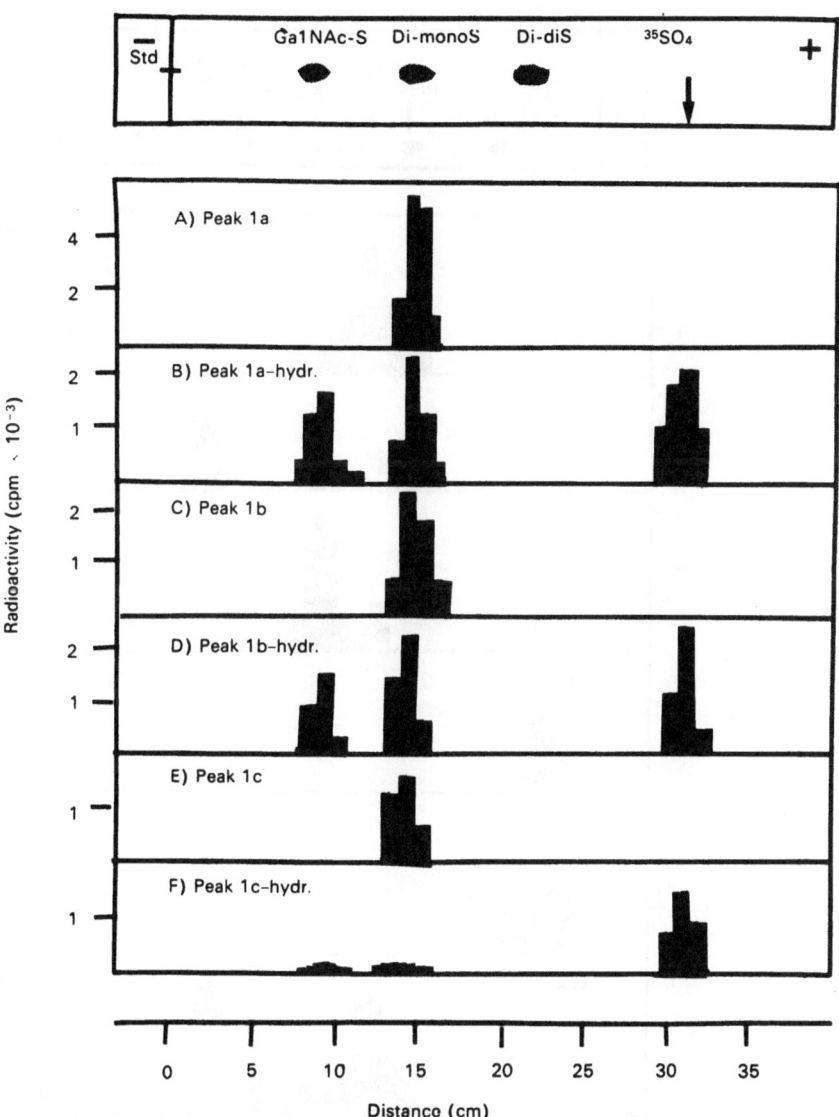

FIG. 7 Paper electrophoresis at pH 5·0 of hydrolysis products of peak (B), 1b (D) and 1c (F).

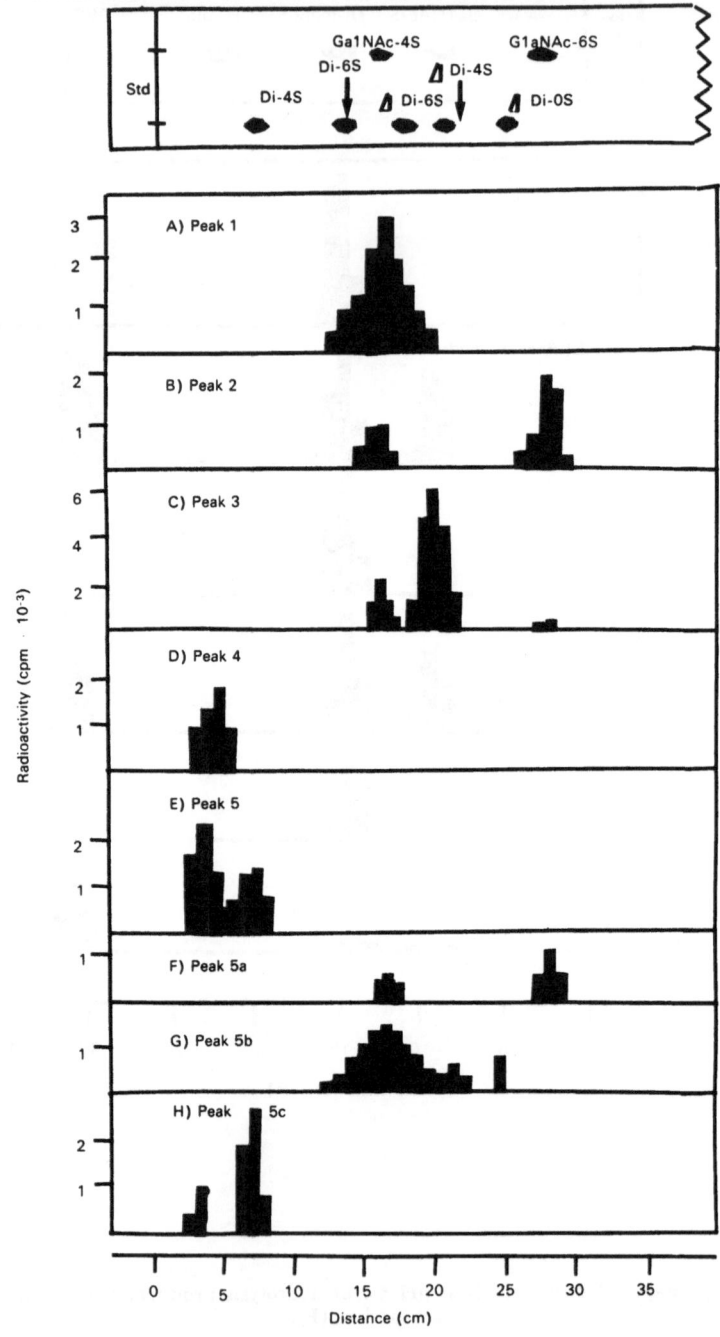

moving, minor component in the electrophoretogram (Fig. 8C) should represent GalNAc-4S. The fact that very little GalNAc-6S is seen in this fraction is consistent with our observation that, although with considerable overlap, GalNAc-4S is eluted later than GalNAc-6S in the ion exchange procedure). (Fransson and Sjöberg, unpublished). The Di-diS fraction (peak 5) was resolved into two components on paper chromatography (Fig. 8E). When the hydrolysis products of Di-diS, i.e. GalNAc-S (5a) and Di-monoS (5b), were chromatographed GalNAc-6S was found to be a prominent product (Fig. 8F). Since the undegraded Di-diS contained more of the fast-moving component (Fig. 8H), it may be concluded that the two peaks observed when the original disaccharide was analyzed (Fig. 8E) represented 6-sulphated and 4-sulphated species. (The slow-moving component was 6-sulphated.) The Di-monoS obtained after hydrolysis of peak 5 (peak 5b) was even more heterogeneous than the original Di-monoS (peak 1). This is not too surprising since these fractions were resolved into two and three components, respectively, upon electrophoresis at pH 3·0 (Fig. 6). Thus, these fractions contained components which differed not only with regard to the sulphate position on the hexosamine residue but also with regard to the nature of the uronosyl moiety.

Summary

The results presented in this communication indicate that normal dermatan sulphate has the following non-reducing terminal sequence: $GalNAc(-SO_4)-[IdUA-GalNAc(-SO_4)]n-IdUA(-SO_4)-$. When this chain is eroded stepwise from the non-reducing end by the action of sulphatases and exoglycosidases a number of intermediates with different termini may be envisaged (Fig. 1). The identification of $IdUA(-SO_4)-GalNAc(-SO_4)$ (peak 5) as a prominent terminal disaccharide of dermatan sulphate accumulated in Hunter fibroblasts is consistent with a lack of sulpho-iduronosyl sulphatase in this metabolic disorder. The disaccharide $IdUA(-SO_4)-GalNAc$ (peak 1c) was also found in Hunter dermatan sulphate. Whether this reflects the activity

FIG. 8 Paper chromatography of various mono- and disaccharides. It should be noted that in this solvent components are separated both according to degree of unsaturation and according to the position of the sulphate substituent. Although it has not been investigated, it seems reasonable to assume that the nature of the uronosyl moiety should also affect the R_F value.

of a sulphohexosamine sulphatase or structural heterogeneity within the polysaccharide cannot be settled at present.

IdUA—GalNAc(—SO_4) (peak 1a) and GalNAc—SO_4 (peak 2) were also present in the chondroitinase-ABC digest of the Hunter poly-saccharide. Since the monosaccharide was more prominent than the disaccharide it is conceivable that they represent terminal units of newly synthesized, undegraded galactosaminoglycan. It is also possible that the dermatan sulphate accumulated within the lyosome might inhibit glycosidases operating in earlier steps of the degradative pathway.

When the Di-diS component, IdUA(—SO_4)—GalNAc(—SO_4) was subjected to partial acid hydrolysis both GalNAc-6S and GalNAc-4S were released, indicating that structures like IdUA(—SO_4)—GalNAc-6-SO_4 are present in human dermatan sulphate. In previous work on the structure of dermatan sulphate from various sources (Fransson *et al.*, 1970) it was regularly observed that L-iduronic acid-containing segments of copolymeric chains were 4-sulphated, while D-glucuronic acid-containing segments were either 4- or 6-sulphated. The presence of 6-sulphated hexosamine adjacent to a sulphated L-iduronic acid residue may indicate that some of the sulphated L-iduronic acid residues are located close to the D-glucuronic acid-containing blocks of the copolymer.

The Di-monoS fraction (peak 1) was resolved into three components by electrophoresis at pH 3·0 (Fig. 6), the fast-moving component was characterized as IdUA(—SO_4)—GalNAc and the slow-moving component as IdUA—GalNAc(—SO_4). The reduced mobility of the latter disaccharide at pH 3·0 is attributable to the weak acidity of the L-iduronic acid (pk_a 3·63) compared to that of D-glucuronic acid (pk_a 3·1) (Mathews, 1961). Most likely this difference is due to the fact that the carboxyl group is axial in L-iduronic acid while it is equatorial in D-glucuronic acid when both sugars assume the C-1 conformation. (Axial carboxyl groups have higher pk_a values than equatorial carboxyl groups in the cyclohexane series (Stolow, 1959).) However, the fast-moving disaccharide, IdUA(—SO_4)—GalNAc, migrated even faster than the D-glucuronic acid-containing standard indicating that its carboxyl group was more acidic than that of IdUA—GalNAc(—SO_4) (peak 1a in Fig. 6). A reasonable explanation to this finding is that sulphated L-iduronosyl units assume the 1-C conformation. In this conformation the carboxylate group would be equatorial and thus more acidic. (The presence of another ionized group on the same sugar residue might also be expected to influence the acidity.) It should be added that X-ray diffraction studies in heparin fibres (Nieduszynski and Atkins, 1973) have led to the proposal that sulphated L-iduronosyl residues assume the I-C conformation.

The Di-diS component (peak 5) IdUA $(-SO_4)-$GalNAc$(-SO_4)$ was partially desulphated by mild acid hydrolysis to yield Di-monoS (peak 5b), IdUA$-$GalNAc$(-SO_4)$. When this material was subjected to electrophoresis at pH 3·0 (Fig. 6a) two components were observed, the major component having the mobility of an IdUA$-$GalNAc$(-SO_4)$ with the uronosyl moiety in the C-1 conformaiton. The minor component had the mobility of a D-glucuronic acid-containing disaccharide. A similar component was also observed in the original Di-monoS (peak 1b in Fig. 6). It is assumed that these components represent the disaccharide IdUA$-$GalNAc$(-SO_4)$ with the uronosyl moiety in the I-C conformation. The latter disaccharide is considered to be the initial hydrolysis product of IdUA$(-SO_4)-$GalNAc$(-SO_4)$; an equilibrium between the energetically more favourable (C-1) IdUA$-$GalNAc$(-SO_4)$ and the (1-C) IdUA$-$GalNAc$(-SO_4)$ would subsequently be established. (It cannot be excluded that the disaccharide GlcUA$-$GalNAc$-SO_4$ was present in peak 1.)

These considerations raise important questions concerning both the biosynthesis and the degradation of dermatan sulphate. It has been observed that sulphation of endogeneously synthesized heparin markedly augmented the rate of epimerization from D-glucuronic acid to L-iduronic acid (Lindahl, Bäckström, Malmström and Fransson, 1972). It is possible that the sulphation process acts as the driving force for alteration of chair conformations (from C-1 to 1-C) which in turn removes (C-1 L-IdUA from the equilibrium (C-1) D-GlcUA$=$(C-1) L-IdUA (both polymer-bound). In this way complete sulphation of L-iduronosyl residues may not be necessary for an effective transformation of D-glucuronosyl to L-iduronosyl residues.

Removal of the sulphate group from a sulphated L-iduronosyl residue during degradation would expose a (1-C) L-IdUA in non-reducing terminal position. This raises the question whether this unit can be released by α-L-iduronidase (Hurler corrective factor) or if a change in chair conformation (from 1-C to C-1) is required. If so, is this equilibrium catalyzed by an enzyme? If not, it is conceivable that this reaction constitutes the rate-limiting step in the degradation of dermatan sulphate.

Acknowledgement

The present work was supported by grants from the Swedish Medical Research Council (B72–13X–139–06C), Gustaf V:s 80–årsfond and the Medical Faculty, University of Lund.

REFERENCES

BACH, G., FRIEDMAN, R., WEISSMANN, B. & NEUFELD, E. F. (1972) *Proceedings of the National Academy of Siences of the U.S.A.*, **69**, 2048.

CANTZ, M., CHRAMBACH, A., BACH, G. & NEUFELD, E. F. (1972) *Journal of Biological Chemistry*, **247**, 5454.

DANES, B. S. & BEARN, A. G. (1966) *Journal of Experimental Medicine*, **123**, 1; **126**, 509.

DISCHE, Z. (1947) *Journal of Biological Chemistry*, **167**, 189.

DORFMAN, A. (1966) In *The Metabolic Basis of Inherited Disease*, pp. 963–94. Eds. J. B. Stanbury, J. B. Wyngaarden & D. S. Fredrickson. New York: McGraw-Hill.

FRANSSON, L.-A. & HAVSMARK, B. (1970) *Journal of Biological Chemistry*, **245**, 4770.

FRANSSON, L.-A., RODEN, L. & SPACH, M. L. (1968) *Analytical Biochemistry*, **23**, 1521.

FRATANTONI, J. C., HALL, C. W. & NEUFELD, E. F. (1968) *Proceedings of the National Academy of Sciences of the U.S.A.*, **60**, 699.

FRATANTONI, J. C., HALL, C. W. & NEUFELD, E. F. (1969) *Proceedings of the National Academy of Sciences of the U.S.A.*, **64**, 360.

KANTOR, T. G. & SCHUBERT, M. (1957) *Journal of the American Chemical Society*, **79**, 152.

KIMMEL, J. R. & SMITH, E. L. (1954) *Journal of Biological Chemistry*, **207**, 515.

LINDAHL, U., BÄCKSTRÖM, G., MALMSTRÖM, A. & FRANSSON, L.-A. (1972) *Biochemical and Biophysical Research Communications*, **46**, 985.

MALMSTROM, A. & FRANSSON, L.-A. (1971) *European Journal of Biochemistry*, **18**, 431.

MATALON, R., CIFONELLI, J. A. & DORFMAN, A. (1971) *Biochemical and Biophysical Research Communication*, **42**, 340.

MATALON, R. & DORFMAN, A. (1966) *Proceedings of the National Academy of Sciences of the U.S.A.*, **56**, 1310.

MATALON, R. & DORFMAN, A. (1972) *Biochemical and Biophysical Research Communications*, **47**, 959.

MATHEWS, M. B. (1961) *Biochimica and biophysica acta*, **48**, 402.

NIEDUSZYNSKI, I. A. & ATKINS, E. D. T. (1973) *Biochemical Journal* (submitted).

PARK, J. T. & JOHNSON, M. L. (1949) *Journal of Biological Chemistry*, **181**, 149.

STOLOW, R. D. (1959) *Journal of the American Chemical Society*, **81**, 5806.

WEISSMANN, B., HADJIIOANNOU, S. & TORNHEIM, J. (1964) *Journal of Biological Chemistry*, **239**, 59.

YAMAGATA, T., SAITO, H., HABUCHI, O. & SUZUKI, S. (1968) *Journal of Biological Chemistry*, **243**, 1523.

DISCUSSION
(of papers by Professor Dorfman and Dr Fransson)

Lutz (Heidelberg). You appear to have dispensed with the use of methylation and silylation as procedures for the elucidation of sulphur position.

Fransson (Lund). All these compounds were radioactively labelled in the sulphate position and are present in only small quantities so we have contented ourselves by only using the radioactive measurements.

Aitkens (Bristol). I was very interested to note the results of the over-sulphate oligosaccharides. Do you have any longer than five monomers?

Fransson. Not yet!

Dean (London). Does Dr Fransson know of a set of conditions for desulphation of iduronic acid without desulphating the remaining sulphated groups?

Fransson. Evaporation, put in water and evaporate down.

Raine (Birmingham). Is there any danger of sulphate groups migrating from one part of the molecule to another or are they quite stable?

Fransson. There have been discussions in the past about this problem but we don't think there are any indications that any of them migrate under these conditions.

Spranger (Keil). Have you had a chance to look at dermatan sulphate in the Maroteaux–Lamy syndrome?

Fransson. No.

Raine. Maroteaux–Lamy seems to be the rarest of the mucopoly-saccharidoses in our experience, is this generally believed?

Spranger. Scheie's is rarer.

Sinclair (London). Would Professor Dorfman elaborate a little further on the correction factors he mentioned previously?

Dorfman (Chicago). I believe that these are identical with the enzymes, the term is used as an operational one until the enzymes are identified.

Saunders (Cardiff). What is the explanation for the low galactosidase enzymes levels previously reported in the fibroblasts from Hunter patients?

Dorfman. I am not sure that I can fully answer that question. There is no doubt that we found about 60 to 70 per cent of normal values in the fibroblasts. Now there are some tricks to this, some of that was limitation by stored polysaccharide and if you raise the salt concentration, the level of galactosidase goes up. We weren't able to confirm the absence of isoenzymes of galactosidase as has been reported. I think that there is a real problem here that none of us understands. We have variations from disease to disease of lysosomal enzymes which are not primary defects, particularly hydrolases. You may have noticed from my slides that the levels of α-N acetylglucosaminidase are somewhat higher in Hurler's than in the normal. There is a whole vast field in the control of lysosomal enzymes which we don't understand at the present time.

Teller (Ulm). I should like to ask Dr Dorfman if he has any explanation why the Morquio fibroblasts store keratan sulphate, isn't keratan sulphate mainly produced in cartilage not in the skin? What does the skin of a Morquio look like? Is it changed morphologically so that we can assume that this is one of the disease situations, that Morquio's store keratan sulphate in the skin?

Dorfman. I don't know of any evidence that Morquio's do store keratan sulphate, we have never found any keratan sulphate in the fibroblasts. Technically this isn't such a simple question, the detection of small amounts which may be present in fibroblast extract. We are at the moment actively working out the structure of keratan sulphate excreted in Morquio cases.

Teller. You speak of keratan sulphate I and II what is the difference between these two, is it one of size?

Dorfman. Keratan sulphate I and keratan sulphate II refer to corneal keratan sulphate as compared with cartilage keratan sulphate and there are many interesting differences between them. The most prominent of which is the linkage to protein. Corneal keratan sulphate has at least one very similar, and it may be the only one, to the glycoprotein linkage to the asparto-N-acetylglucosamine linkage while in cartilage the primary linkage is a hydroxyamino acid one (threonine or serine). It is not absolutely certain that there are no other linkages in the cartilage one. There are some differences in the amount of mannose you may find.

Now Dr Dawson recently isolated keratan sulphate fragments excreted in GM1 gangliosidosis, the so called keratan sulphate like material. He found at least one of the fragments to be the linkage fragment of cartilage keratan sulphate showing the linkage of N-acetylgalactosamine to threonine.

Raine. This question of keratan like substance that Suszuki said was occurring in the organs of GM1 gangliosidosis cases. When he first said that his evidence was largely based on the fact that the mucopolysaccharide he extracted contained galactose, and keratan sulphate was the only one we knew about that contained galactose. Even he admitted that this was rather flimsy evidence. Would you say, and this is a double question to Dr Fransson and Dr Dorfman, that there is much evidence for dermatan sulphate and heparan sulphate from different sources within the body or the animal species, being chemically different? More important still is there any evidence that these same things from different animal species are different. I particularly ask in this connection, are the keratans worse than say dermatan and heparatan sulphates in chemical variation? It seems to me that they well might be.

Dorfman. I think they are 'worse' at the moment because we don't understand them so well.

As far as the question about organ specificity is concerned certainly we know that there is a difference what we tend to call microheterogenicity, differences in the amount of sulphation and frequently the position of sulphate occur from tissue to tissue and between species. I think that one of the striking things about this type of compound is that they are very conservative compounds from an evolutionary point of view. So you find such similar structures in even invertebrates not only in mammals, the structures are very very similar. Dr Matthews who has spent years studying the question has written an extensive monograph on the subject which is to be published shortly, dealing with the evolutionary significance of comparative structure.

Now the compound which is most troublesome, in this respect, is heparan sulphate, in that we have isolated, at various times, everything from scratches that appear to be isomers of hyaluronic acid back to heparin with that variation from no sulphate to 2·5 sulphate residues per repeating disaccharide repeating unit. As I have said we don't know much about sources in the body.

Finally in terms of trying to understand what is excreted. I think there are some real problems that have caused a great deal of confusion as to the differences in degradation in different tissues, we have tried by the most certain of techniques known to us to find any evidence of the end of glycosidase-hyaluronidase action in fibroblasts, we didn't find any. I believe that what happens in fibroblasts when they re-ingest or degrade substances that have not been excreted is an almost completely exoglycosidase reaction. Now any of the material that gets away from the fibroblasts and gets into the circulation has quite a different fate. Once it gets into the reticulo-endothelial system, into liver, spleen, white cells, there is hyaluronidase activity easily demonstrated and therefore it is degraded to oligosaccharides and appears quite differently. Now I think the reason why in the β-glucosidase deficiency, as appears from data I have seen, the material excreted is dermatan sulphate, because dermatan sulphate when acted upon by hyaluronidase gives rather large fragments. Chondroitin sulphate and hyaluronic acid give very small fragments and they may be readily missed and it would be very interesting now to look into this more carefully for smaller oligosaccharides. Years ago at the origin of our collaboration with Dr Fransson we found large amounts of oligosaccharides in Hurler urine.

Fransson. I should mention that there were differences in tissue in the same animal. In dermatan sulphate the variation of hyaluronic acid: glucuronic acid ratio is a guide. Take skin dermatan sulphate, 95 per cent of the population had something like 10:1 for this ratio. Some 5 per cent had a ratio of 50:50. We like to believe that this is a reflection of the alternate degradation, that part of the dermatan sulphate chains, the hyaluronic acid residues, can to some extent be converted back to chondroitin like fragments, back polymerization as we call it. If these segments become of sufficient size they can subsequently be acted upon by hyaluronidase and this comes back to what Professor Dorfman just said. If dermatan sulphate comes out in the circulation and reaches other tissues where hyaluronidase present, the combined action of reverse epimerase and hyaluronidase can bring about fragmentation of the dermatan sulphate to the oligosaccharides present in Hurler's urine.

Marshall (London). The possibility of intracellular change in the conformation from C1 in the iduronic acid moiety of dermatan sulphate to IC as the sulphated iduronic acid is of considerable interest. Would you care to comment on the stage at which this conformation change occurs, because the change might be expected to lead to a very considerable alteration in the three dimensional structure of the whole macromolecule in which iduronic acid occurs?

Fransson. We have been thinking along these lines and have also studied the biosynthesis of hyaluronic acid in collaboration with a colleague from Uppsala University. We have done this in heparan as well as dermatan sulphate. We find a striking dependence on sulphation, there is no epimerization, to put it briefly, if you use microsomal preparations and make an endogenous product adding both of the nucleotide sugars. You can make a chondroitin like chain, there is no hyaluronic acid in it until you add PAPS to the system and allow for a certain sulphation. The degree of sulphation goes along with the rate of epimerization. So where there's sulphate there is also hyaluronic acid. We are not sure of the connection between these events but we have to have sulphation to get epimerization. It could be that sulphation goes on first and makes a site for the epimerase or vice versa the epimerase has an equilibrium and this is in favour of glucuronic acid rather than hyaluronic acid. So that you have to have a pool with other reactions removing hyaluronic acid from this equilibrium in order to get an efficient transformation. Then the sulphation of hyaluronic acid with the change in chair configuration could constitute such a reaction and lead to a sufficient pool.

Renwick (London). Do blood group antigens accumulate in patients with deficiency of any of the glycosidases we have been hearing about?

Dorfman. This I think is a very interesting question; that was one of the things I was referring to in a general manner. So far there has been no demonstration of this accumulation, the closest thing to that is the evidence that a fucose containing compound in the fucosidoses has H activity. This has been isolated by Dr Dawson who is looking for such compounds right now.

14

The treatment of genetic
mucopolysaccharidoses

Ulrich N. Wiesmann

The treatment of genetic disorders has been attempted in recent years and in some of them it has yielded an encouraging success. Especially so in disorders of amino acid metabolism where dietary restrictions are an effective therapy, normal psychomotor development of the otherwise severely damaged children has been reported (Bickel, Gerrard and Hickmann, 1954). However, in most other syndromes of inborn errors of metabolism the outcome of human treatment experiments has been unconvincing (Crocker and Farber, 1962; Green, Hug and Schubert, 1969; Hug and Schubert, 1967; Clausen and Melchior, 1967) even in disorders where the underlying biochemical defect has been known. Treatment of genetic mucopolysaccharidoses by means of dietary restrictions and by use of drugs has been attempted before the biochemical background of the different clinical syndromes has been elucidated (Crocker, 1968; Levin, Fajerman and Jacoby, 1971; DeJong, Robertson and Schafer, 1968). In recent years the biochemical defects have been worked out for a number of different types of mucopolysaccharidoses (Kresse and Neufeld, 1972; Cantz, Chramach and Neufeld, 1970; Neufeld and Cantz, 1971; Matalon and Dorfman, 1972; O'Brien, 1973) and the basis for the substitution of the deficient enzymes has been partially elaborated in tissue culture. (Neufeld *et al.*, 1971; Wiesmann, Rossi and Herschkowitz, 1972). Partially based on this recent biochemical work therapeutic trials have been performed in patients with mucopolysaccharidoses (Di Ferrante *et al.*, 1971; Knudson, Di Ferrante and Curtis, 1971; Dean, Muir and Benson, 1973). The present paper will review the therapeutic efforts in patients with MPS-oses and will analyse the possibilities for successful treatment of these disorders. Special emphasis will be placed on the problem of enzyme substitution and the prospects of gene therapy will be discussed.

Clinical aspects of the mucopolysaccharidoses

Acid mucopolysaccharides are high molecular weight compounds containing large carbohydrate chains consisting of repeated units of uronic acids and partially sulphated hexosamines. In native state they are usually attached to a protein backbone. Mucopolysaccharidoses (MPS-oses) are a group of inherited disorders of mucopolysaccharide metabolism involving mostly a defective degradation of the carbohydrate chains. The classical MPS-oses are characterized by moderate to severe skeletal deformities, typical somatic changes and a significantly increased excretion of urinary mucopolysaccharides (MPS). Mental retardation may or may not be a prevalent symptom of this disorder, but is very typical for the Hurler and the Sanfilippo syndrome. Comprehensive reviews have been published by McKusick (1969), Dorfman (1972) and Rampini (1969). The Atypical mucopolysaccharidoses are a number of disorders that share some clinical symptoms with the classical MPS-oses but do not excrete excessive amounts of urinary MPS.

Biochemistry of the stored products

Originally described as a lipid storage disorder, Hurler's syndrome was recognized by Brante (1952) to be a mucopolysaccharide storage disease. Dorfman and Lorincz (1957) discovered that the urine of patients with this disorder contained large amounts of heparan and dermatan sulphates. For review of the results of the analyses of stored MPS in organs and also in the urine of the patients, see Dorfman and Matalon (1972). Chains of acid mucopolysaccharides in the connective tissue are covalently bound to proteins and intimately interwound with collagen fibres (Muir, 1964). The material which is stored in excess or excreted in the urine was identified as heparan sulphate and dermatan sulphate and found to have a much smaller molecular weight than the intact and functional proteoglycan molecules in the tissue. The protein core seems to be removed and the carbohydrates made water soluble by partial degradation (Knecht, Cifonelli and Dorfman, 1967; Neufeld and Frantantoni, 1970). Some of the aspects of the pathophysiology of the degradation of acid mucopolysaccharides are summarized in Fig. 1.

Normally the newly synthetized proteomucopolysaccharide is secreted from the cells and incorporated into extracellular structures. Vit. C

Therapy of MPS-oses

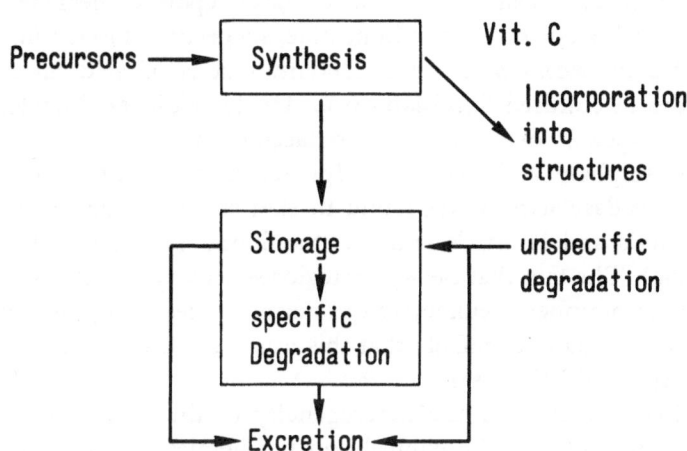

FIG. 1   Pathophysiology of MPS metabolism.
(For explanation see text)

is necessary for the fixation and the formation of insoluble complexes with collagen. A small portion of the MPS never leaves the cells but is readily broken down in the lysosomal storage pool. Partial extracellular degradation of the protein-MPS complex seems to take place and results in water soluble, but still fairly high molecular MPS. This fraction can either be taken up into the cells by pinocytosis or excreted into the urine. In the cells it undergoes specific degradation by lysosomal digestion to products that can either be re-utilized or excreted in the urine. In MPS-oses the portion of the soluble MPS is increased, because of congestion of the cells, due to the block in the specific degradation, and is therefore excreted in excess into the urine. Small molecular fragments may result from further unspecific degradation of the macromolecular soluble fraction and therefore be proportionally increased in MPS-oses.

The underlying defects in classical MPS-oses and the phenomenon of 'correction'

Van Hoof and Hers (1964) first presented evidence 'indicating that the diseases known as mucopolysaccharidoses, were due to the primary defect of one acid hydrolase normally present in lysosomes and resulted in the accumulation of incompletely degraded mucopolysaccharides'.

In cultured fibroblasts grown from skin biopsies of patients with Hurler's syndrome Danes and Bearn (1965) reported metachromatic granules which stained with toluidine blue, suggesting stored mucopolysaccharides in excess of normal. Determinations of acid mucopolysaccharides in cultured fibroblasts from Hurler patients (Matalon and Dorfman, 1968a) demonstrated an accumulation of intracellular dermatan sulphate and heparan sulphate. A profound deficiency of beta-galactosidase activity was found in skin and in organs of patients with Hurler's and Hunter's and also Sanfilippo syndrome (McBrinn *et al.*, 1969). The fact that beta-galactosidase activity in cultured fibroblasts and in peripheral leukocytes was normal (Wiesmann, unpublished results, 1971), made it unlikely that this was the primary defect for the different types of MPS-oses.

The first evidence for the heterogeneity of the lysosomal enzyme defects responsible for the clinical and biochemical expression of the different types of MPS-oses came from the laboratory of Dr E. F. Neufeld (National Institute of Health). There Fratantoni, Hall and Neufeld (1968a) could demonstrate that the abnormal accumulation of MPS; labelled with $^{35}SO_4$, in Hunter and in Hurler cells could be reverted to normal by a protein like substance produced by normal cells and recovered from the medium in which the cells had been growing for several days ('conditioned medium'). Mutual correction of the abnormal degradation of $^{35}SO_4$–MPS in Hurler and in Hunter fibroblasts could be achieved by mixing both cell-lines, or by addition of conditioned media concentrates from one genotype to the cells of the other genotype (Fratantoni, Hall and Neufeld, 1968b). Later it was found by Kresse, Wiesmann, Cantz, Hall and Neufeld (1971) that on the basis of mutual correction of cultured fibroblasts from patients with Sanfilippo syndrome, this disorder could be separated into two biochemically distinct subtypes. On the other hand, the biochemical defect in Hurler and Scheie syndrome seemed to be identical (Wiesmann and Neufeld, 1970). Recent work to uncover the underlying enzyme deficiencies has produced the expected success. Kresse *et al.* (1972) identified Sanfilippo A factor as heparan sulphate-sulphatamidase, O'Brien (1973) showed that the missing enzyme in Sanfilippo B was a N-acetyl-alpha-glucosaminidase. Matalon *et al.* (1972) found that alpha-L-iduronidase activity was absent in Hurler's disease. This enzyme was also missing in the Scheie syndrome as had been suspected previously by Bach, Friedman, Wiesmann and Neufeld (1973). Very recently the deficient enzyme in Hunter's syndrome has been identified as a dermatan sulphate-sulphatase (Cantz, Chrambach and Neufeld, 1973). A summary of the underlying defects of classical MPS-oses is shown in Table I.

TABLE I *Enzyme defects in classical mucopolysaccharidoses*

Disorder	MPS stored	Enzyme defect
Hurler	DS, HS	α-L-iduronidase
Scheie	DS	α-L-iduronidase
Hunter	DS, HS	Iduronate sulphatase
Sanfilippo A	HS	Heparan sulphate-sulphatase
Sanfilippo B	HS	N-acetyl-α-glucosaminidase
Maroteaux–Lamy	DS	N-acetylgalactos-amine-4-sulphatase
Morquio	KS, DS	?

DS=Dermatan sulphate
HS=Heparan sulphate
KS=Keratosulphate

Therapy of any storage disorder can be attempted either by reducing the synthesis of the substance stored or by enhancing the rate of its breakdown by specific or by unspecific degradation. The rationale of the therapy will be influenced by the current knowledge of the primary defect. In MPS-oses as long as the primary defects were obscure, therapeutic efforts were emphasized on the control of synthesis and on the fixation of the MPS in the tissues or in the cells. Now, that we know about the enzyme deficiencies, enzyme replacement seems to be an effective therapy.

Evaluation of the therapy in patients (*Table II*)

Exact diagnosis of the type of the MPS-oses is a prerequisite for the therapeutic trials. Although the specific enzyme defects are known in Hurler, Hunter and Sanfilippo's syndromes, the determination of the enzymes is far from being a routine procedure. Typing of MPS-oses

TABLE II   *Criteria in the evaluation of the effect of a treatment*

1. Diagnosis of the type of the mucopolysaccharidosis.
2. Natural history of the disorder.
3. Clinical findings:
   —Physical handicap.
   —Brain dysfunction.
4. Biochemical findings:
   —MPS excretion.
   —Morphology of skin, and of liver biopsies.
   —Lymphocyte inclusions.
5. Long-term effect of the treatment.

by means of the mixed cell culture (Fratantoni *et al.*, 1968b), at least in our hands, is still a valid tool to diagnose unclassified cases of MPS-oses. Typing also can be achieved by testing the corrective effect of urinary protein concentrates of patients on reference cell lines with known types of MPS-oses. Noncorrection of the $^{35}SO_4$-MPS degradation under well controlled conditions suggests identity of the patients genotype with that of the reference well culture. Before a disorder or a special patient is selected for a therapeutic experiment the natural course (onset, variation and duration) of the untreated disease should be known, to evaluate any long-term effects. If a patient is treated from a family, where other patients have demonstrated an exceptionally mild course of the disease and longevity, no conclusions really can be drawn on the effect of the therapy in patients with a more severe form of the same genetic type.

Thorough clinical examinations preferentially at monthly intervals (depending on the age of the patient) should be performed prior to the onset of the treatment. This allows for evaluation of the rate of progression and the fluctuations of the clinical symptoms. The same clinical criteria, of course, should always be applied before, during and after treatment. The crucial criteria of the short-term effects of the therapeutic trials seem to be the biochemical analyses of the urinary MPS and the different molecular fractions thereof. Of some help in the evaluation also could be the morphological, histochemical and if possible biochemical analyses of repeated tissue biopsies or white blood cell preparations.

Therapeutic efforts based on the reduction of the synthesis of MPS, or on extruding intracellular MPS

This section is of historical interest only. The therapeutic efforts described have been greatly stimulated by the assumption, that storage of MPS in classical MPS-oses resulted from an overload of the cells by an increased synthesis of normal MPS or by a synthesis of an abnormally built MPS resistant to total degradation (Matalon and Dorfman 1968b). Table III reviews the literature on these efforts.

None of these human experiments resulted in a lasting effect on the urinary MPS excretion or on the clinical course of the disorder.

Effective reduction of synthesis of a substance so widely distributed in the ground tissue of the organism proves to be difficult to achieve and if possible, would probably be deleterious to the patient.

TABLE III   *Therapeutic trials with drugs or diet*

'Therapy'	Hypothesis	Object	Reference
Corticosteroids	Reduction of MPS synthesis and fixation	Patients	Whitehouse and Bostrom (1961) Wolfson, Davidson, Harris, Kahana and Lorinz (1963) Rennert and Dekaban (1966)
Vitamin A	Reduction of intracellular MPS	Fibroblasts Patients	Danes and Bearn (1966) Rennert *et al.* (1966) Danes and Bearn (1967) Madson and Linker (1969)
Avoidance of Vitamin C	Reduction of intracellular MPS	Fibroblasts Patients	Schafer *et al.* (1968) DeJong *et al.* (1968)
Dietary Galactose reduction	Reduction of MPS synthesis	Patient	Levin *et al.* (1971)

Therapeutic efforts based on increasing the rate of degradation of stored MPS

Tissue culture has been both a model for the study of the mucopoly-saccharidoses, displaying storage of acid sulphated mucopolysaccharides (Danes *et al.*, 1965) as well as a pacemaker for the therapeutic efforts in the patients. The observation by Hors-Cayla that human serum (Hors-Cayla, Maroteaux and DeGrouchy, 1968) resulted in the dis-appearance of metachromasia in Hurler fibroblasts and the experiments of Neufeld *et al.* (1970) demonstrating a faulty degradation to be the cause of the abnormal MPS accumulation, prompted Di Ferrante to infuse fresh human plasma into patients with Hurler and Hunter disease (Di Ferrante and Nichols, 1972). Dr Neufeld and her group also have provided the preliminary evidence for the possibility of sub-stitution therapy in cultured fibroblasts from Hurler, Hunter and Sanfilippo syndrome, using as a source of enzymes or factors urinary protein concentrates (Neufeld *et al.*, 1971). Normal serum significantly reduces the accumulation of $^{35}SO_4$-MPS in Hurler and Hunter fibro-blasts (Wiesmann, 1972) (unpublished results) and increases the rate of disappearance of the labelled MPS in chase experiments.

The patients Di Ferrante had chosen for infusion therapy were a 15-month-old Hurler boy and two Hunter patients 3 and 5 years of age from a family with a very mild course of the disease (Di Ferrante *et al.*, 1972). 150–200 ml of fresh frozen human plasma were infused at a rate of 3 ml/min. Four hourly intervals were maintained between one infusion and the next one. The total amount of plasma infused varied between 20–80 ml per kg body weight. This was given over a period of 32–68 h.

The criteria of the therapeutic effect were the urinary excretion patterns of the large molecular glycosamino-glycans (GAG) and the small molecular GAG (GAG fragments). In untreated patients there was an excess of large GAG over the smaller fragments. According to Di Ferrante the large molecular fraction represents the material that normally would have been degraded by specific enzymes. By infusing fresh plasma the proportion of large molecular GAG decreases and that of the small fragments increases. However quantitatively the increase in small fragment GAG does not fully account for the decrease of the large molecular GAG.

A clinical improvement of the patient treated with plasma infusion also was reported, but the clinical criteria applied were less well documented than the biochemical ones. Infusion of 5 per cent dextrose instead of plasma had no effect on the GAG excretion. Summarizing their experiences with plasma infusions the authors state that 'the striking, but transitory, clinical and biochemical changes observed in patients affected by mucopolysaccharidoses I and II after infusion of normal human plasma lend hope to the possibility of influencing the course of these diseases once purified preparation of corrective factors become available'.

Recently another group of workers have treated three Sanfilippo patients with fresh plasma infusions. In all three patients there was an increase in total urinary GAG of between 50 and 1,000 per cent after infusion of fresh plasma equivalent to eight pints of blood (Dean *et al.*, 1973). There was little difference in the molecular size distribution of the polymeric material isolated from each patient before and after plasma infusion. The GAG fragments in one patient appeared to have undergone further degradation to even smaller fragments. In the two other patients belonging to the same sibship no such phenomenon was observed. In the one patient a decrease in the ratio of sulphate to uronic acid during and shortly after the infusion was observed, indicating desulphation of the small molecular GAG. In the two others an increase in the ratio of sulphate to uronic acid was demonstrated, indicating the possible cleavage of the latter from the GAG. The data are compatible with the assumption that one patient was of Sanfilippo A type (heparan sulphate-sulphatase deficiency) and the two siblings were of the Sanfilippo B type (N-acetyl-hexosaminidase deficiency). No clinical data on the patients before and after the plasma infusion was given.

Leukocyte transfusion

Knudson *et al.* (1971) have reported on the favourable effects of leukocyte transfusions in a child with Hunter's syndrome. The therapeutic reasoning for this trial was that lymphocytes could be a source of corrective factors similar to the ones provided with the infusion of fresh plasma. It also was speculated that lymphocyte transfusions could stimulate *de novo* synthesis of the missing enzymes. The criteria used for evaluation of the effect of the therapy were the same as for the plasma infusion Leukocytes were collected with a IBM-NCI blood cell separator. 70–90 per cent of the leukocytes collected were lymphocytes. In the first series of ten daily infusions the patients received cells from his father, fourteen days before the series of transfusions started the father was sensitized to the antigen Keyhole limpet hemocyanin (KLH). Immunity to KLH was successfully transferred to the patient as indicated by the delayed hypersensitivity to this antigen seven days after the last leukocyte transfusion from the patient's father. The changes in the GAG excretion pattern were more marked than with plasma infusions alone. The increase of the small GAG fragments, as well of the high molecular GAG excretion, rose to considerable amounts averaging an increase of 200–250 per cent over a period of twelve days.

The clinical effects were described as beneficial, similar to the ones after plasma infusions. No adverse reactions, except fever, immediately after the transfusion were reported. Reduction of metachromatic staining material in skin biopsies and a decrease in liver size were noted. According to the authors the clinical changes lasted several months, indicating 'that a rate of two or three lymphocyte transfusions per year might afford sustaining benefits'. It seems that these results give some hopes for future therapy of the patients with classical mucopolysaccharidoses. However, although nothing, except for fever reactions, has been reported indicating any adverse effects of plasma and or lymphocyte transfusions, it should be cautioned, that plasma infusions *per se* might be hazardous, because of circulatory overload and increased risk of serum hepatitis.

The mechanisms by which the described effects were produced are hitherto not very well understood. Unspecific effects could be explained by the action of an active acid hyaluronidase (DeSalegui and Pigman, 1967) present in human serum. However, because of its acidic pH optimum, extracellular action of this enzyme seems to be unlikely. Even if we consider specific enzyme substitution on a cellular level, we might wonder how much of the specific enzymes reached their destination in the lysosomes and how they should cross the blood brain barrier which would be necessary to improve brain function in the patients. Ethical problems arise from the fact that we might arise hopes in the parents of such children without being able to reassure them that the treatment really is effective in the long run and without harm to the children.

Tissue culture as a model for therapy

Now that we know the deficient enzymes responsible for producing the different types of mucopolysaccharidoses, we could think of infusing enriched or purified enzyme preparations from human sources into the patients. However we think that, since tissue culture has served us so far so well in studying the defects in these disorders, we should consider the use of these cells as a model for therapy even more extensively. In the last few years we have been interested in the substitution of lysosomal enzymes in the enzyme deficient cultured cell. Since at that time the mucopolysaccharide degrading enzymes were only known as corrective factors we have chosen arylsulphatase A deficient fibroblasts from patients with metachromatic leukodystrophy as a model for lysosomal enzyme substitution (Wiesmann *et al.*, 1972). Crude aryl-sulphatase A was prepared from normal human male urine by ammonium sulphate precipitation at 80 per cent saturation. After extensive dialysis against 0·9 per cent saline the arylsulphatase A preparation was added to the culture medium of normal fibroblasts and fibroblasts from patients with MLD, for three days. The cells were harvested by trypsin-ization and after sonication arylsulphatase A activity was measured. The results were expressed as μg p-nitrocatechol produced per h and per mg of cell protein. The results are shown in Table IV. In both normal and arylsulphatase deficient cells an increase in the activity of arylsulphatase A was noted. Intracellular location of the enzyme was demonstrated by

TABLE IV   *Enzyme substitution in fibroblasts from patients with meta-chromatic leukodystrophy*

	Intracellular arylsulphatase A activity (U^* per mg cell protein)	
		After enzyme substitution
MLD–1	5·1	30·5
MLD–2	4·0	45·2
MLD–3	6·3	28·6
Normal–1	182·5	250·0
Normal–2	200·1	220·0
Normal–3	169·2	180·0

*U=nMols p-nitrocatecholsulphate per hour

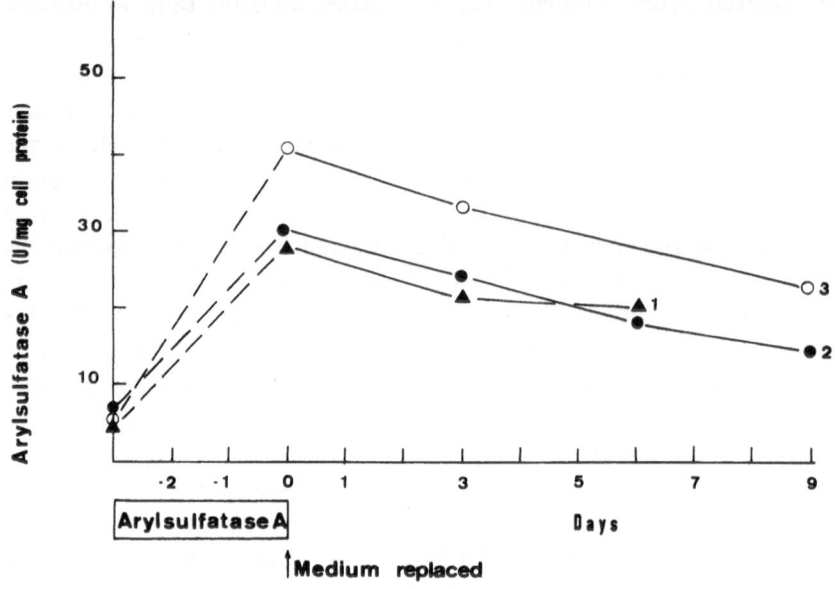

FIG. 2   Enzyme replacement in fibroblasts: Decrease of substituted arylsulphatase A
activity in MLD cells. MLD-1/MLD-2/MLD-3.
(From WIESMANN *et al.*, 1972, with the courtesy of *Acta paediatrica Scandinavica*.)

the fact that the substituted enzyme had a half life of more than ten
days (Fig. 2) as compared to the half life of the enzyme in the culture
medium of two to three days. In preliminary experiments the substituted enzyme could be located in the electron microscopy level in the
vacuoles of the treated cells by a staining reaction based on the precipitation of the sulphate produced as barium sulphate (Bischof *et al.*,
1972, unpublished results). Substitution of the arysulphatase A in
MLD cells also resulted in a shift of the pH optimum of the residual
enzyme at pH 6·0 to the regular pH optimum at pH 5·0. In order to
show the effect of the enzyme substitution on cerebroside, we have
prelabelled normal and MLD fibroblasts with ^{35}S-sulphatide, added
to the culture medium prior to the substitution of the cells with arylsulphatase A. A complete reversal of the defective degradation of
^{35}S-sulphatide in treated MLD cells could be achieved as shown in
Table V, thus proving the beneficial effect of enzyme substitution on
the faulty degradation of sulphatide. Similar experiments successfully
were performed by Porter, Fluharty and Kihara (1971).

It should be mentioned, that neither fresh human serum with an

TABLE V *Correction of abnormal ^{35}S-sulphatide metabolism by enzyme substitution*

Per cent degradation* in 'Chase' experiment of ^{35}S-sulphatide previously accumulated by the cells

	%	After enzyme substitution %
MLD–1	0·0	52
MLD–2	18·6	61
MLD–3	21·6	61
Normal–1	68·0	57
Normal–2	65·0	60
Normal–3	60·0	49

* Degradation measured as free ^{35}S in the medium.

arylsulphatase activity of 50 μg/ml/h nor concentrated media fractions of about the same activity had any effects on the ^{35}S-sulphatide degradation nor did they result in an increase of intracellular aryl-sulphatase A (Wiesmann *et al.*, 1971, unpublished results). Both preparations however produced, if added to fibroblasts from classical MPS-oses, a considerable correction of the abnormal $^{35}SO_4$-MPS degradation. The results of experiments with normal human AB plasma are summarized in Table VI (Wiesmann *et al.*, 1972, unpublished results). Figure 3 shows the corrective effect of 20 per cent human serum on $^{35}SO_4$-MPS degradation in Sanfilippo A and B fibroblasts. The typing of the fibroblasts was done by mixed cell culture with reference cell lines, kindly provided by Dr E. F. Neufeld, according to Kresse *et al.* (1971). A dose responsive correction of Sanfilippo A and B fibroblasts could be achieved by fresh serum dialysed against Eagel minimal essential medium (MEM). Analyses of the results from correction experiments using the serum of a Sanfilippo B patient in increasing doses on fibroblasts from Sanfilippo A and B patients (Fig. 4) cautiously can be interpreted as a dose responsive correction of $^{35}SO_4$-MPS degradation in Sanfilippo A fibroblasts, whereas the small but significant correction on Sanfilippo B fibroblasts seems to be an unspecific effect not related to the amount of serum added to the cultures. This

TABLE VI   *Effect of 20 per cent human AB serum on the 'degradation'*
of $^{35}SO_4$-MPS in prelabelled fibroblasts

Fibroblasts		Increase of 'degradation' over control*
		%
Hurler	N=3	50 ±5
Hunter	N=3	72 ±5
Sanfilippo A	N=2	50
Sanfilippo B	N=2	80
Maroteaux–Lamy		45 ±3
I-Cell	N=4	55 ±10

*Test cultures received 10 per cent fetal calf serum + 20 per cent human serum, control cultures only 10 per cent fetal calf serum.

observation suggests that Sanfilippo B factor or N-acetyl-alpha-glucos-aminidase activity is not present in the serum of Sanfilippo B patients.

In a preliminary set of experiments we also tried to evaluate the effect of sonicated leukocyte supernatant on the degradation of $^{35}SO_4$-MPS in Sanfilippo A and B fibroblasts. To our surprise only fibroblasts from Sanfilippo A but not those from Sanfilippo B were corrected. This finding seems to be confirmed by a personal communication from Dr Giesbert in Leyden, Holland, that he was unable to find activity of N-acetyl-alpha-glucosaminidase in peripheral leukocytes homogenates (Giesbert, personal communication).

Further experiments for the study of the mechanism involving pinocytosis and retention of lysosomal enzymes should be stressed, since there is accumulating evidence that unless lysosomal enzymes are taken up into the cells no specific functional enzyme substitution seems to be possible.

In Fig. 6 two of the possibilities of enzyme pinocytosis are demonstrated. (a) Native proteins like functional enzymes either could be pinocytosed as solutes in the fluid ingested. This way of entering the cells would be highly inefficient and would require high concentrations of enzymes in the extracellular fluid. (b) The other mechanism proposed suggests an affinity of the enzymes towards the cell membrane resulting in a very efficient pinocytosis of the proteins adherent to the membrane. We are inclined to give priority to the mechanism (b), which we would

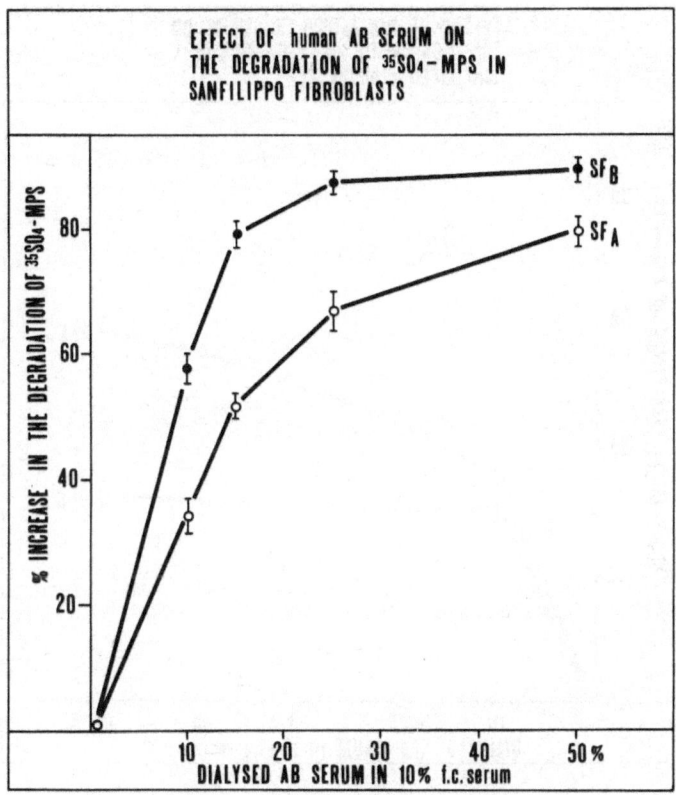

FIG. 3 Effect of human AB serum on the degradation of $^{35}SO_4$-MPS in Sanfilippo fibroblasts. The fibroblasts from patients with Sanfilippo A and B were prelabelled for four days with 5 μCi carrier-free $^{35}SO_4$ per ml of Eagle MEM with 10 per cent fetal calf serum. After thorough washing the cells with saline *in situ*, unlabelled fresh medium containing 0 (control), 10, 15, 25 and 50 per cent of AB serum, dialysed against Eagle MEM was added to the cells. Two days after the beginning of the chase, the cells were harvested and the intracellular $^{35}SO_4$-MPS was measured according to Fratantoni *et al.* (1968a). The increase in reduction of $^{35}SO_4$-MPS in serum treated cells was expressed as a percentage of the control.

call preferential pinocytosis, as the way lysosomal enzymes are taken up into the cells. Evidence for a highly specific uptake mechanism is derived from the fact, that in I-cell disease, or Mucolipidosis type II, the enzymes found in large quantities in the extracellular fluids (Wiesmann, Lightbody, Vassella and Herschkowjtz, 1971a; Wiesmann, Vassella and Herschkowjtz, 1971b) are no longer able to be pinocytosed intracellularly as shown by the experiments of Hickman and Neufeld (1972) and ourselves (Wiesmann *et al.*, in press).

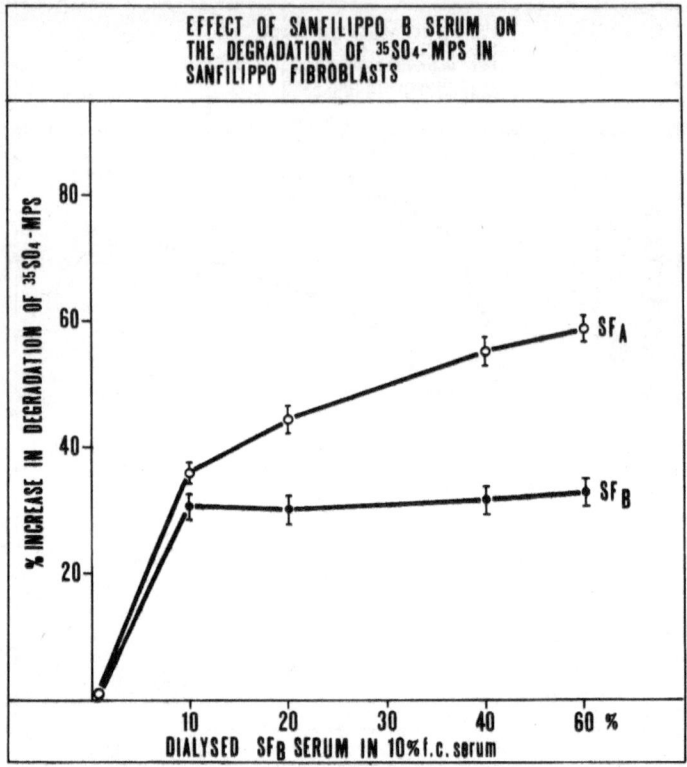

FIG. 4   Effect of Sanfilippo B serum on the degradation of $^{35}SO_4$-MPS in Sanfilippo
fibroblasts.
(For explanation see legend to Fig. 3.)

Prospects of enzyme therapy

Infusion of purified lysosomal enzyme preparation could be an effective way to substitute the cells from patients with lysosomal storage disorders, especially MPS-oses. Sources of human enzymes might be urine which contains a great number of these hydrolases, and also placentas. Here the problem of having enough material would be solved. Purification however of lysosomal enzymes has to be paralleled by *in vitro* culture substitution experiments, since it can be shown that purified enzymes from human urine may lose the privilege of preferential pinocytosis although they remain fully active against natural and artificial substrates (Wiesmann, unpublished results).

Artificial lysosomes in which lysosomal enzymes are wrapped into

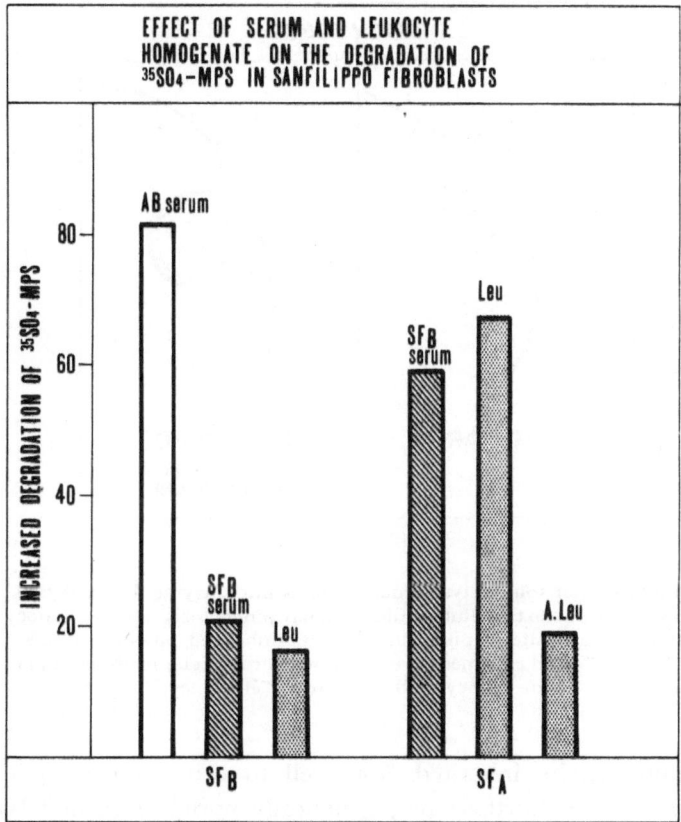

FIG. 5   Effect of serum and leucocyte homogenate on the degradation of S[35]-MPS in the Sanfilippo fibroblasts.

artificial membranes, like liposomes, could facilitate enzyme substitution in patients. They even might provide a means to overcome the blood brain barrier by being ingested into migratory cells by phagocytosis. These cells are supposed to be able to leave the blood capillaries on their way into the tissue and even when they have been destroyed, they could still be a source of enzyme for other phagocyting cells in the brain.

Gene therapy still far remote from being applied to patients has made some recent contributions to the future possibilities of therapy of inborn errors of metabolism. Here again tissue culture has provided tools to study these very dramatic possibilities (Freese, 1972). There is evidence that human cells can express some genetic information contained in the DNA or RNA of animal or bacterial viruses and that the transferred

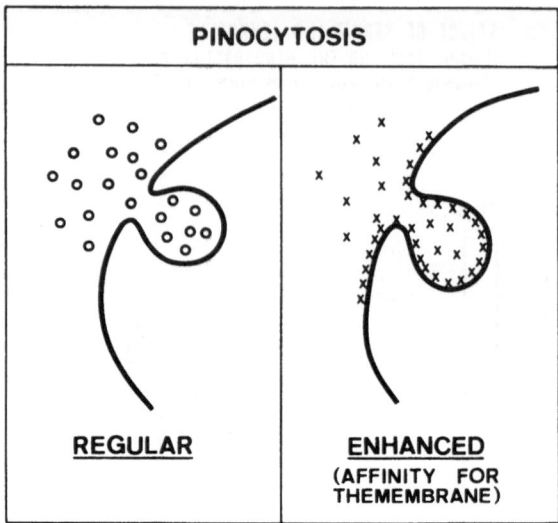

FIG. 6   Pinocytosis of soluble lysosomal enzymes into enzyme deficient cells. O, +, soluble enzymes in the extracellular fluid. Regular pinocytosis refers to pinocytosis of native proteins as a solute in pinocytosed fluid. Enhanced pinocytosis refers to the possibility that lysosomal enzymes have an affinity for the cell membrane and therefore are pinocytosed with greater efficiency.

information can be inherited from cell to cell (Merril, Geier and Petricciani, 1972). Furthermore, genetically normal human DNA can be taken up by human cells either directly or packed into a virus coat (Ostermann, Waddell and Aposhian, 1971). However, I quote from Ostermann, 'The introduction of new genetic material into a cell may cause completely unpredictable results in cellular growth of differentiation. We are convinced that carefully controlled application of molecular biology to the treatment of human diseases should be of great benefit to humanity and should result in the creation of useful lives for many people handicapped by genetic deficiencies.'

REFERENCES

BACH, G., FRIEDMAN, R., WEISSMANN, B. & NEUFELD, E. F. (1972) The defect in the Hurler and Scheie syndromes: Deficiency of α-L-iduronidase. *Proceedings of the National Academy of Sciences of the U.S.A.*, **69,** 2048.
BICKEL, H., GERRARD, J. & HICKMANN, E. M. (1954) Influence of phenylalanine intake on the chemistry and behaviour of a phenylketonuric child. *Acta Pediatrica*, **43,** 64.
BRANTE, C. (1952) Gargoylism: a mucopolysaccharidosis. *Scandinavian Journal of Clinical and Laboratory Investigation*, **4,** 43.

CANTZ, M. J., CHRAMBACH, A. & NEUFELD, E. F. (1970) Characterisation of the factor deficient in the Hunter syndrome by polyacrylamide gel electrophoresis. *Biochemical and Biophysical Research Communications,* **39,** 936.

CANTZ, M. J. (1973) *Biochemical and Biophysical Research Communications* (in press).

CLAUSEN, J. & MELCHIOR, J. C. (1967) Treatment of metachromatic Leukodystrophy. *Lancet,* **ii,** 834.

CROCKER, A. C. & FARBER, S. (1962) Therapeutic approaches to the lipidoses. In *Cerebral Sphingolipidoses,* p. 421, Eds. S. M. Aronson & B. W. Volk. New York: Academic Press.

CROCKER, A. C. (1968) Therapeutic trials in the inborn errors. An attempt to modify Hurler's Syndrome. *Pediatrics,* **42,** 887.

DANES, B. S. & BEARN, A. G. (1965) Hurler's syndrome: demonstration of an inherited disorder of connective tissue in cell culture. *Science,* **149,** 987.

DANES, B. S. & BEARN, A. G. (1966) Hurler's syndrome: Effect of retinol (Vit. A alcohol) on cellular mucopolysaccharides in the cultured human skin fibroblasts. *Journal of Experimental Medicine,* **124,** 1181.

DANES, B. S. & BEARN, A. G. (1967) The effect of retinol (Vit. A alcohol) on urinary excretion of mucopolysaccharides in the Hurler syndrome. *Lancet,* **ii,** 1029.

DEAN, M. F., MUIR, H. & BENSON, P. F. (1973) Mobilization of glycosaminoglycans by plasma infusion in mucopolysaccharidosis III—two types of response. *Nature,* **243,** 143.

DEJONG, B. P., ROBERTSON, W. VAN B. & SCHAFER, I. A. (1968) Failure to induce scurvy by ascorbic acid depletion in a patient with Hurler's syndrome. *Paediatrics,* **42,** 889.

DESALEGUI, M. & PIGMAN, W. (1967) The existence of an acid-active hyaluronidase in serum. *Archives of Biochemistry and Biophysics,* **120,** 60.

DI FERRANTE, N., NICHOLS, B. L., DONALLY, P. V., NERI, G., HRGOVCIC, C. & BERGLUND, R. K. (1971) Induced degradation of glycosaminoglycans in Hurler's and Hunter's syndromes by plasma infusions. *Proceedings of the Academy of Sciences of the U.S.A.,* **68,** 303.

DI FERRANTE, N. & NICHOLS, B. L. (1972) A case of the Hunter syndrome with progeny. *Johns Hopkins Medical Journal,* **130,** 325.

DORFMAN, A. & LORINZ, A. E. (1957) Occurrence of urinary acid mucopolysaccharides in the Hurler syndrome. *Proceedings of the Academy of Sciences of the USA.* **43,** 443.

DORFMAN, A. (1972) Die molekulare Grundlage der Mucopolysaccharidosen: Der gegenwärtige Stand unserer Kenntnisse. *Trinagel,* **11,** 43.

DORFMAN, A. & MATALON, R. (1972) The Mucopolysaccharidoses. In *The metabolic basis of inherited disease,* p. 1218. Eds. J. B. Stanbury, J. B. Wyngarden & D. S. Frederickson. New York: McGraw-Hill.

FRATANTONI, J. C., HALL, C. W. & NEUFELD, E. F. (1968a) The defect in Hurler's and Hunter's syndromes: Faulty degradation of mucopolysaccharide. *Proceedings of the National Academy of Sciences of the U.S.A.,* **60,** 699.

FRATANTONI, J. C., HALL, C. W. & NEUFELD, E. F. (1968b) Hurler and Hunter syndromes mutual correction of the defect in cultured fibroblasts. *Science,* **162,** 570.

FREESE, E. (1972) Prospects of gene therapy. *Science,* **175,** 1024.

GREEN, H. L., HUG, G. & SCHUBERT, W. K. (1969) Metachromatic leukodystrophy: Treatment with arylsulphatase A. *Archives of Neurology,* **20,** 147.

HICKMAN, S. & NEUFELD, E. F. (1972) A hypothesis for I-cell disease: Defective hydrolases that do not enter lysosomes. *Biochemical and Biophysical Research Communications,* **49,** 992.

HORS-CAYLA, M. C., MAROTEAUX, P. & DE GROUCHY, J. (1968) Fibroblasts en culture au cours de mucopolysaccharidoses: Influence du sérum sur la métachromasie. *Annales de Genetique,* **11,** 265.

HUG, G. & SCHUBERT, W. K. (1967) Lysosomes in type II glycogenosis: Changes during administration of extracts from aspergillus niger. *Journal of Cell Biology,* **35,** 1.

KNECHT, J., CIFONELLI, J. A. & DORFMAN, A. (1967) *Journal of Biological Chemistry,* **242,** 4652.

KNUDSON, A. G., DI FERRANTE, N. & CURTIS, J. E. (1971) Effect of leukocyte transfusion in a child with type II mucopolysaccharidosis. *Proceedings of the National Academy of Sciences in the U.S.A.,* **68,** 1738.

KRESSE, H., WIESMANN, U. N., CANTZ, M., HALL, C. W. & NEUFELD, E. F. (1971) Biochemical heterogenicity of the Sanfilippo syndrome: Preliminary characterisation of two deficient factors. *Biochemical and Biophysical Communications,* **42,** 28.9

KRESSE, H. & NEUFELD, E. F. (1972) The Sanfilippo A corrective factor. *Journal of Biological Chemistry*, **247**, 2164.
LEVIN, B., FAJERMAN, J. & JACOBY, N. M. (1971) Mucopolysaccharidosis. *Proceedings of the Royal Society of Medicine*, **65**, 339.
MADSON, J. A. & LINKER, A. (1969) *Journal of Pediatrics*, **75**, 843.
MATALON, R. & DORFMAN, A. (1968) Intracellular mucopolysaccharides of fibroblasts cultured from Hurler's syndrome. *Federation Proceedings, Federation of American Societies for Experimental Biology*, **27**, 719.
MATALON, R. & DORFMAN, A. (1972) Hurler's syndrome, an alpha-L-iduronidase deficiency. *Biochemical and Biophysical Research Communications*, **47**, 959.
McBRINN, M., OKADA, S., WOOLACOTT, H., PATEL, V., WAN HO, M., TAPEL, A. L. & O'BRIEN, J. S. (1969) Betagalactosidase deficiency in the Hurler syndrome. *New England Journal of Medicine*, **281**, 338.
McKUSICK, V. A. (1969) The nosology of mucopolysaccharidoses. *American Journal of Medicine*, **47**, 730.
MERRIL, C. R., GEIER, M. R. & PETRICCIANI, J. C. (1972) Bacterial virus gene expression in human cells. *Nature*, **233**, 398.
MUIR, H. (1964) Chemistry and metabolism of connective tissue glycosaminoglycans. *International Reviews of Connective Tissue Research*, **2**, 101. Ed. D. A. Hall.
NEUFELD, E. F. & FRATANTONI, C. J. (1970) Inborn errors of mucopolysaccharide metabolism. *Science*, **169**, 141.
NEUFELD, E. F. & CANTZ, M. J. (1971) Corrective factors for inborn errors of mucopolysaccharide metabolism. *Annals of the New York Academy of Science*, **179**, 514.
O'BRIEN, J. S. (1973) Sanfilippo syndrome: Profound deficiency of alpha-acetyl-glucosaminidase activity in organs and in skin fibroblasts from type B patients. *Proceedings of the National Academy of Sciences of the U.S.A.* (in press).
OSTERMAN, J. V., WADDELL, A. & APOSHIAN, H. V. (1971) Gene therapy systems: the need, experimental approach and implications. *Annals of the New York Academy of Science*, **179**, 514.
PORTER, M. T., FLUHARTY, A. L. & KIHARA, H. (1971) Correction of abnormal cerebroside sulphate metabolism in cultures of metachromatic leukodystrophy fibroblasts. *Science*, **172**, 1263.
RAMPINI, S. (1969) Das Sanfilippo-syndrom (polydystrophe oligophrenie, HS-mucopolysaccharidose). *Helvetica pediatrica Acta*, **24**, 55.
RENNERT, O. M. & DEKABAN, A. S. (1966) Modification of urinary mucopolysaccharide excretion in patients with Hurler's syndrome. *Clinical Pharmacology and Therapy*, **7**, 783.
SCHAFER, I. A., SULLIVAN, J. C., SVEJCAR, J., KOFOED, J. & ROBERTSON, W. VAN B. (1968) Study of the Hurler syndrome using cell culture: Definition of the biochemical phenotype and the effect of ascorbic acid on the mutant cell. *Journal of Clinical Investigation*, **47**, 321.
VAN HOOF, F. & HERS, H. G. (1964) L'ultrastructure des cellules hepatiques dans la maladie de Hurler (Gargoylism). *Comptes rendu hebdomadaire des seances de l'Academie des Sciences* (Paris), **259**, 1281.
WIESMANN, U. N. & NEUFELD, E. F. (1970) Scheie and Hurler syndromes: Apparent identity of the biochemical defect. *Science*, **169**, 72.
WIESMANN, U. N., LIGHTBODY, J., VASSELLA, F. & HERSCHKOWITZ, N. N. (1971a) Multiple lysosomal enzyme deficiency due to enzyme leakage? *New England, Journal of Medicine*, **284**, 109.
WIESMANN, U. N., VASSELLA, F. & HERSCHKOWITZ, N. N. (1971b) I-cell disease: Leakage of lysosomal enzymes into extracellular fluids. *New England Journal of Medicine*, **285**, 1090.
WIESMANN, U. N., ROSSI, E. E. & HERSCHKOWITZ, N. N. (1972) Correction of the defective sulphatide degradation in cultured fibroblasts from patients with metachromatic leukodystrophy. *Acta pediatrica Scandinavica*, **61**, 296.
WIESMANN, U. N., VASSELLA, F. & HERSCHKOWITZ, N. N. (1973) Mucolipidosis II (I-cell disease): A clinical and biochemical study. *Acta pediatrica Scandinavica* (in press).
WHITEHOUSE, M. W. & BOSTROM, H. (1961) Studies on the action of some anti-inflammatory agents in inhibiting the biosynthesis of mucopolysaccharide sulphates. *Biochemical Pharmacology*, **7**, 135.
WOLFSON, S. L., DAVIDSON, E., HARRIS, J. S., KAHANA, L. & LORINCZ, A. E. (1963) Longterm corticosteroid therapy in Hurler's syndrome. *American Journal of Diseases of Childhood*, **106**, 3.

DISCUSSION
(of paper by Dr Wiesmann)

Spranger (Kiel). Thank you, Dr Wiesmann, for reviewing the clinical data on what you have chosen to call human experimentation on patients with mucopolysaccharidoses. We note the fine difference between the original title of your paper and the subject you have chosen to talk about which is human experimentation rather than treatment.

Brenton (London). I wonder if you could clarify something for me? When the enzyme enters the cell in culture does the entry of the enzyme into the cell depend on the fact that the cell has recently been trypsinized or not, will it go into the cell if it has been in culture several days?

Wiesmann. Yes. Just the same. If anything just the reverse. We have noted that in cells kept for three to four days in culture, trypsin reduced the ability to take up these molecules.

Brenton. The reason I asked was that I think that there was some evidence in the past that long trypsinization damaged membranes. I wondered if it leaked in rather than actively being taken up.

Wiesmann. If that was so then we wouldn't have observed this kind of enhanced take up, if it leaked in by diffusion anything that leaked in better would do better than the enzyme, but this is not so, all molecules large enough to be pinocytosed are different in this respect from the iso-enzyme in that they are taken up much less efficiently.

Raine (Birmingham). Arylsulphatase is an artificial substrate and it is testing the enzyme that we would really like to estimate, i.e. cerebroside sulphatase, it has been shown that these enzymes are not really the same thing, for example the rate of maturation of these two enzymes in the rabbit after birth is different. A heat stable factor is concerned, which when added to arylsulphatase really makes it into cerebroside sulphatase. I wonder if it were possible that in some of your inclusion experiments into cells the results were being affected by this and other factors. It all depends really on how you prepare your material from human urine, before adding it to your cell culture medium.

Wiesmann. When you analyse for arysulphatase A according to Dobson and Baron, the result is total arylsulphatase with either natural or artificial substrate the same curve is obtained.

We think that the enzyme which really enters the cell is really arylsulphatase A because when you analyse the effect of the substrate (we don't take any artificial substrate we take normal substrate), by loading the cells prior or afterwards with the sulphated cerebroside sulphatide and you are then really dealing with the natural substrate for the natural enzyme. The preparation we use is simply precipitation of urine with ammonium sulphate at 40 per cent saturation. Arylsulphatase A is precipitated leaving back arylsulphatase B. Further purification of the crude preparation doesn't improve its capacity.

Raine. My second point was going to be kept until later but Professor Spranger's remarks after Dr Wiesmann's talk really brings it to the fore. I mean the ethical considerations of this kind of experimentation. I wanted to say that I thought Dr Wiesmann's emphasis on the careful planning of this type of study was one of the more valuable things he put across. If I may express a personal point of view about this, first of all one has to deal with the straight ethical problem. We are really inhibited in this country because the official advice comes from a Medical Research Council document which says that it is unethical to do any experiment on any child because the child cannot give informed consent, being legally incompetent to do so, neither can the parent or guardian give it on behalf of the child. This is undoubtedly inhibiting this kind of investigation in Britain. I took part in a discussion on the subject which was eventually published in the *British Medical Journal* a couple of months ago. I would draw your attention to this publication, not for any words of wisdom, but for the fact that three fairly seriously minded people were unanimous that something had to be done about it, if we were to make any progress.

My other point is that if we're to do this kind of study we want to plan them most carefully. I think it is terrible if you read something in the latest journal and dash off to try it on the patient where it is concerned with the treatment area. Certainly not the sort of thing where you can do a small trial and expect to switch it off and the patient and his parents then not to worry about it. I do think this ought to have a great deal of thought given to it and in that light I would like to mention the sort of thing we are doing in association with Dr Stevenson in Glasgow on metachromatic leucodystrophy. We have infused white cells into the patient, who was in a fairly terminal state because he had first had Vit. A deficiency diet treatment, and it had been decided that this wasn't going to be successful. Just to consider the problem of infusing white cells, first you have polymorphs, you have lymphocytes then you have the immunological problem that might arise from infusing cells. As I understand it these are greater with respect to lymphocytes, so the first thing we did was to find out if the enzyme we wanted to give was normally in lymphocytes or polymorphs. It turned out that it was normally in polymorphs, and at least we had the option of not infusing lymphocytes by separating out the polymorphs. However that was not the first approach we made. The first approach was to infuse a whole mixture of cells but to irradiate the cells to suppress the antigenic reaction of the cells. We studied white cell and plasma enzyme levels over the course of a few weeks. We decided to work out a regime which would be given monthly not three-monthly as you suggested and the pattern of activity that we got with these whole, but irradiated cells, was that the enzyme activity went up and then came down to fairly low levels and was pretty well over by three weeks and certainly by four.

Spranger. Activity in plasma?

Raine. In white cells taken from patient after infusion so really a mixture of his own cells and infused cells. Next time we decided to risk the antigenic problem and not irradiate the cells. The number of cells infused were fewer than we would have liked but although the level was lower it was more evenly spread over four weeks. So we would like now to go on using non-irradiated cells and if we look like running into antigenic problems we would just use polymorphs separating out the lymphocytes. I would not like this to be quoted as the sort of experiment worth pursuing but I am pointing out that you have to work out a number of technical problems before embarking on anything that could legitimately be called treatment.

Benson (London). You mentioned that dextran infusion in patients with the mucopolysaccharidosis produced similar effects to plasma. Do you mean that dextran causes a mobilization of total glycosaminoglycans or does it actually cause degradation of high molecular weight glycosaminoglycans?

Wiesmann. No.

Dean (London). May I make the point that the results of our treatment of mucopolysaccharidoses are probably attributable to two factors:

1. Non-specific affect of infusing large plasma volumes.
2. Specific effect due to the enzyme within the plasma, reflected in the size change in small molecular weight fragments resolved on Sephadex G25.

LABORATORY ASPECTS OF THE MUCO-POLYSACCHARIDOSES INCLUDING DIAGNOSIS AND SCREENING

15

The laboratory diagnosis of the mucopolysaccharidoses

P. W. Lewis, J. F. Kennedy, and D. N. Raine

The recognition of the mucopolysaccharidoses in the laboratory has hitherto been based on simple urine tests dependent upon the poly-anionic nature of the glycosaminoglycans excreted in these disorders. The chemistry and biochemistry of these substances has recently been reviewed by Kennedy (1973).

The first of these methods (Berry and Spinanger, 1960) was to stain a spot of urine on filter paper with the blue dye toluidine blue which, in the presence of an acid mucopolysaccharide, was converted to a purple colour a phenomenon known as 'metachromasia'. The chemistry of metachromasia, both in this form and in the form of histological staining, has been the subject of considerable discussion (Danes, Scott and Bearn, 1970; Matalon and Dorfman, 1972a). The toluidine blue test, however, is not specific for glycosaminoglycans as it also gives positive results with nucleic acids in tissues and in urine containing cellular material such as leucocytes associated with renal infection. To over-come this, the dye alcian blue, used under defined conditions, was recommended (Carson and Neill, 1962). Although this improved the specificity of the test and is widely used (Procopis, Turner, Ruxton and Brown, 1968; McDonald, Lozzio and Lotkin, 1970) no substantial studies have been made to determine the diagnostic efficiency of the test either for mucopolysaccharidoses as a whole or for the individual diseases as these have been progressively defined. More recently a spot test using paper impregnated with azure A has been described (Berman, Vered and Bach, 1971).

A further approach (Dorfman, 1958) depends on the fact that urine when mixed with a solution of albumin results in turbidity proportional to the amount of acid mucopolysaccharide present. This can be meas-ured and this test too has found wide application (Steiness, 1961; Carter, Wan, and Carpenter, 1968).

Another test based on the formation of a similar insoluble complex, this time with a quaternary ammonium compound cetylpyridinium chloride (CPC) was devised by Manley and Hawksworth (1966) and found favour for some time. Because of the number of false positive results the test in its original form is not now so widely used, but similar tests using quaternary ammonium salts in buffered solutions are reported to be more reliable (Renuart, 1966; Pennock, Mott and Batstone, 1970).

Some glycosaminoglycans are normally excreted in urine: these are hyaluronic acid and chondroitin 4- and 6-sulphates. The glycosaminoglycans associated with the mucopolysaccharidoses are dermatan sulphate, heparan sulphate and keratan sulphate. All but the last of these contain uronic acid, so that if these substances are precipitated by cetylpyridinium chloride and the total uronic acid determined in the precipitate a quantitative measure of the excretion can be made and abnormal concentrations recognized (Di Ferrante, 1967). This has proved a useful investigation and has been applied to a large number of normal children and to a number of patients with the more common forms of mucopolysaccharidosis. (Teller, Burke, Rosevear and McKenzie, 1962; Pennock, White and Wharton, 1972.)

Finally, Whiteman (1973a) has made the reaction of glycosaminoglycans with alcian blue quantitative and applied it to urine (Whiteman, 1973b). This investigation, unlike the determination of CPC-precipitable uronic acid, measures all the pathological glycosaminoglycans since it includes keratan sulphate.

So far there has been no comprehensive investigation of the reliability and consistancy of these several tests for the recognition of mucopolysaccharidoses as a group and certainly not for the individual forms of the disease. The present report is concerned with this.

The tests so far described are designed to evaluate the total excretion of glycosaminoglycan without regard to the individual types of mucopolysaccharidosis (Table I, see Spranger, 1972). Attempts to separate and quantitate the different mucopolysaccharides have met with varying degrees of success.

Paper chromatographic separation of dermatan and heparan sulphates has been applied to urine from patients with the Hunter and Hurler syndromes (Terry and Linker, 1964; Good, 1967; McDonald *et al.*, 1970). At first it seemed that more dermatan sulphate was excreted by the Hurler patients and more heparan sulphate by the

Hunter patients, but this has not been supported by subsequent investigations.

Purified preparations of glycosaminoglycans have been separated by thin-layer chromatography using silica, cellulose and other media (Wusteman, Lloyd and Dodgson, 1966; Bischel, Austin, Kemeny, Hubble and Lear, 1966; Havass and Szabo, 1972) but the resolution was poor. Marzullo and Lash (1967) obtained good separation of six glycosaminoglycans using silica gel plates developed with n-propanal, concentrated ammonia and water but this does not appear to have been used to examine glycosaminoglycans in urine. Teller and Ziemann (1969) distinguished Hunter and Sanfilippo patients using isopropanol in a formate buffer to develop cellulose plates, and more recently Humbel and Chamoles (1972) using the method of Lippiello and Mankin (1971) obtained different patterns of urinary glycosaminoglycans from patients with the Hunter and Hurler syndromes, which could not be distinguished from each other, and from Sanfilippo, Morquio and Maroteaux-Lamy patients. This technique involves dipping the cellulose plate in a succession of solutions of calcium acetate in decreasing concentrations of ethanol and allowing each to run a particular distance from the origin. Reports indicate that it provides the most promising separations so far achieved.

Glycosaminoglycans have been fractionated into non-sulphated and sulphated groups on Ecteola cellulose ion-exchange columns (Wessler, 1967) and have been further fractionated by elution from strong anion-exchange columns with increasing concentrations of sodium chloride (Schiller, Slover and Dorfman, 1961; Di Ferrante, 1967; Blackham and Raine, 1969). Elution from columns of cellulose saturated with cetylpyridinium chloride using varying concentrations of magnesium chloride in cetylpyridinium chloride is also claimed to separate a number of glycosaminoglycans (Svejcar and Robertson, 1967). Resolution by ion-exchange procedures is, however, limited by the heterogeneous nature of some glycosaminoglycans. (Pearce, Mathieson and Grimmer, 1968).

Separation of purified preparations of glycoasaminoglycans by electrophoresis on paper (Foster and Pearce, 1961) and starch gel (Brookhart, 1965) has been achieved and tissue glycosaminoglycans have been separated by electrophoresis on polyacrylamide-agarose gel (McDevitt and Muir, 1971). Electrophoretic analysis of urinary glycosaminoglycans has been most rewarding when cellulose acetate was used. Several electrolyte systems have been recommended, viz. barium acetate and cadmium acetate (Wessler, 1968), hydrochloric acid (Wessler, 1971) and zinc sulphate (Kimura and Tsurumi, 1969). Resolution of chondroitin 4- and 6-sulphates and dermatan sulphate is claimed using calcium acetate as the electrolyte (Seno, Anno, Kondo, Nagase and Saito, 1970). Cellulose acetate has also been used for two-dimensional electrophoretic separation of the chondroitin sulphate isomers, heparan sulphate, keratan sulphate, hyaluronic acid and heparin (Hata and Nagai, 1972).

Since two glycosaminoglycans, dermatan sulphate and heparan sulphate are excreted in varying proportions in five of the six types of mucopolysaccharidosis, such separation techniques may still not, by themselves, allow the several mucopolysaccharidoses to be differentiated. (The original classification into six types has since been revised, see McKusick, 1966 and 1972.)

In spite of this we are able to present an electrophoretic technique which qualitatively differentiates at least four types of mucopolysaccharidosis.

The most recent and so far the most specific approach to differential diagnosis is the effect of growing skin fibroblasts from different patients in a common culture. When the cells are from patients with the same disease, metachromasia and the abnormal utilization of radioactive sulphate persists, but when they are from patients with different diseases these abnormalities are corrected (Frantantoni, Hall and Neufeld, 1968). This work has been extended to five types of mucopolysaccharidosis and patients may now be classified by culturing skin fibroblasts with those from a bank of known type specimens (Neufeld and Cantz, 1970; Kresse, Wiesmann, Cantz, Hall and Neufeld, 1971; Barton and Neufeld, 1972).

Patients studied

Two hundred and sixteen urine specimens from 169 patients within the Midland area have been examined for mucopolysaccharide excretion. These comprise 149 patients in whom a mucopolysaccharidosis was suspected clinically or needed to be excluded: 30 of these were eventually diagnosed as such on clinical and biochemical findings. Twenty further patients were studied because they did not have any connective tissue disorder and serve as a control group. This same group of 20 patients together with all those in whom an excessive excretion of glycosaminoglycan was found by the quantitative assays and those patients definitely diagnosed as Morquio disease on clinical grounds (even though some of the latter did not show excessive excretion of glycosaminoglycan) were examined by a cellulose acetate electrophoretic technique based on a method of Wessler (1968).

Screening tests

In the present study urine has been examined by a modification of the alcian blue spot test (Carson *et al.*, 1962) and by the bovine albumin turbidity test (Steiness, 1961). This latter test, as originally described, did not include a urine blank. However, in some instances it seemed that the result of this test differed from the clinical and other findings. It was observed that, even after dialysis, some urines retained a degree of turbidity which contributed to the final result in the bovine albumin turbidity test. When the turbidity produced by urine with buffer alone, in place of the buffered albumin reagent, was subtracted from that produced with albumin, the result appeared to be more in accord with the clinical observations. We, therefore, have examined the value of including a blank whenever this test was applied.

Fig. 1 shows the distribution of these urine blank values, and shows that omission of the blank can lead to a substantial and variable error. It may be necessary, if a blank is regularly included in the test, to lower

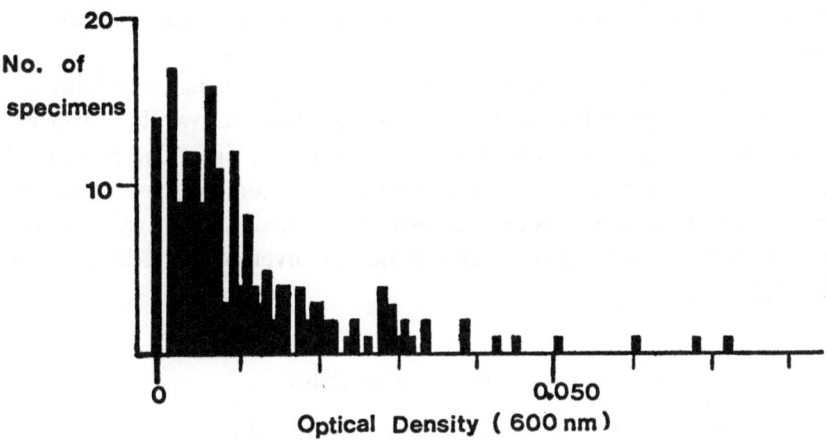

FIG. 1   Blank values in the bovine albumin turbidity test: results from 192 specimens.

the optical density (0·04) regarded as the upper limit of normal. This more discriminating limit will be established as more known mucopolysaccharidosis patients are studied but it seems that this will be an optical density about 0·01 lower than that used hitherto.

The urinary glycosaminoglycans were quantitatively determined by two different techniques: precipitation with cetylpyridinium chloride (CPC) followed by determination of uronic acid in the precipitate (Di Ferrante, 1967) and the quantitative alcian blue test of Whiteman (1973b).

Value of short-term urine specimens

Di Ferrante and Lipscomb (1970) report that when random urine specimens, as distinct from 24h collections, are tested for glycosaminoglycan excretion, the results may falsely indicate either normality or abnormality and they recommend that even with these collections over a longer period the mucopolysaccharide excretion should be related to urinary creatinine.

We have examined 41 random urine specimens and related the findings to those on 24 h collections from the same patients. So far all of the subjects studied in this way have proved by biochemical and clinical criteria to be suffering from something other than a mucopolysaccharidosis. In one subject abnormal results were obtained with both qualitative screening tests but examination of a 24 h specimen was normal. Similarly, one patient whose random urine specimen was negative by both qualitative screening tests produced a rather concentrated 24 h specimen on which these tests were positive but here the quantitative assays were normal.

A similar study of random urine specimens from patients with the several mucopolysaccharidoses is in progress but meanwhile it appears to be safer to work only with 24 h collections of urine. The additional precaution of keeping these cold during collection, to avoid bacterial breakdown of the macromolecular form of the acid mucopolysaccharides on which the tests depend, should not be overlooked (Manley and Hawksworth, 1966).

Screening tests in different mucopolysaccharidoses

It is of interest to consider the extent to which these several screening tests will detect any patient with a mucopolysaccharidosis of whatever type and also the possibility that, if some of the tests are positive in one of the types and negative in others, whether they provide a pattern that will differentiate one or more of these disorders. The results have, therefore, been considered in relation to the clinical diagnosis where this was confidently expressed. Where the clinical diagnosis was in doubt the results of the screening tests have been analyzed separately.

In nine patients with either the Hunter or Hurler syndromes the alcian blue spot test and the bovine albumin turbidity test were positive in all instances. In two of these patients a further 24 h collection was made and, except for the alcian blue spot test in one of these, the results were again positive. In the case of the exception the urine was very dilute (24 h volume 900 ml, creatinine concentration 11 mg/100 ml compared with 275 ml and 15 mg/100 ml on the previous specimen) so it would seem wise to ensure that, when collections are made, an excessive fluid intake is avoided.

These same tests were also consistently positive in three patients with the Morquio syndrome, but were negative in six others. These correspond to McKusick's (1972) classification of the Morquio syndrome into those with and those without mucopolysacchariduria. Four Sanfilippo patients gave positive alcian blue spot tests, but in three of these the turbidity test was normal. One patient with Scheie's syndrome gave normal results with both tests. However, the specimen was extremely dilute (24 h volume 2200 ml, cretinine concentration 17 mg/100 ml) and it will be necessary to repeat this before the value of the tests in this disease can be assessed. We have had the opportunity to study two sisters with minimal skeletal deformities, similar to the patients described by Horton and Schimke (1970). In both cases the albumin turbidity test was positive but only one was positive by the alcian blue spot test.

Twenty normal subjects were examined as controls. Two of these gave equivocal alcian blue spot tests, but further investigation of these established that they were quite normal. Four subjects gave abnormal albumin turbidities when this test was performed without including a urine blank. When this was included the results became normal (OD less than 0·04).

The excretion of uronic acid precipitable by cetylpyridinium chloride was unequivocably increased in all Hurler, Hunter, Sanfilippo, Scheie and Morquio-with-mucopolysacchariduria cases and the values in the Hunter and Hurler patients were distinctly higher than in all others.

Similarly clearly abnormal results were given by the quantitative alcian blue assay in patients with these diseases but in two cases the results were only just abnormal when compared with the normal findings, published elsewhere in this volume and by Dr P. Whiteman. Some Morquio patients showed a raised excretion by the quantitative alcian blue assay whilst others did not. This variation supports the findings of other groups who have failed to detect excessive excretion of mucopolysaccharides in some Morquio patients (Bitter, Muir, Mittwoch and Scott, 1966; Norum, 1969).

The glycosaminoglycan excretion as measured by both the CPC-precipitable uronic acid excretion and the quantitative alcian blue test in the two sisters with the Horton and Schimke disease, though abnormal, was not as high as that in any of the Hunter or Hurler patients.

The CPC-precipitable uronic acid assay, when applied to the group of normal subjects, confirmed that this, when related to urinary creatinine, falls with age up to the mid-teens. All but three of the results fell within the limits defined by Teller *et al.* (1962) and only three out of 17 were slightly higher than the upper limits of Pennock *et al.* (1972). Similarly, the quantitative alcian blue test, when related to creatinine excretion, shows that the upper limit of the normal range declines with age. In three of the 20 subjects chosen as normal controls, although the alcian blue spot test and the albumin turbidity test were normal, the CPC-precipitable uronic acid and the quantitative alcian blue test were abnormal. In all three, urine was collected within two days of extra-corporeal-circulation for cardiac surgery. The explanation of this anomoly is not yet apparent.

Electrophoretic separation of urinary glycosaminoglycans

Although all four screening tests allow the detection of patients with the Hunter, Hurler and Morquio-with-mucopolysacchariduria syndromes and with rather less confidence the Sanfilippo and Scheie syndromes, they do not offer any help in the differentiation of these from each other. To this end an electrophoretic separation of urine glycosaminoglycans was examined.

As a preliminary it is necessary to concentrate the urine sample using Carbowax and Visking tubing. The concentrate is applied to cellulose acetate and run alongside a standard preparation containing chondroitin 4-sulphate, chondroitin 6-sulphate, dermatan sulphate, heparan sulphate, keratan sulphate and hyaluronic acid (provided by Dr M. B. Matthews, Chicago). These standards are from tissues and may not have the same degree of sulphation or polymerization as the material in human urine; they, therefore, serve only as a control of the reproducibility and quality of each electrophoretic run. Electrophoresis is carried out in barium acetate, 0·1 mol/1 (Wessler, 1968) at 5 v/cm for 4·5 h. The strips are stained in alcian blue, 1 g/100 ml in 2 per cent (v/v) aqueous acetic acid and washed in the same strength of acetic acid.

This was applied to 36 patients in whom the screening tests were abnormal or who were confidently diagnosed as cases of Morquio disease. These represent six disease types: Hurler, Hunter, Sanfilippo, Scheie and Morquio with and without mucopolysacchariduria. In addition the 20 normal subjects were examined in the same way. Examination of the electrophoretic separations allowed five (Lewis, Kennedy and Raine, 1973) and later a sixth pattern to be defined. These are shown as A to F in Fig. 2.

Where there was a confident clinical diagnosis there was a valuable correlation between the mucopolysaccharidosis type and one of the electrophoretic patterns. All Hurler and Hunter patients showed the three banded type A pattern. The three Morquio-with-mucopolysacchariduria patients had the two banded type C pattern. A different two banded pattern, type D, was observed in a patient with the Scheie syndrome. Pattern E has only been observed in normal subjects and patients with Morquio disease without mucopolysacchariduria. Our first patient with the Sanfilippo syndrome showed a different pattern again, type B, but later three patients, confidently diagnosed as having the Sanfilippo syndrome, showed the new pattern type F. It is interesting that the two sisters with the very mild affection which Horton *et al.* (1970) reported to be associated with the excretion of dermatan and heparan sulphates have fallen into the type A pattern characteristic of the Hunter and Hurler syndromes. Fig. 2 also shows the results in a number of patients who have been assigned to an electrophoretic pattern but of whom a critical clinical examination has not yet been made. The results in the 20 normal subjects used as a control are shown in Fig. 3. All gave the same electrophoretic pattern, type E.

Conclusion

As a result of these studies it would seem that the simple screening

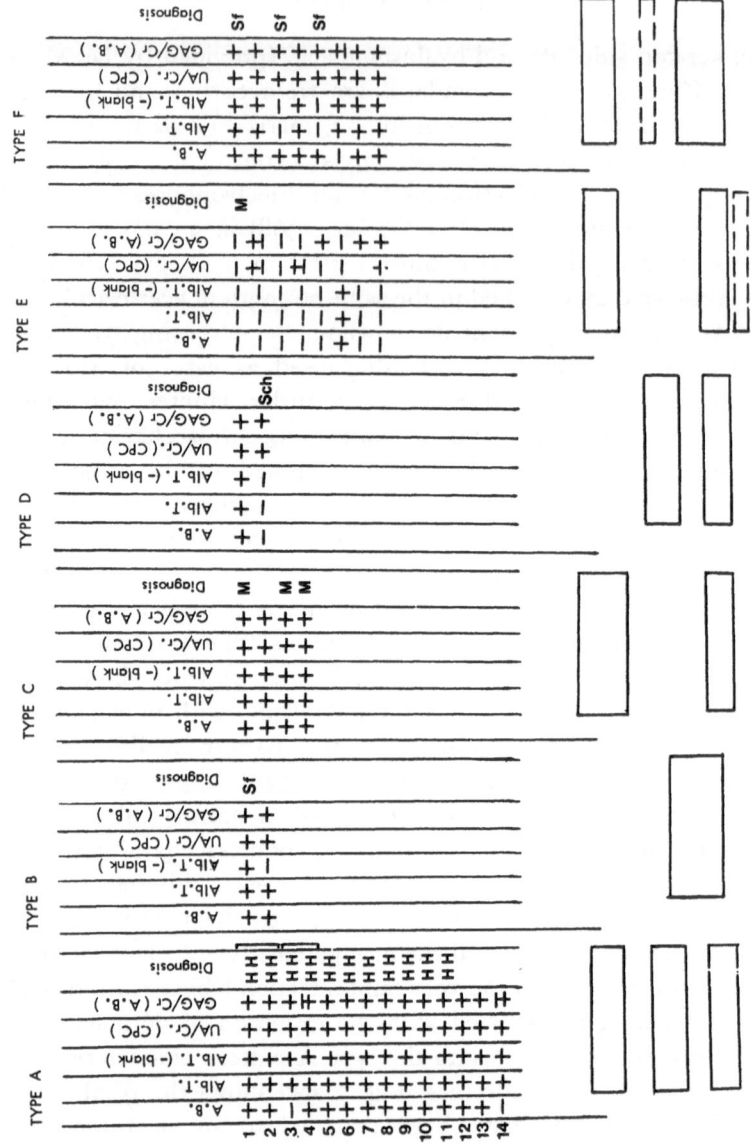

tests are reliable in detecting the Hunter, Hurler, Morquio-with-mucopolysacchariduria and Sanfilippo syndromes but that these are less reliable in the Morquio syndrome without mucopolysacchariduria and in some patients at present regarded as cases of the Sanfilippo syndrome with the three banded electrophoretic pattern. Some of these equivocal cases have been resolved by the determination of urinary glycosaminoglycan in terms of the CPC-precipitable uronic acid and the quantitative alcian blue test. The technical simplicity of the latter compared with the determination of uronic acid, together with the ability of the alcian blue test to include keratan sulphate commends this as the method of choice for the detection of abnormal mucopolysacchariduria.

The electrophoretic separation of urinary glycosaminoglycans presented here still does not allow all patients to be assigned to a specific type of mucopolysaccharidosis. It does, however, permit a greater degree of discrimination than any other laboratory investigation available hitherto. Without this, except for some complex separation procedures, it has been necessary to rely wholly on clinical findings in assigning particular patients to one or other of the disease categories and, more recently, to confirm these by cross-culturing the fibroblasts from the patients with those of known cases of the several diseases. At least with the electrophoretic technique as described, patients can be said to belong to the Hunter and Hurler group (further differentiation will require fibroblast cross-culture studies and genetic analysis); the Morquio-with-mucopolysacchariduria syndrome; the Scheie syndrome; and the Sanfilippo syndrome which in our hands appears to fall into two categories. The full significance of this last observation has yet to be explored. It is useful to know that negative biochemical tests in patients clinically believed to belong to the Morquio group do not exclude this diagnosis.

FIG. 2   Results of the chemical investigation of glycosaminoglycans in 24 h urine specimens from 36 patients.
Types A-F represent the six electrophoretic patterns found. Type E was given by the 20 normal urines examined.
Results of the other determinations are represented as + abnormal, ± borderline, — normal. A.B. = Alcian Blue spot test; Alb. T. = bovine albumin turbidity; UA/Cr. (CPC) = cetylpyridinium chloride precipitable uronic acid to creatinine ratio; GAG/Cr. (A.B.) = glycosaminoglycan to creatinine ratio determined by the quantitative Alcian Blue technique. Where a confident clinical diagnosis was made it is indicated by: HH = Hurler or Hunter; Sf = Sanfilippo; M = Morquio; Sh = Scheie. Results bracketed together are for different specimens from the same patient.

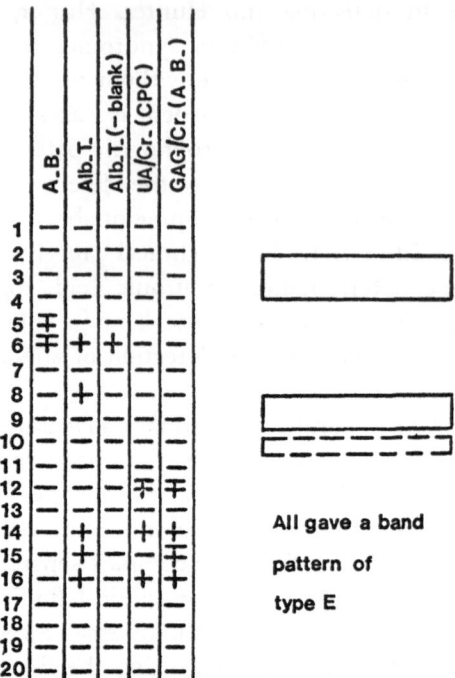

FIG. 3   Results of the chemical investigation of glycosaminoglycans in 24 h urine specimens from 20 non-mucopolysaccharidosis patients. For symbols and headings see Fig. 2.

This technique is capable of further diagnostic value since it should be possible to elute the different bands from the electrophoretic strip and characterize these by qualitative determination of their aminohexose and uronic acid components.

The definitive diagnostic procedure for the mucopolysaccharidoses would be the demonstration of the specific enzyme deficiency and several of these are now known, Table I. Using skin fibroblasts, deficiency of α-L-iduronidase has been demonstrated in the Hurler and Scheie syndromes (Matalon and Dorfman, 1972b; Bach, Friedman, Weissmann and Neufeld, 1972) and in patients thought to represent a mixture of these two syndromes (McKusick, 1972) and also in the unusual patients of Horton and Schimke (McKusick, 1972). Cross-correction experiments with cultured fibroblasts have indicated the existence of two clinically indistinguishable forms of the Sanfilippo syndrome, types A and B. This finding is supported by the demonstra-

TABLE I *Biochemical characteristics of the several mucopolysaccharidoses*

Mucopolysaccharidosis	Urinary glycosaminoglycans	Enzyme deficiency
I-Hurler syndrome	Dermatan sulphate Heparan sulphate	α-L-iduronidase
II—Hunter syndrome	Dermatan sulphate Heparan sulphate	Iduronate sulphatase
IIIA—Sanfilippo syndrome A	Heparan sulphate	Heparan sulphate sulphatase
IIIB—Sanfilippo syndrome B	Heparan sulphate	N-actyl-α-D-glucos-aminidase
IV—Morquio syndrome	Keratan sulphate	Not known
V—Scheie syndrome	Dermatan sulphate Heparan sulphate	α-L-iduronidase
VI—Maroteaux–Lamy syndrome	Dermatan sulphate Heparan sulphate	N-acetylgalactos-aminc-4-sulphatase

tion of two enzyme deficiencies in the fibroblasts from Sanfilippo patients; N-acetyl-D-glucosaminidase in type B (O'Brien, 1972) and heparan sulphate sulphatase in Type A (Kresse and Neufeld, 1972). Clearly this complex group of diseases is on the verge of ultimate classification but there is still evidence that the group may be fragmented still further before this is achieved.

Acknowledgements

This work has been supported by grants from The Research Committee of the United Birmingham Hospitals Endowment Fund. We are most grateful to all of the clinicans who have allowed us to study their patients and to their nursing and laboratory colleagues who have made possible the urine collections from these difficult patients. We record our thanks to Dr Paul Whiteman of the Hospital for Sick Children, London, for making available to us unpublished information concerning his quantitative alcian blue test.

REFERENCES

BACH, G., FRIEDMAN, R., WEISSMANN, B. & NEUFELD, E. F. (1972) The defect in the Hurler and Scheie syndromes: deficiency of α-L-iduronidase. *Proceedings of the National Academy of Sciences of the U. S. A.*, **69**, 2048.
BARTON, R. W. & NEUFELD, E. F. (1972) A distinct biochemical deficit in the Maroteaux–Lamy syndrome (mucopolysaccharidosis v). *Journal of Pediatrics*, **80**, 114.
BERMAN, E. R., VERED, J. & BACH, G. (1971) A reliable spot test for mucopolysacchridosis. *Clinical Chemistry*, **17**, 886.
BERRY, A. K. & SPINANGER, J. (1960) A paper spot test useful in study of Hurler's syndrome. *Journal of Laboratory and Clinical Medicine*, **55**, 136.

BISCHEL, M., AUSTIN, J. H., KEMENY, M. D., HUBBLE, C. M. & LEAR, R. K. (1966) Separation and identification of acid polysaccharides by thin-layer chromatography. *Journal of Chromatography*, **21**, 40.

BITTER, T., MUIR, H., MITTWOCH, U. & SCOTT, J. D. (1966) A contribution to the differential diagnosis of Hurler's disease and forms of Morquio's syndrome. *Journal of Bone and Joint Surgery*, **48-B**, 637.

BLACKHAM, G. A. & RAINE, D. N. (1969). The biochemistry of the mucopolysaccharidoses. *Annals of Clinical Biochemistry*, **6**, 49.

BROOKHART, J. H. (1965). Separation of acid polysaccharides by starch gel electrophoresis. *Journal of Chromatography*, **20**, 191.

CARSON, N. A. J. & NEILL, D. W. (1962) Metabolic abnormalities detected in a survey of mentally backward individuals in Northern Ireland. *Archives of Disease of Childhood*, **37**, 505.

CARTER, C. H., WAN, A. T. & CARPENTER, D. G. (1968) Commonly used tests in the detection of Hurler's syndrome. *Journal of Pediatrics*, **73**, 217.

DANES, B. S., SCOTT, J. E. & BEARN, A. G. (1970) Further studies on metachromasia in cultured human fibroblasts. *Journal of Experimental Medicine*, **132**, 765.

DI FERRANTE, N. (1967). The measurement of urinary mucopolysaccharides. *Analytical Biochemistry*, **21**, 89–106.

DI FERRANTE, N. & LIPSCOMB, H. S. (1970) Urinary glycosaminoglycans versus creatinine excretion; a used and abused parameter. *Clinica chimica acta.*, **30**, 69–72.

DORFMAN, A. (1958) Studies on the biochemistry of connective tissue. *Pediatrics*, **22**, 576–89.

FOSTER, T. S. & PEARCE, R. H. (1961) Zone electrophoresis of acid mucopolysaccharides. *Canadian Journal of Biochemistry and Physiology*, **39**, 1771–82.

FRANTANTONI, J. C., HALL, C. W. & NEUFELD, E. F. (1968). Hurler and Hunter syndromes; mutual correction of the defect in cultured fibroblasts. *Science*, **162** 570–2.

GOOD, T. A. (1967) Ascending paper chromatography of sulphated acid mucopolysaccharides. *Analytical Biochemistry*, **19**, 109–18.

HATA, R. & NAGAI, Y. (1972) A rapid and micro method for separation of acidic glycosaminoglycans by two-dimensional electrophoresis. *Analytical Biochemistry*, **45**, 462–8.

HAVASS, Z. & SZABO, L. (1972) Thin-layer chromatographic separation of glycosaminoglycans. *Journal of Chromatography*, **71**, 580–4.

HORTON, W. A. & SCHIMKE, R. N. (1970) A new mucopolysaccharidosis. *Journal of Pediatrics*, **77**, 252–8.

HUMBEL, R. & CHAMOLES, N. A. (1972) Sequential thin-layer chromatography of urinary acidic glycosaminoglycans. *Clinica chimica acta*, **40**, 290–3.

KENNEDY, J. F. (1973) The chemistry of the acidic mucopolysaccharides (glycosaminoglycans). *Biochemical Society Transactions*, 1,000.

KIMURA, A. & TSURUMI, K. (1969) An improved method for the electrophoretic separation of acid mucopolysaccharides on cellulose acetate sheets. *Journal of Biochemistry*, **65**, 303.

KRESSE, H., WIESMANN, U., CANTZ, M., HALL, C. W. & NEUFELD, E. F. (1971) Biochemical heterogeneity of the Sanfilippo syndrome; preliminary characterization of two deficient factors. *Biochemical and Biophysical Research Communications*, **42**, 892–8.

KRESSE, H. & NEUFELD, E. F. (1972) The Sanfilippo A corrective factor. Purification and mode of action. *Journal Biological Chemistry*, **247**, 2164–70.

LEWIS, P. W., KENNEDY, J. F. & RAINE, D. N. (1973) Investigation of urinary glycosaminoglycans in the mucopolysaccharidoses. *Biochemical Society Transactions*, 1,000.

LIPPIELLO, L. & MANKIN, H. J. (1971) Thin-layer chromatographic separation of the isomeric chondroitin sulphates, dermatan sulphate and keratan sulphate. *Analytical Biochemistry*, **39**, 54–8.

McDEVITT, C. A. & MUIR, H. (1971) Gel electrophoresis of proteoglycans and glycosaminoglycans on large pore composite polyacrylamide-agarose gels. *Analytical Biochemistry*, **44**, 612–22.

McDONALD, T. P., LOZZIO, C. & LOTKIN, P. (1970) Rapid detection and identification of mucopolysaccharides in urine. *Clinical Pediatrics*, **9**, 272–6.

McKUSKICK, V. A. (1966) The Mucopolysaccharidoses. In *Heritable disorders of connective tissue*. 3rd Ed. pp. 325–99. Saint Louis; Mosby.

McKusick, V. A. (1972) The Mucopolysaccharidoses. In *Heritable disorders of connective tissue*. 4th ed., pp. 521–686. Saint Louis; Mosby.

Manley, G. & Hawksworth, J. (1966). Diagnosis of Hurler's syndrome in the hospital laboratory and determination of its genetic type. *Archives of Disorders of Childhood*, **41**, 91–6.

Marzullo, G. & Lash, J. W. (1967) Separation of glycosaminoglycans on thin layers of silica gel. *Analytical Biochemistry*, **18**, 575–8.

Matalon, R. & Dorfman, A. (1972a) Acid mucopolysaccharides in cultured human fibroblasts. *Lancet*, ii, 838–41.

Matalon, R. & Dorfman, A. (1972b) Hurler's syndrome, an α-L-iduronidase deficiency. *Biochemical Biophysical Research communications*, **47**, 959–63.

Neufeld, E. F. & Cantz, M. J. (1970) Corrective factors for inborn errors of mucopolysaccharide metabolism. *Annals of the New York Academy of Sciences*, **32**, 580–7.

Norum, R. A. (1969) Nonkeratosulphate-excreting Morquio syndrome. In *Clinical delineation of birth defects*, Vol. **IV**, p. 334. Edited by D. Bergsma, National Foundation—March of Dimes; New York.

O'Brien, J. S. (1972). Sanfilippo syndrome; profound deficiency of alpha-acetyl-glucosaminidase activity in organs and skin fibroblasts from type B patients. *Proceedings of National Academy of Sciences of the United States of America*, **69**, 1720–2.

Pearce, R. H., Mathieson, J. M. & Grimmer, B. J. (1968) Investigation of anionic glycosaminoglycans by ion-exchange chromatography. *Analytical Biochemistry*, **24**, 141–56.

Pennock, C. A., Mott, M. G. & Batstone, G. H. (1970) Screening for mucopolysaccharidoses. *Clinica chimica acta*, **27**, 93–7.

Pennock, C. A., White, F. & Wharton, B. A. (1972) CPC precipitable uronic acid: creatinine ratio in random urine samples collected from normal children. *Acta pediatrica Scandinavica*, **61**, 125–7.

Procopis, P. G., Turner, B., Ruxton, J. T. & Brown, D. A. (1968) Screening tests for mucopolysaccharidosis. *Journal of Mental Deficiency Research*, **12**, 13–17.

Renuart, A. W. (1966) Screening for inborn errors of metabolism associated with mental deficiency or neurologic disorders or both. *New England Journal of Medicine*, **274**, 384–7.

Schiller, S., Slover, G. A. & Dorfman, A. (1961) A method for the separation of acid mucopolysaccharides: its application to isolation of heparin from the skin of rats. *Journal of Biological Chemistry*, **236**, 983–7.

Seno, N., Anno, K., Kondo, K., Nagase, S. & Saito, S. (1970) Improved method for electrophoretic separation and rapid quantitation of isomeric chondroitin sulphates on cellulose acetate strips. *Analytical Biochemistry*, **37**, 197–202.

Spranger, J. (1972) The Systemic Mucopolysaccharidoses. *Ergebnisse der Inneren Medizin Kinderheilkunde*, **32**, 165–265.

Steiness, I. (1961) Acid mucopolysaccharides in urine in Gargoylism. *Pediatrics*, **27**, 112–7.

Svejcar, J. & Robertson, W. van B. (1967) Micro separation and determination of mammalian acidic glycosaminoglycans (mucopolysaccharides). *Analytical Biochemistry*, **18**, 333–50.

Teller, W., Burke, E. C., Rosevear, J. W. & McKenzie, B. F. (1962) Urinary excretion of acid mucopolysaccharides in normal children and patients with gargoylism. *Journal of Laboratory and Clinical Medicine*, **59**, 95–101.

Teller, W. & Ziemann, A. (1969) Thin-layer chromatography of urinary glycosaminoglycans as a screening procedure for mucopolysaccharidosis. *Hormone Metabolism Research*, **1**, 32–5.

Terry, K. & Linker, A. (1964) Distinction among four forms of Hurler's syndrome. *Proceedings of Society for Experimental Biology* (N.Y.), **115**, 394–402.

Wessler, E. (1967) Determination of acidic glycosaminoglycans (mucopolysaccharides) in urine by an ion-exchange method. Application to collagenoses, gargoylism, the nail patella syndrome and Farber's disease. *Clinica chimica acta*, **16**, 235–43.

Wessler, E. (1968) Analytical and preparative separation of acidic glycosaminoglycans by electrophoresis in barium acetate. *Analytical Biochemistry*, **26**, 439–44.

Wessler, E. (1971) Electrophoresis of acidic glycosaminoglycans in hydrochloric acid: A micro method for sulphate determination. *Analytical Biochemistry*, **41**, 67–9.

WHITEMAN, P. (1973a) The quantitative measurement of Alcian Blue-glycosamino-glycan complexes. *Biochemical Journal*, **131**, 343–50.

WHITEMAN, P. (1973b) The quantitative determination of glycosaminoglycans in urine with Alcian Blue 8GX. *Biochemical Journal*, **131**, 351–7.

WUSTEMAN, F. S., LLOYD, A. G. & DODGSON, K. S. (1966) Thin-layer chromatography and the rapid identification of common acidic glycosaminoglycans. *Journal of Chromatography*, **21**, 32–9.

16

Screening newborns for mucopolysaccharidoses

Juan Sabater

The screening of newborns for inborn errors of metabolism is carried out in many countries, and amongst the diseases that most frequently figure in these diagnostic programmes are phenylketonuria in the first place followed by galactosaemia, histidinemia, maple syrup urine disease and tyrosinosis.

We have also carried out the screening for mucopolysaccharides.

Material

Pieces of 3MM Whatman or similar paper, sized 5 by 3 cm, were given to the parents of the newborns in the maternity clinic. The mother was told to insert the paper in the baby's napkin when he was 20 days old, and when it was wet with urine to allow the paper to dry and send it by mail to the laboratory in the special envelope provided by us. In the laboratory, discs 6 mm diameter were cut out with a paper punch. Then using sheets of 3MM chromatographic Whatman paper measuring 20 by 6 cm, 40 holes were made in four rows of 10. A disc of each urine was inserted in each hole, and the reference number was marked with a pencil.

Methods

All 40 samples inserted in the support paper are immersed for one minute in a solution of toluidine blue (toluidine blue, 1 g: acetone 400 ml: distilled water 100 ml.). They are then washed in three consecutive baths of 10 per cent acetic acid, each bath lasting five minutes and being agitated by means of oscillation. The discs corresponding to urine with normal mucopolysaccharides excretion assume a pale blue colour, the same as the rest of the paper used as support. If there is an increase in the urinary elimination of these substances, the discs take on a violet colour. This technique is a personal adaptation, for use with urine impregnated filter paper, of Berry's urinary metachromasia reaction (Berry and Spinanger, 1960) for the detection of mucopoly-saccharides in urine.

Enzyme determinations in urine—the methods followed were those described by Van Hoff and Hers (1968).

Beta-Galactosidase: The substrate used was 4-methylumbelliferyl-beta-D-galactopyranoside (Sigma) in a M citrate buffer (pH$=3\cdot6$) with fluorimetric reading (Aminco-Bowman spectrophotofluorometer) at 360 nm for excitation and 448 nm for emission.

Alpha-fucosidase: The substrate used was p-nitrophenyl-alpha-L fucopyranoside (Sigma) in an acetate buffer (pH$=5\cdot5$ and $0\cdot5$ M) with colorimetric reading at 405 nm (Eppendorf-photometer).

Arylsulphatase: The substrate used was o-nitrocatechol-sulphate (Sigma) in an acetate buffer (pH$=5$ and $0\cdot5$ M) with colorimetric reading at 546 nm (Eppendorf-photometer).

Results

In Table I, we describe the results obtained in the first 15,000 tests carried out on newborn babies.

TABLE I

Number of newborns analysed	15,000
Positive at 20 days of age	103
Percentage positive	0·68
New control sample at 3 months of age	78
Positive at 3 months	5
Positive at 12 months	2

The urine sample corresponding to the 20th day after birth was positive for the metachromasia test in 103 cases, i.e. 0·68 per cent in these positive cases, another urine sample was requested at three months and 78 were received, of these 78 samples five were still positive. At six months of age, a new check was made on these five cases, and they all still gave positive results with the urinary metachromasia test.

Between eight and twelve months of age, liquid samples of urine were requested, and with these the metachromasia test with toluidine-blue was repeated and the cetylpridinium chloride turbidity test was carried out as well as the values for beta-galactosidase, alpha-fucosidase and arylsulphatase activity. The results are summarized in Table II

TABLE II

Case	Age (months)	Berry's Test	β-Galactosidase	α-Fucosidase	Aryl-sulphatase
1.M	8	+	No activity	No activity	4·22
1.M	10	—	24·88	3·65	7·32
2.V	11	++	No activity	0·98	4·90
2.V	14	+	No activity	1·20	5·30
3.R	12	—	27·26	2·67	4·80
4.S	10	—	33·22	3·16	5·00
5.C	12	+++	No activity	0·30	10·12

Enzymatic activities in urine expressed as mu/mg protein.
Our normal values (children up to 24 months).
β-Galactosidase   mean = 13·35 (range 3.3–24.7)
α-Fucosidase   mean = 1.76   (range 0·45–3·65)
Arylsulphatase   mean = 8·07 (range 1·4–21.3)

in cases 3.R and 4.S the Berry's test was negative and the enzyme activities in urine were normal at 12 and 10 months of age respectively. In case 1.M Berry's test still gave a positive result at 8 months of age and no beta-galactosidase and alpha-fucosidase activity was detectable, however, all these results became normal with another sample sent at 12 months of age. In case 2.V and 5.C the abnormalities persisted at 9 and 10 months respectively. Now, at 14 months in the case 2.V, a positive Berry's test persists as does the absence of beta-galactosidase. Similarly, for case 5.C, now at 12 months, the Berry's test persists strongly positive and there is a deficit of beta-galactosidase activity. So far both children are clinically normal.

Discussion. The clinical symptoms of the mucopolysaccharidoses usually become evident between the second and third years of life, and very little is known as to when the urinary elimination of mucopolysaccharides in these diseased children rises to an abnormal level as measured by common screening methods. Maroteaux and Lamy (1966) and Steinbach, Preger, Williams and Cohen (1968) have even described clinically typical forms of mucopolysaccharidoses without an abnormal elimination of mucopolysaccharides in urine.

If the accumulation of mucopolysaccharides at abnormal levels takes place from the first days of life, it should be possible to make an early diagnosis in newborns. This possibility is borne out by the fact that, as we found, there may be transient enzyme deficits which are accompanied by an unusually high urinary elimination of mucopolysaccharides, which, when enzyme activity appears is reduced to normal. As an example, we can quote case 1.M, in which at 8 months of age Berry's test was positive and no urinary activity was detected for beta-galactosidase and fucosidase, whilst at 10 months the screening test became negative and at the same time normal enzyme activity appeared in the urine.

In principle, this would back up the possible existence of transient enzyme deficits because of the immaturity of lysosomal hydrolases just as transient enzyme deficits have been demonstrated in other groups of diseases (transient tyrosylemia, transient hyperphenylalaninemia, increased proline elimination in newborns because of the immaturity of the renal transport systems), if in such transient forms an increase in the elimination of mucopolysaccharides in the urine can be detected, it may be logical to assume that the classical syndromes that arise with a genetic deficit for a specific hydrolase could be also detected earlier in newborns.

We believe it is of great importance to be able to establish when the abnormal urinary elimination of mucopolysaccharides begins in this group of diseases, and therefore we consider it is very necessary to include this screening in the early diagnostic programme for inborn errors of metabolism. We have filed all the samples of urine-impregnated filter paper from the newborns on whom we have carried out the tests in our screening programme for PKU and other inborn errors of metabolism, to see in a few years' time, retrospectively, if the Berry's test carried out at 20 days of age had been positive in children affected with mucopolysaccharidoses. This present study has been conducted only on a part of the 60,000 samples received in our screening programme during its first two and a half years' operation.

There is also the problem of mucopolysaccharidoses which occur without any apparent enzyme deficit. In such cases it is possible that the elimination of mucopolysaccharides in urine takes place later on and follows an evolution parallel to the clinical evolution of the patients. There are no certain data on this possibility and it is only by carrying out the screening test on great numbers of newborns that we may have more definite criteria at some time in the future.

The exact genetical classification of mucopolysaccharidoses, the precise biochemical understanding and the real significance of urinary elimination of mucopolysaccharides are not yet well established and it would therefore be of great clinical and scientific value to be able to detect possibly affected babies before the clinical symptoms appear.

REFERENCES

BERRY, H. K. & SPINANGER, J. A. (1960) A paper spot test useful in study of Hurler's syndrome. *Journal of Laboratory and Clinical Medicine*, **55**, 136.

MARGOLIS, R. U. (1969) Mucopolysaccharides, in *Handbook of Neurochemistry*, vol. **1**, Ed. Lajtha. Plenum Press, pp. 245–60.

MAROTEAUX, P. & LAMY, M. (1966) La pseudo polydystrophie de Hurler. *Presse médicale*, **74**, 2889–2892.

MAROTEAUX, P. & HORS-CAYLA, M. C. (1970) Le probleme biologique des mucopolysaccharidoses. *Annales de Biologie Clinique*, **28**, 11–114.

McKUSICK, V. A., KAPLAN, D., WISE, D., BRIAN HANLEY, W., SUDDARTH, S. B., SEVICK, M. E. & EDWARD MAUMANEE, A. (1965) The genetic mucopolysaccharidoses. *Medicine*, **44**, 445–42.

Rapports of the XII Congres de l'Association des Pediatres de Langue Francaise. Tome 3 (1969) Expansion Scientifique Francaise.

STEINBACH, H. L., PREGER, L., WILLIAMS, H. E. & COHEN, P. (1968) The Hurler syndrome without abnormal mucopolysacchariduria. *Radiology*, **90**, 472–8.

VAN HOFF, F. & HERS, H. G. (1967) L'ultrastructure du foie dans certaines thésaurismoses. *Revue International Hepat*, **17**, 815–26.

VAN HOFF, F. & HERS, H. G. (1968) The abnormalities of Lysosomal enzymes in mucopolysaccharidoses. *European Journal of Biochemistry*, **7**, 34–44.

VAN HOFF, F. (1969) Acid Hydrolases in Mucopolysaccharidoses. *FEBS Symposium*, **19**, 339–46.

17

Acid glycosaminoglycan excretion in the mucopolysaccharidoses. Determination of glycosaminoglycans in urine and amniotic fluid using new microanalytical techniques

Paul Whiteman

The demonstration of excessive mucopolysacchariduria strongly supports a clinical diagnosis of mucopolysaccharidosis. In the past difficulties have arisen due to the unreliability of some of the screening procedures, from equivocal methods of expressing results and from failure to compile adequate control ranges. For the purposes of routine screening, it is essential to have a relatively simple and yet reliable procedure for the quantitative determination of urinary glycosamino-glycans. The glycosaminoglycan : creatinine ratio is a useful index of glycosaminoglycan excretion. Although 24 h collections of urine are preferable, they are not easily obtained from severely handicapped patients. Pennock, White and Wharton (1972) have shown that if early morning urine specimens and those with creatinine concentrations under 15 mg/100 ml are excluded, the uronic acid : creatinine ratios of random daytime specimens are comparable to the values obtained using 24 h urine collections.

Qualitative analysis of urinary glycosaminoglycans may be helpful in differentiating some of the different types of mucopolysaccharidosis. The present report describes some simple new techniques for the analysis of urinary glycosaminoglycans and assesses their usefulness in the diagnosis of mucopolysaccharidosis.

Assessment of Mucopolysacchariduria

The total glycosaminoglycan content of the urine was determined by a technique involving complex formation with the cationic dye Alcian Blue 8 GX (I.C.I. Ltd).

The basic principles and methodology of this technique have been described in detail elsewhere (Whiteman, 1973a, b). In the standard procedure glycosaminoglycan standard solution (20 μl containing 1–10 μg glycosaminoglycan) or centrifuged urine (20 μl for patients with mucopolysaccharidosis; 50 μl for control subjects) was mixed with 1 ml of a freshly prepared reagent containing 0·05 per cent w/v Alcian Blue 8 GX and 50mM-MgCl$_2$ in a 50mM-sodium acetate buffer (pH 5·8). After equilibration for 2 h at room temperature the Alcian Blue-glycosaminoglycan complex was separated by centrifugation at 2,000 g for 15 minutes. After the precipitate had been washed with ethanol (2 ml) and again isolated by centrifugation, it was dissociated with 1 ml of 40 per cent w/v solution of Manoxol IB (dibutyl ester of sodium sulphosuccinic acid; B.D.H. Chemicals Ltd, Poole, Dorset, U.K.). The E_{620} of the resulting clear blue solution was measured in 1 cm microcuvettes.

The glycosaminoglycan content of urine was determined by reference to a calibration curve constructed by using sodium chondroitin 4-sulphate as standard. The results are expressed in terms of mg glycosaminoglycan per litre of urine.

Urine specimens (mainly 24-h collections) from 27 patients with mucopolysaccharidosis were examined using the above technique. Although the concentration of glycosaminoglycans in the urine of these patients tended to be higher than that in the urine of control subjects, there was nevertheless a moderate degree of overlap between the two groups. Infants and young children gave the highest concentrations of urinary glycosaminoglycans in the control groups whereas adult patients with mucopolysaccharidosis tended to have lower concentrations than children with mucopolysaccharidosis. This emphasizes the care that is necessary in the interpretation of spot tests for mucopolysacchariduria. Infants and young children may give false positive spot tests and some older patients with mucopolysaccharidosis may give false negative spot tests. This is, of course, more likely to happen when random urine specimens are collected.

There was good correlation between the results obtained by the Alcian Blue method and by the determination of the cetyl pyridinium-precipitable uronic acid (Fig. 1). The standard chondroitin 4-sulphate used in the Alcian Blue method contained 34 per cent w/v uronic acid. This factor was used to calculate the theoretical value for uronic acid in urine analysed by the Alcian Blue method.

In order to allow for the normal physiological changes in renal function the excretion of glycosaminoglycans can be expressed as:

$$\frac{\text{Urinary glycosaminoglycan concentration (mg/l)} \times 100}{\text{Urinary creatinine concentration (mg/100 ml)}}$$

Table I shows the variation of glycosaminoglycan : creatinine ratio with age for random daytime specimens of urine from hospitalised control patients who had none of the stigmata of the mucopolysacchari-doses. A small group of healthy children with ages ranging from 6 to 10 years gave values comparable to the hospitalized controls of the same age range.

The results of analysis of urine specimens from 27 patients with mucopolysaccharidosis are summarized in Table II. The diagnosis of

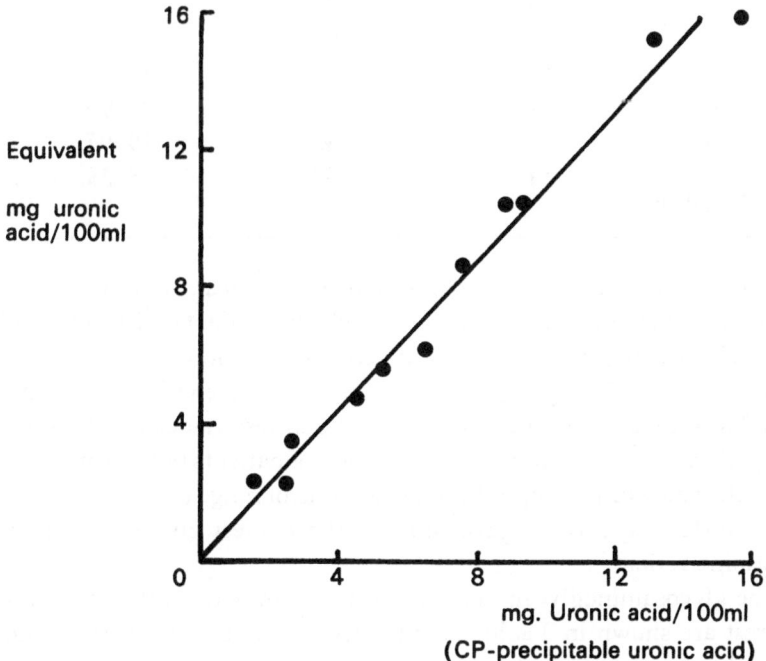

FIG. 1 Comparison of different procedures for the determination of urinary glycosaminoglycans.
The total glycosaminoglycan content of eleven urine specimens from control subjects and patients with mucopolysaccharidosis was determined by using two different methods. The results obtained using the Alcian Blue method are shown by the ordinate (chondroitin sulphate as standard) and the cetyl pyridinium precipitable-uronic acid is shown by the abscissa (glucuronic acid as standard).

TABLE I   *Control Range for Glycosaminoglycan : Creatinine Ratio*
Urine was collected from patients in the Hospital for Sick Children,
London, who had none of the stigmata of the mucopolysaccharidoses.

Age Range	Number of Patients	Glycosaminoglycan : creatinine ratio	
		Mean	Range (±2 SD)
0–4 weeks	14	278	196–361
1–3 months	6	212	81–343
3–6 ,,	7	205	105–305
6–12 ,,	6	154	37–270
1–2 years	8	126	60–192
2–3 ,,	8	129	86–173
3–5 ,,	14	96	55–136
5–7 ,,	15	81	55–107
7–9 ,,	14	66	36–96
9–11 ,,	15	68	40–96
11–13 ,,	14	59	25–92
13–15 ,,	7	43	19–67
18–50 ,, (healthy adults)	14	29	15–39

mucopolysaccharidosis was supported by clinical, radiological and
sometimes histochemical evidence. In all the patients with mucopolysaccharidosis the glycosaminoglycan : creatinine ratio was greatly elevated
above the control range (±2 SD) for the same age (Fig. 2). A patient
with Morquio's syndrome gave one of the lowest values for the glycosaminoglycan : creatinine ratio in this group of patients but this was nearly
twice the value of the upper limit of the control range (+2 SD). Patients
with Hurler's syndrome gave some of the highest glycosaminoglycan:
creatinine ratios.

The glycosaminoglycan : creatinine ratios in a few other diseases of
interest are shown in Table III. Slightly elevated values were found in
Type I GM_1-ganglio-sidosis and in osteogenesis imperfecta. A patient
with osteopetrosis had a moderately raised ratio which perhaps is not
surprising in view of the gross disturbance in bone metabolism which
occurs in this condition. However, marked elevation of glycosaminoglycan excretion is a particular feature of the mucopolysaccharidoses
which helps to differentiate these conditions from others which are not

TABLE II   *Analysis of Glycosaminoglycans in Urine from Patients with Mucopolysaccharidosis*

Patient	Age	Major	Minor	mg GAG/L* (Alcian Blue method)	GAG : creatinine ratio
SH	3	HS	CS	536	462
SB	5	HS	CS	445	485
SN	12	HS	CS	201	575
TS	9/12	HS	CS	282	414
FW	6	HS	CS	176	400
NP	3	HS	CS	127	552
KA	9	HS	CS	268	284
JS	14	DS, HS	CS	243	419
WL	14	DS, HS	CS	93	388
RM	4	DS, HS	CS	144	600
DD	3	DS, HS	CS	364	910
VC	4	DS, HS	CS	202	577
CO	1	DS	CS, HS	306	900
MT	5	DS	CS, HS	419	953
NW	7	DS	CS, HS	575	820
AR	1	DS	CS, HS	265	651
CG	20	DS	CS	156	208
LG	15	DS	CS	159	274
MW	4	DS	CS	763	898
JB	13	DS	CS	256	448
SM	3	DS	CS	163	542
LB	20	DS	CS	155	408
BG	2	DS	CS	128	609
CL	3	DS	CS	420	769
DB	22	DS	CS	68	454
DW	8	CS	KS	183	197
TN	3	CS	KS	127	354

CS = chondroitin sulphate   DS = dermatan sulphate
HS = heparan sulphate   KS = keratan sulphate
* Expressed in terms of sodium chondroitin 4-sulphate which was used as a standard for the method.

primary disorders of glycosaminoglycan metabolism. Patients with renal disease in the form of the nephrotic syndrome and acute glomeru-lonephritis gave normal glycosaminoglycan : creatinine ratios.

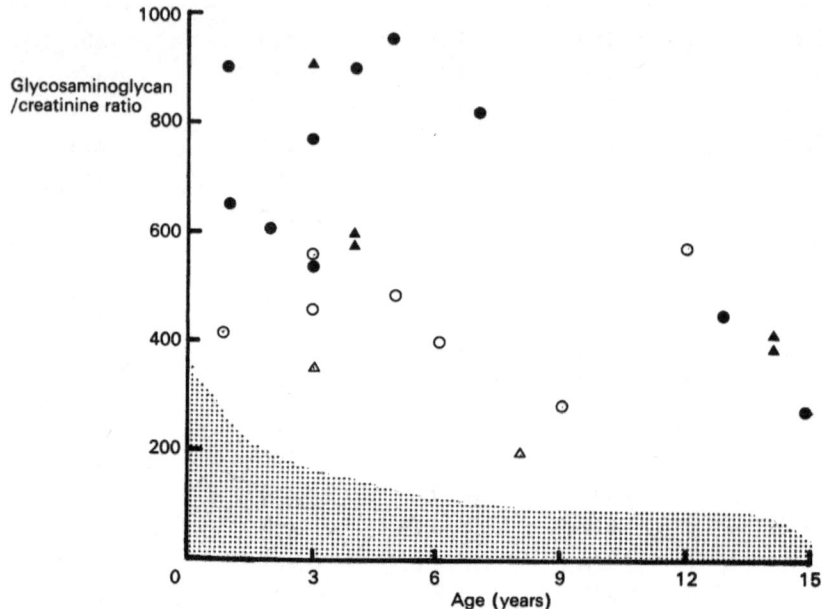

FIG. 2   Glycosaminoglycan:creatinine ratio in patients with mucopolysaccharidosis. The stippled area defines the upper level of the control range (+2 SD).
Key: ● = Dermatan sulphate excretors.
▲ = Patients excreting large amounts of both dermatan and heparan sulphates.
△ = Keratan sulphate excretors.
○ = Heparatan sulphate excretors.

The Alcian Blue method for the determination of total urinary gly-cosaminoglycans has proved to be useful and reliable as a procedure for screening the mucopolysaccharidoses provided that certain pre-cautions are observed. Urine should be preserved with merthiolate (e.g. in 5,000 w/v) and stored deep frozen. Alkaline urine should be neutralized or made slightly acid with acetic acid. Although the sul-phated glycosaminoglycans in urine appear to be fairly stable, it is pointless to attempt to analyse putrefying urine since organisms such as proteus vulgaris can degrade these substances.

TABLE III   *Glycosaminoglycan Excretion in Conditions Other than the Mucopolysaccharidoses*

Patient	Clinical details	GAG: Creatinine ratio	Normal range of ratio for age of patient ± 2 SD
JD	GM$_1$-ganglio-sidosis, Type 1	295	37–270
SMc	„ Type 2	85	40–96
AS	Metachromatic leukodystrophy	83	55–136
AJ	Sea blue histiocyte syndrome	49	19–67
DK	Ehlers–Danlos syndrome	92	55–136
ND	Osteogenesis imperfecta	175	55–136
WI	Osteopetrosis	174	55–107
DG	Nephrotic; —300 mg protein/100 ml urine	60	19–67
SN	Nephrotic; —300 mg protein/100 ml urine	84	25–92
RC	Acute glomerulonephritis; —haematuria+270 mg protein/100 ml urine	47	36–96

Qualitative analysis of urinary glycosaminoglycans

Qualitative analysis of urinary glycosaminoglycans should be carried out in all patients with raised glycosaminoglycan : creatinine ratios. Electrophoresis provides a simple means of analysis and is less affected by molecular weight variations than are many other methods.

A new method of preparing urinary glycosaminoglycans for electrophoresis by forming complexes with Alcian Blue has been described elsewhere (Whiteman, 1973b). This has since been modified according to the brief account given below.

Urine, 1–2 ml, is mixed with 20 volumes of Alcian Blue reagent (the same as that used for the determination of total urinary glycosaminoglycans). After 2 h equilibration at room temperature the Alcian Blue-glycosaminoglycan complex is isolated by centrifugation and washed with ethanol (2 ml). After centrifugation, the ethanolic supernatant is discarded and the complex dissociated by vigorous shaking for 3 minutes in a mixture of 4M-NaCl and methanol (2 : 1 v/v; 0·3 ml).

The mixture is transferred to a small plastic tube and 0·1 ml of 0·1M-Na_2CO_3 and 0·3 ml water are added and the contents mixed. After 30 minutes the denatured Alcian Blue is removed by centrifugation and the glycosaminoglycans are precipitated from the clear supernatant by the addition of 3 volumes of ethanol. After the precipitate has been isolated and dried it is taken up in 25–50 μl of water and the preparation is now ready for electrophoresis.

For routine purposes Wessler's barium acetate system of electrophoresis is preferred because this separates the urinary glycosaminoglycans into three clinically useful groups (Wessler, 1970). The actual procedure adopted in our laboratory was described in detail elsewhere (Whiteman, 1973b). The same Alcian Blue reagent used to isolate the glycosaminoglycans is also used to stain the cellulose acetate electrophoresis strips. Figure 3 shows some typical separations of urinary glycosaminoglycans on cellulose acetate by one-dimensional electrophoresis in barium acetate (0·1M). The urinary glycosaminoglycans run at rates almost identical to those of the equivalent standard glycosaminoglycans. Patients with Types II and III mucopolysaccharidoses give fairly characteristic patterns but it is not so easy to differentiate the other types of mucopolysaccharidosis excreting dermatan sulphate with little or no heparan sulphate. If attempts are made to quantitate the fractions it is most important that overloading of the sample does not occur. This leads to loss of staining in the centres of the bands and grossly underestimates the true glycosaminoglycan content.

The single fast-moving band seen in the Type IV mucopolysaccharidosis resembles that found in normal children. One of the limitations of this system of electrophoresis is the failure to separate chondroitin sulphate and keratan sulphate.

Two-dimensional electrophoresis using a pyridine acetic acid buffer (pH 6·0) and a barium acetate solution is useful for a more detailed study of glycosaminoglycans in urine and amniotic fluid (Whiteman, 1973c). This method is preferred to the two-dimensional system of electrophoresis advocated by Hata and Nagai (1972) which used a formic acid pyridine buffer (pH 3·0) and a barium acetate solution.

Figure 4a shows a typical separation of six standard glycosaminoglycans using two-dimensional electrophoresis. A standard marker is routinely included in the second run and this allows accurate identification of the positions of glycosaminoglycans according to Wessler's method. During the first run chondroitin sulphate, dermatan sulphate

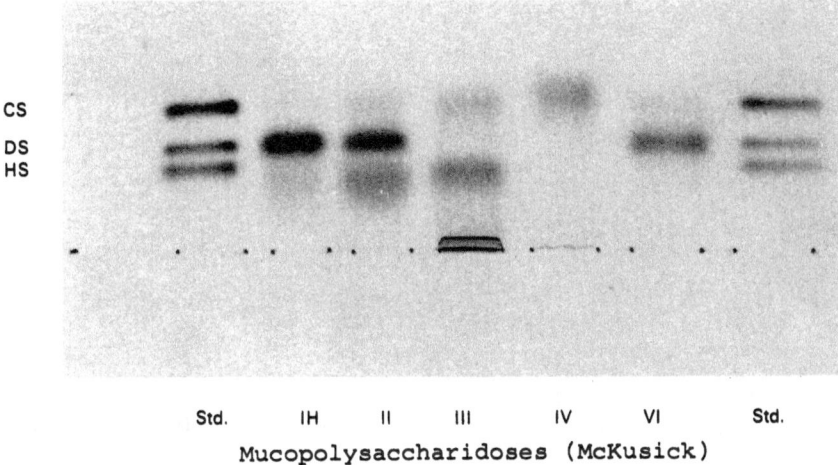

CS
DS
HS

Std.   IH   II   III   IV   VI   Std.

Mucopolysaccharidoses (McKusick)

FIG. 3 Electrophoresis of urinary glycosaminoglycans in o·1M barium acetate (3 hours at 7·5 V/cm). Standard markers: CS, chondroitin sulphate; DS, dermatan sulphate; HS, heparan sulphate.

and heparin, the components with the highest charge densities, run ahead of keratan sulphate, hyaluronic acid and heparan sulphate respectively, The peculiar oblique appearance of the keratan sulphate spot is probably related to the known polydisperse nature of this substance. Figure 4b illustrates the separation of urinary keratan sulphate from chondroitin sulphate in a patient with Morquio's syndrome. In normal children only a single round spot of chondroitin sulphate is seen using this system.

Two-dimensional electrophoresis of urinary glycosaminoglycans from patients with Hunter and Sanfilippo syndromes are also shown (Figs. 4c and 4d). These results are of academic interest in that the heparan sulphate fractions have been resolved into two components. One of these has a mobility in the first buffer which suggests that it is of high sulphate content. Knecht, Cifonelli and Dorfman (1967) described the presence of heparin-like components in the urine of patients with Hurler's syndrome and suggested that these were degradation products. The heparin-like component seen in our system has diffused further into the surrounding cellulose acetate than the other components indicating that this might be of low molecular weight. In addition, the critical electrolyte concentration of this fraction is low whereas that of a standard heparin preparation is high.

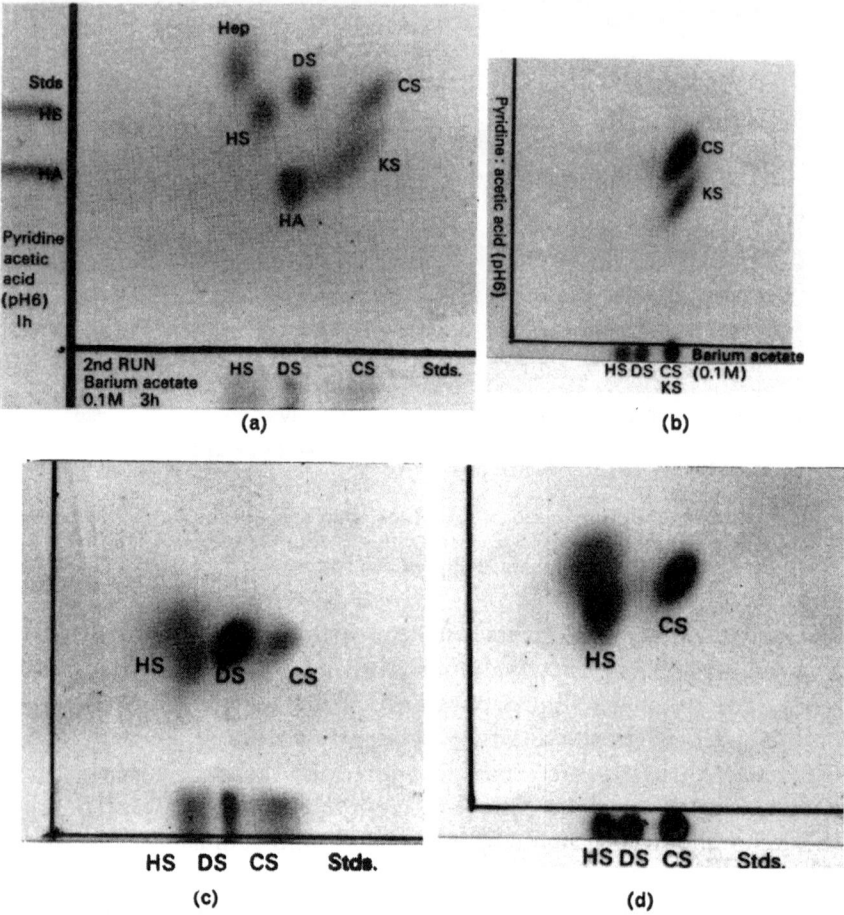

FIG. 4(a) Two-dimensional electrophoresis of standard glycosaminoglycans on cellulose acetate.

1st run: pyridine-acetic acid-water (100:10:890, v/v; pH6), 1 hour at 7·5 V/cm.
2nd run: 0·1M barium acetate, 3 hours at 7·5 V/cm.

Standard glycosaminoglycans were included in the first and second runs.

Key: CS, chondroitin sulphate; KS, keratan sulphate; DS, dermatan sulphate; HA, hyaluronic acid; HEP, heparin; HS, heparan sulphate.

FIG. 4(b) Two-dimensional electrophoresis of urinary glycosaminoglycans from a patient with Morquio's syndrome.

Standard glycosaminoglycans were included in the second run and are shown near the abscissa. Key: as for Fig. 4(a).

FIG. 4(c) Two-dimensional electrophoresis of urinary glycosaminoglycans from a patient with Hunter's syndrome.

Key: as for Fig. 4(a).

FIG. 4(d) Two-dimensional electrophoresis of urinary glycosaminoglycans from a patient with Sanfilippo's syndrome.

Key: as for Fig. 4(a).

For routine screening purposes the two-dimensional method is best reserved for special purposes such as the demonstration of keratan sulphate in urine or the analysis of amniotic fluid glycosaminoglycans.

It is also possible to quantitate each individual component of the electrophoretogram by measuring the extinction of the Alcian Blue component of each spot in dimethyl sulphoxide (in press).

Profiles of interaction of Alcian Blue 8 GX and urinary glycosaminoglycans

Scott (1955, 1970) has shown that the critical electrolyte concentration for a particular polyanion that is the molarity of a salt at which there is an abrupt decrease in interaction between the polyanion and the precipitating cation (e.g. Alcian Blue 8 GX), is related to the molecular weight of the polyanion and the nature of its ionic charges. By using a simple modification of the Alcian Blue method described in the present report it is possible to construct profiles of interaction of Alcian Blue 8 GX and urinary glycosaminoglycans in different concentrations of $MgCl_2$ (Whiteman, 1973a, b). Figure 5 shows typical profiles in patients with different types of mucopolysaccharidosis. Patients with Sanfilippo syndrome who excrete large amounts of low molecular weight heparan sulphate have Alcian Blue-glycosaminoglycan interaction profiles strikingly different to those found in other types of mucopolysaccharidosis. This method is not reliable for differentiating most of the other types of mucopolysaccharidosis although patients with Morquio's syndrome may be an exception since the presence of keratan sulphate causes an extended critical electrolyte concentration. It might therefore be possible to screen for the Sanfilippo syndrome by measuring the ratio of the amount of glycosaminoglycan-Alcian Blue complex formed using a reagent containing $0.05M$-$MgCl_2$ (i.e. as in the routine screening method for total glycosaminoglycan determination) to that formed using a reagent containing $0.2M$-$MgCl_2$. In patients with Sanfilippo syndrome, this figure would be about 4 and in other mucopolysaccharidoses it would be much lower (usually under 2). A similar procedure might be used to screen for the presence of excessive amounts of keratan sulphate in the urine by measuring the ratio of complex formation in the presence of $0.05M$-$MgCl_2$ and $0.5M$-$MgCl_2$. However, there are two practical points to be noted in these procedures. Firstly, the volume of the urine sample should be sufficient to give a reading (E_{620}) between 0.7 and 1.0 for the reaction in $0.05M$-$MgCl_2$. Secondly, a reagent blank

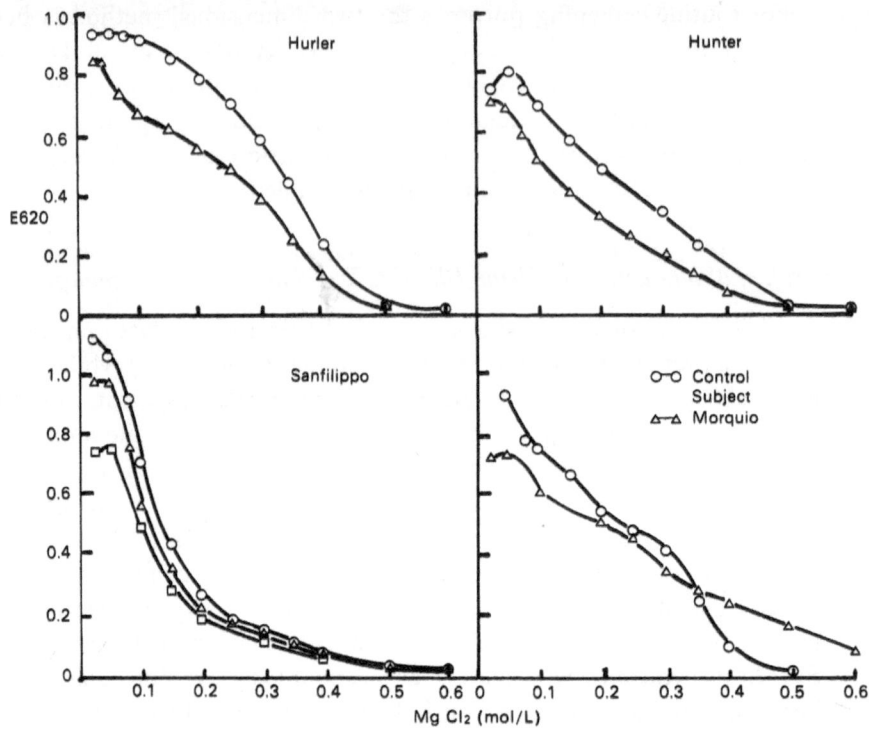

FIG. 5   Effect of $MgCl_2$ concentration on interaction of Alcian Blue and urinary
glycosaminoglycans of patients with mucopolysaccharidoses.
The ordinate shows the extinction of Alcian Blue released from Alcian Blue-glycosaminoglycan complexes, which were formed in different concentrations of $MgCl_2$.
Top left: two patients with Hurler's syndrome. Top right: two patients with Hunter's
syndrome. Bottom left: three patients with Sanfilippo's syndrome. Bottom right:
one patient with Morquio's syndrome and one control subject (age 2 years).

must be set up for each Alcian Blue reagent used (blank values should
be low if freshly prepared reagents are used).

Differential staining of electrophoretograms in Alcian Blue reagents
containing different concentrations of magnesium chloride also allows
an assessment to be made of the molecular weights of the individual
glycosaminoglycans.

The differential diagnosis of the types of mucopolysaccharidosis
depends initially on a careful assessment of the clinical, radiological
and histochemical features of the patient in question together with a
quantitative and qualitative analysis of the urinary glycosaminoglycans.
When all these factors are considered it is possible in many cases to

make an accurate diagnosis. A minority of patients with mucopolysaccharidosis still defy accurate classification. This situation will exist until all the relevant enzyme deficiencies have been discovered.

Analysis of glycosaminoglycans in amniotic fluid

Recent findings suggested that the analysis of glycosaminoglycans of amniotic fluid is unreliable for the pre-natal diagnosis of the mucopolysaccharidoses. Theoretically, it should be possible to measure the glycosaminoglycans of foetal urine in amniotic fluid by about the fourteenth week of pregnancy. At that time, hyaluronic acid is the predominant glycosaminoglycan in amniotic fluid and abnormal components from foetal urine would represent only a small proportion of the total glycosaminoglycan content. In these circumstances, measurement of the total glycosaminoglycan content or the percentage of hyaluronidase resistant glycosaminoglycan may lead to false conclusions. For this, and other reasons (Whiteman, 1973c) the individual glycosaminoglycans should be determined if this method of pre-natal diagnosis is to be fairly assessed. This approach has recently been investigated using new micro-analytical techniques (Whiteman, 1973c) and some of the preliminary results are included in this report.

Glycosaminoglycans were isolated from amniotic fluid using a modification of the method previously described for their isolation from urine and separated by two-dimensional electrophoresis on cellulose acetate strips. After staining with Alcian Blue, areas of strip containing individual spots were cut out, dissolved in dimethyl sulphoxide and the relative proportions of glycosaminoglycan components determined from the extinctions of Alcian Blue in these solutions (Newton, Scott and Whiteman—submitted for publication).

Amniotic fluid obtained at 21 weeks in a terminated pregnancy which produced an affected Hurler foetus contained dermatan sulphate, heparan sulphate, chondroitin sulphate and hyaluronic acid (Fig. 6a). Amniotic fluid obtained at 25 weeks' gestation in a case associated with a Sanfilippo sibling contained a large amount of heparan sulphate (Fig. 6b). The foetus was subsequently found to be affected with the Sanfilippo syndrome (Ferguson-Smith *et al.*, 1973). In control amniotic fluids (9–25 weeks' gestation) the concentration of hyaluronic acid was found to decrease with increasing gestation time, whereas chondroitin sulphate gradually increased in concentration until it became the major

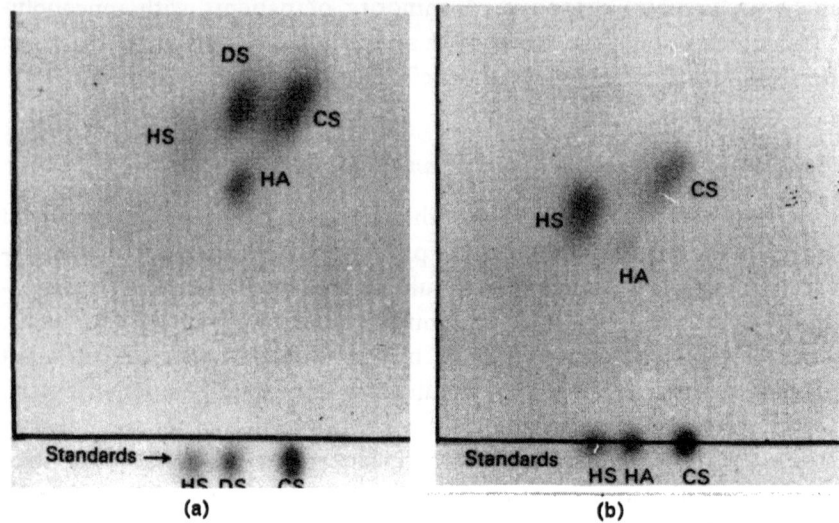

(a)   (b)

FIG. 6(a) Two-dimensional electrophoresis of glycosaminoglycans in Hurler
amniotic fluid (21 weeks' gestation).
HA, hyaluronic acid; CS, chondroitin sulphate; DS, dermatan sulphate; HS, heparan
sulphate.
FIG. 6(b) Two-dimensional electrophoresis of glycosaminoglycans in Sanfilippo
amniotic fluid (25 weeks' gestation).
HA, hyaluronic acid; CS, chondroitin sulphate; HS, heparan sulphate.

TABLE IV   *Qualitative Analysis of Glycosaminoglycans in Amniotic
Fluid*

	Amniotic fluid at 21 weeks		Amniotic fluid at 25 weeks	
	Hurler	Control	Sanfilippo	Control
	%	%	%	%
Hyaluronic acid	19	63	5	13
Chondroitin sulphate	40	37	43	87
Dermatan sulphate	33	—	—	—
Heparan sulphate	8	—	52	—

Results are expressed as percentages of the total glycosaminoglycan
content.
— Not detected by two-dimensional electrophoresis.

glycosaminoglycan component after about 21 weeks. The important difference between the affected amniotic fluids and controls of comparable gestation was in the presence of excessive amounts of dermatan or heparan sulphates. Examples of typical analyses are shown in Table IV.

A more precise method of defining the presence of abnormal amounts of dermatan and heparan sulphates in amniotic fluid is to express them in ratio to the chondroitin sulphate component (Whiteman, 1973c). Results would then be less affected by the hyaluronic acid content, which changes considerably with gestational age, and by changes in the water content of amniotic fluid.

Wherever possible, independent methods of pre-natal diagnosis should be used in conjunction with the method described, here until the reliability of the latter has been established. This applies particularly to the earlier weeks of pregnancy for which little information is available.

Acknowledgements

I wish to record my appreciation of the help and encouragement given by Professor Barbara Clayton, Dr A. D. Patrick and Dr J. E. Scott. Thanks are also due to Dr Rosemary Stephens and the other physicians at the Hospital for Sick Children who allowed me to study the patients under their care.

I thank the Medical Research Council for a Junior Research Fellowship.

REFERENCES

FERGUSON-SMITH, M. A., DUNCAN, D. M., LOGAN, N. W., HALL, F., WUSTEMAN, F. S. & HARPER, P. S. (1973) *Lancet*, **ii**, 45–46.

HATA, R. & NAGAI, Y. (1972) *Analytical Biochemistry*, **45**, 462.

KNECHT, J., CIFONELLI, J. A. & DORFMAN, A. (1967) *Journal of Biological Chemistry*, **242**, 4652.

NEWTON, D. J., SCOTT, J. E. & WHITEMAN, P. (in press).

PENNOCK, C. A., WHITE, F. & WHARTON, B. A. (1972) *Acta Paediatrica*, **61**, 125.

SCOTT, J. E. (1955) *Biochimica et biophysica acta*, **18**, 428.

SCOTT, J. E. (1970) In *Chemistry and Biology of the Intercellular Matrix*, Vol. **2**, pp. 1105–19. Ed. E. A. Balazs, London: Academic Press.

WESSLER, E. (1970) *ACTA Univ. Ups. Abstr. Upps. Diss. Med.*, 85

WHITEMAN, P. (1973a) *Biochemical Journal*, **131**, 343.

WHITEMAN, P. (1973b) *Biochemical Journal*, **131**, 351.

WHITEMAN, P. (1973c) *Lancet*, **i**, 1249 (letter).

18

An evaluation of methods suitable for a clinical laboratory study of abnormal glycosaminoglycan excretion

Charles A. Pennock

The study of urinary glycosaminoglycan (GAG) excretion usually involves time-consuming complex methods of isolation and analysis quite unsuited to the routine hospital laboratory. In Bristol an attempt has been made to develop simple techniques which require the minimum of technician time and still provide useful diagnostic information.

The first requirement is a screening test which will detect abnormal excretors without false negative results and with the minimum of false positive results. Ideally this test should be simple to perform and applicable to random samples of urine since a 24 h collection frequently presents difficulty in childhood. A number of simple screening tests, based on the interaction of GAG with acidified albumin, quaternary ammonium salts or a variety of dyes, have been described. A method based on the work of Scott (1960) which involves the measurement of the turbidity produced by a complex formed between cetylpyridinium chloride (CPC) and GAG (Manley and Hawksworth, 1966) has been modified (Pennock, 1969) by using CPC in citrate buffer at pH 4·8 to overcome the critical effects of pH, ionic strength and time dependence of the reaction using an aqueous solution of CPC which is not buffered. The turbidity of the test sample is compared with that of a standard solution of chondroitin sulphate under the same conditions. Results are expressed as CPC units per gram of urinary creatinine and the test may be used on random samples of urine. The test gives a low incidence of false positive results and no false negative results have been found so far. It has been compared with other screening tests (Pennock, Mott and Batstone, 1970) and has been found to be either more reliable or easier to perform. Denny and Dutton's (1962) modification of Dorfman's (1958) acidified bovine albumin test gave no false positive results but false negative results have been found in patients with Sanfilippo and Hurler's syndrome (Pennock, White, Murphy, Charles and Kerr, 1973).

A test using cetyltrimethyl ammonium bromide and visually assessing the density of the flocculent precipitate formed (Renuart, 1966) is difficult to interpret without considerable experience and also gives false negative results (Procopsis, Turner, Buxton and Brown, 1968). A toluidine blue spot test (Berry and Spinanger, 1960) while giving a few false positive results, gave a false negative result in a patient with Hurler's syndrome due to protein interference with the development of metachromasia, while an Alcian Blue spot test gave too many false positive results (25 per cent). The measurement of non-dialysable hexuronic acid (Segni, Romano and Tortorolo, 1964) has the disadvantages of false positive results arising due to non-specific chromogens, or false negative results due to losses of urinary GAG in patients with mucopolysaccharidoses (up to 50 per cent according to Constantopoulos, 1968).

The estimation of CPC precipitable hexuronic acid (Di Ferrante, 1967) is a more time-consuming but very reliable procedure which is probably best used as a confirmatory test when the CPC-citrate test is positive. Neither of these tests may be positive in patients with Morquio's disease since they excrete excess keratosulphate which does not contain hexuronic acids (Pedrini, Lennzi and Zambotti, 1962) and may not precipitate with CPC under certain conditions. It is possible that the Alcian Blue test described by Whiteman (1973) will be a more reliable test in this condition. However, positive CPC-citrate screening tests have usually been found in patients with Morquio's disease who actually have abnormal excretion (vide infra). This is probably because keratosulphate (KS) is usually excreted as a protein complex with chondroitin sulphate (CS) (Kaplan, McKusick, Trebachi and Lazarus, 1968; Dean, Muir and Ewins, 1971) which will precipitate with CPC thus giving a positive screening test and raised CPC precipitable hezuronic acid.

The major advantage of the CPC citrate screening test is that it takes urine concentration into account, which most other tests do not, and is easy and quick to perform. The reagent has a shelf life at room temperature of several years, the method is controlled by the inclusion of a standard and the only significant interfering substances are glycoproteins which may be co-precipitated with GAG and give false positive results, especially in patients with renal disease. The majority of false positives are probably due to drugs and usually revert to a negative result when drugs are withdrawn or the child recovers (Pennock *et al.*, 1970).

There is a progressive fall in CPC units/gram of creatinine with age which is confirmed by a similar fall in CPC precipitable hexuronic acid. The latter follows the same pattern when random urines are used (Pennock, White and Wharton, 1972) as when 24 h collections are studied (Teller, Burke, Rosevear and McKenzie, 1962). A diurnal rhythm in GAG excretion exists (Di Ferrante and Lipscomb, 1970) but, provided mid-morning samples are used, random samples will give results in the same range as 24 h results (Pennock *et al.*, 1972). CPC precipitable hexuronic acid per gram of creatinine (UA/C ratio) shows a sharp increase shortly after birth reaching a peak in the third week of life and declining thereafter (Pennock, Wharton and White, 1971).

This may account for the higher incidence of positive screening tests in the first year of life and may make interpretation difficult at this age.

Further qualitative examination can be done on GAG isolated from 50–100 ml of urine by the method of Di Ferrante (1967) using CPC. The proportion of isolated material which is resistant to testicular hyaluronidase digestion (HyalR per cent) can be estimated by incubation of a solution of isolated GAG in $0.1M$ acetate buffer (pH 5.6) in $0.15M$ sodium chloride with (test) or without (control) bovine testicular hyaluronidase (1 mg/ml) for 18 h at $37°C$. The amount digested is measured by using the CPC citrate screening test reagent. The turbidity is measured and the results expressed as a percentage of the control. (Pennock *et al.*, 1973). Normal individuals excrete mainly CS which is digested and thus gives a result usually below 30 per cent. Patients with mucopolysaccharidoses excrete heparan sulphate (HS), dermatan sulphate (DS) or keratosulphate (KS) in excess and, since these are resistant to testicular hyaluronidase digestion, the HyalR per cent is usually above 70 per cent. Patients with Hurler's syndrome may give a test turbidity which is greater than the control value, presumably due to splitting of some DS molecules at the glucuronyl residues into large fragments which still precipitate with CPC.

The next step in qualitative examination is to define the pattern of GAG excretion. Kaplan (1969) has shown that abnormal GAG excretors can be divided into four main groups: (1) predominantly DS excretors (Hurler's and Scheie's syndrome) with ratio of DS to HS of about 3:1; (2) excretors of equal amounts of DS and HS (Hunter's syndrome); (3) excretors of HS (Sanfilippo syndrome); and (4) excretors of DS (Maroteaux–Lamy syndrome). Since HS contains glucosamine (gluN) and DS contains galactosamine (galN) as principal hexosamine (hexN) it is possible to separate these four groups on the basis of hexN analysis. However, as Kaplan, points out, separation of the two hexosamines is difficult and involves time-consuming column chromatography. Furthermore, he emphasizes the difficulties of separating DS and HS by a number of currently available column chromatographic methods. In an attempt to overcome these problems, Murphy,

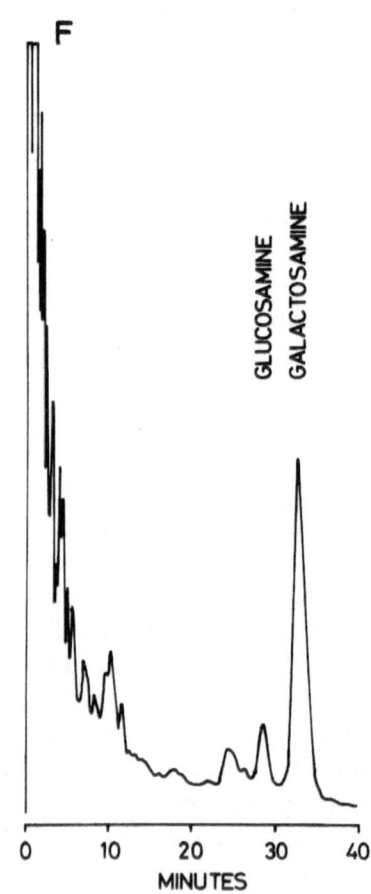

FIG. 1   GLC tracing of hexosamine analysis on a sample from a patient with Hurler' syndrome.

Pennock and Longdon (1973) have developed a gas-liquid chromato-graphic (GLC) method which separates gluN and galN as single deriva-tive peaks. A solution of isolated GAG (after estimation of hexuronic acid by the method of Bitter and Muir, 1972) is hydrolysed without separation of the constituent GAG or removal of other substances which might interfere in colorimetric hexosamine assays. The hexosamines released are reduced and converted to their alditol acetates which can be separated isothermally at 220°C within 40 minutes. The use of an autosolid injection system on a Pye 104 gas chromatograph enables a large number of samples to be analysed in a single batch. A typical separation is shown in Figs. 1 and 2 which show results obtained in patients with Hurler's syndrome and Sanfilippo syndrome respectively.

Additional confirmation of the GAG pattern may be obtained by electrophoresis or thin layer chromatography (TLC) but none of these methods gives perfect separations of various GAG although two methods may be useful in combination. Electrophoresis in a barbitone buffer at pH 9·2 (Manley and Hawksworth, 1966) relies on the different charge density of individual GAG to achieve separation. It thus suffers from the disadvantage that mobility of urinary GAG may not be the same as reference samples due to de-sulphation and partial degradation of urinary material. It does not separate all of the different GAG molecules but this has one advantage if it is used to support data obtained by the methods described above since DS migrates with CS and KS migrates with HS (Manley, Severn and Hawksworth, 1968). Thus the galN-containing molecules and the gluN-containing mole-cules migrate as separate bands. (Hyaluronic acid and heparin are not usually present in significant amounts.) Scanning of the separation (after staining with Alcian Blue) and expressing the two major bands as a percentage of the total, usually correlates well with the GLC result. If the material is resistant to hyaluronidase digestion this clearly sug-gests that the CS/DS band is mainly DS.

Other electrophoretic methods rely on the 'backbone' structure of GAG to achieve separation. A number of methods using cupric acetate as electrolyte medium have been described but do not give good separa-tion. A method using zinc sulphate (Hardingham and Phelps, 1970) gives good separation of HS and DS but not of KS. Separation of all three from other GAG can be achieved using barium acetate (Wessler, 1968) but even in this method the bands migrate very close together even after a three hour electrophoresis and interpretation often remains difficult.

A valuable alternative to electrophoresis is the TLC method described by Lipiello and Mankin (1971) and modified by Humbel and Chamoles (1972). This method relies on the relative solubility of calcium salts

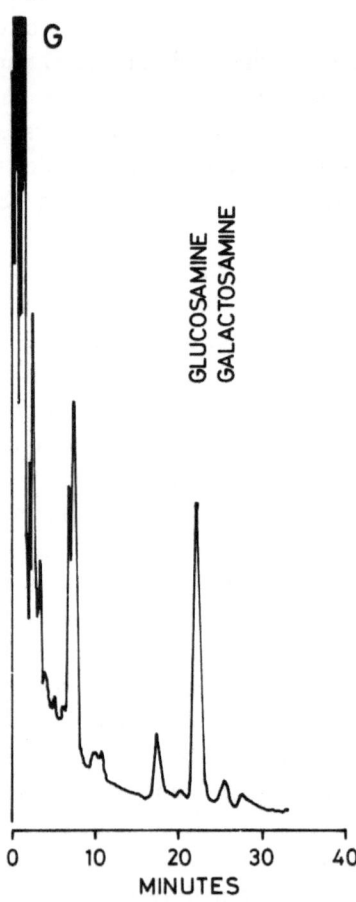

FIG. 2   GLC tracing of hexosamine analysis on a sample from a patient with Sanfilippo syndrome.

of different GAG in ethanol and is easily and rapidly performed. It has the great advantage that it clearly separates KS from other GAG which is valuable in the diagnosis of Morquio's disease. In this laboratory it has been found to give occasional bizarre patterns in other mucopolysaccharidoses mainly because urinary DS migrates as two or three bands instead of one. This method and electrophoresis in barbitone buffer appear to be the best combination for confirmation of results of the other analyses described above. The methods used are summarized in Table I.

A study using these methods and involving the screening of four thousand infants and children with abnormal development gave 5 per cent positive results in the first year of life and 2·6 per cent in childhood

TABLE I   *A simple programme for analysis of urinary glycosaminoglycans*

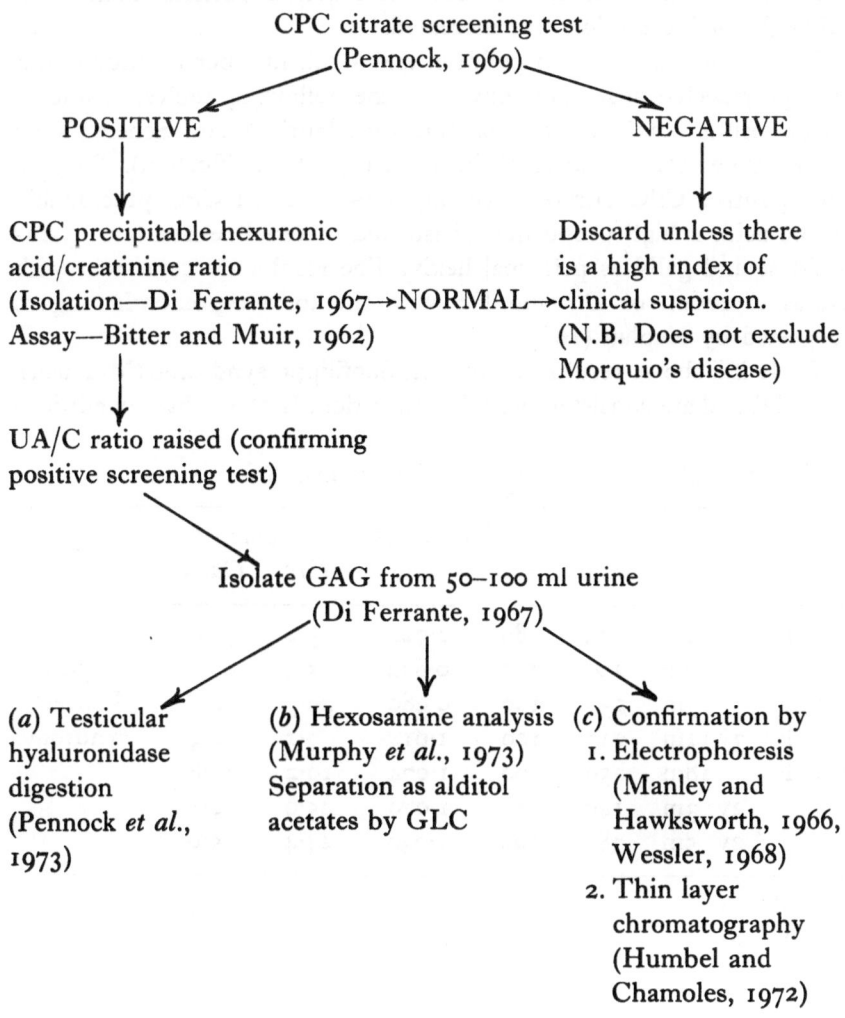

CPC citrate screening test
(Pennock, 1969)

POSITIVE   NEGATIVE

CPC precipitable hexuronic   Discard unless there
acid/creatinine ratio   is a high index of
(Isolation—Di Ferrante, 1967→NORMAL→clinical suspicion.
Assay—Bitter and Muir, 1962)   (N.B. Does not exclude
                                              Morquio's disease)

UA/C ratio raised (confirming
positive screening test)

Isolate GAG from 50–100 ml urine
(Di Ferrante, 1967)

(*a*) Testicular   (*b*) Hexosamine analysis (*c*) Confirmation by
hyaluronidase   (Murphy *et al.*, 1973)   1. Electrophoresis
digestion   Separation as alditol   (Manley and
(Pennock *et al.*,   acetates by GLC   Hawksworth, 1966,
1973)   Wessler, 1968)
                                                     2. Thin layer
                                                        chromatography
                                                        (Humbel and
                                                        Chamoles, 1972)

(Pennock *et al.*, 1973). (Another study using the same screening method (Valdivieso, 1973) to screen one thousand children gave 3·2 per cent positive results.) Many of these results returned to normal when the child had recovered from a current illness or drugs had been withdrawn. In all cases where sufficient urine was available for more detailed analysis, children giving false positive results were found to have a qualitatively normal excretion pattern. Twenty-one per cent of all positive results were from children with bone dysplasias including the mucopolysaccharidoses, but, with the exception of the latter, these patients were shown to excrete GAG of a normal pattern (mainly CS) although total excretion was increased.

The results obtained on children and small number of adults with mucopolysaccharidoses are shown in the following tables. Table II shows results obtained from patients with Hurler's and Scheie's syndomes (types IH and IS of McKusick's (1972) classification). They all gave positive CPC citrate screening tests, a raised CPC precipitable uronic acid, a high proportion of isolated material resistant to hyaluronidase and galN as principal hexN. The results are consistent with excess excretion of DS and HS with the former predominating as suggested by Kaplan (1969).

Table III shows results obtained in Sanfilippo syndrome (McKusick type III) and are consistent with HS excretion. In these three conditions

TABLE II   *Type IH and IS (Hurler and Scheie syndromes)*

Ref No.	Sex	Age	UA/C ratio	HyalR %	Hex/UA ratio	Hexosamine % GluN	GalN	Diagnosis
1	F	13m	183	89	0·924	25·0	75·0	
80	M	1y 2m	104	100	0·852	15·5	84·5	Type IH
111	F	17m	254	100	0·980	29·5	70·5	Hurler's
182	F	3y 11m	217	100	1·014	7·1	92·4	syndrome
215	F	18m	259	100	1·074	19·2	80·8	
		2y 3m	146	82	1·070	25·9	74·1	
		2y 5m	382	100	1·030	24·4	75·6	
91	M	11y	90	100	0·935	29·6	70·4	Type IS
92	M	8y	74	100	0·860	26·2	73·8	Scheie's syndrome

TABLE III   *Type III (Sanfilippo Syndrome)*

Ref No.	Sex	Age	UA/C ratio	HyalR %	Hex/UA ratio	Hexosamine % GluN	GalN
2	M	15 2m	50	100	0·980	100	—
4	F	7y	119	100	0·757	76·9	23·1
		11y	290	83	0·590	83·1	16·9
59	M	9y	76	100	0·900	83·3	16·7
70	M	2y 8m	60	78	0·805	67·0	33·0
		4y 8m	76	100	0·970	75·8	24·2
84	M	12y 10m	104	100	0·880	78·8	21·2
220	M	6y 1m	49	100	1·020	77·3	22·7

therefore, an analytical approach which is easier than previously described methods has given reliable definition of the excretion pattern and distinguished these patients from normal. In all cases the conclusions drawn were confirmed by electrophoresis or thin layer chromatography.

Three other groups of patients require special comment. They include patients with Hunter's syndrome, Morquio's disease and patients with atypical or bizarre results using the above methods.

Results from three patients with Hunter's syndrome (McKusick type II) are shown in Table IV, which clearly shows that, while they all gave a positive screening test, a raised UA/C ratio and raised HyalR per cent, the distribution of hexosamines is not equal as suggested by Kaplan. One patient (No. 199) has definite Hunter's syndrome clinically and electrophoresis and thin layer chromatography showed roughly equal amounts of DS and HS with a small amount of CS. The latter

TABLE IV   *Type II (Hunter's Syndrome)*

Ref No.	Sex	Age	UA/C ratio	HyalR %	Hex/UA ratio	Hexosamine % GluN	GalN
180	M	3y 9m	129	92	1·120	18·5	81·5
		4y 5m	52	83	1·340	21·4	78·6
199	M	24y	23	100	1·460	34·1	65·9
212	M	5y 4m	62	57	0·870	16·6	83·4
		5y 9m	108	83	0·920	29·6	70·4

probably explains the excess of galN over gluN and why the hexN ratio is not the same as Kaplan's results. Another patient (212) shows similar results with a hexN distribution consistent with Hurler's syndrome (see Table II). However the HyalR per cent was low and this was explained by a significant band of CS on electrophoresis and thin layer chromatography which would account for an increase in galN. Even when allowance is made for this however, there was still a preponderance of DS over HS. Clinical features in this patient are intermediate between types IS and II and further studies are necessary before definite comment can be made about the diagnosis and the urinary findings.

The third patient in this group (No. 180) also gave results which were consistent with Hurler's syndrome but many clinical features were in keeping with a diagnosis of Hunter's syndrome. Furthermore, this patient was studied by Dr Rosemary Stephens at the Institute of Child Health, London, and fibroblast cultures studied in Professor Neufeld's department clearly showed deficiency in Hunter corrective factor. (The nature and specificity of the corrective factors in the mucopolysaccharidoses have been reviewed by Cantz, Chrambach, Bach and Neufeld, 1973.)

Although Kaplan (1969) has shown equal amounts of HS and DS in Hunter's syndrome, Maroteaux (1970) found that the proportions are not equal and do not differ significantly from those found in Hurler's syndrome. The results presented here clearly support the latter statement and the simple methods used cannot differentiate Hunter's syndrome from Hurler's syndrome.

The second group of patients presenting difficulty are patients with Morquio's disease (McKusick type IV) who excrete excessive amounts of keratosulphate (KS) usually in the form of a KS-CS-Protein complex (Kaplan *et al.*, 1968). There are two aspects to this problem; one concerns the difficulty of differentiating Morquio's disease from other spondyloepiphsial dysplasias in which GAG excretion is normal (Maroteaux and Lamy, 1967) and the other concerns the problem of KS excretion even in patients with definite clinical and radiological features of Morquio's disease. Adults with this disease may not show any abnormality of GAG excretion (Maroteaux and Lamy, 1967).

One might expect, since KS is resistant to testicular hyaluronidase digestion, contains gluN as principal hexN and galactose in place of hexuronic acid residues, that the results by the methods described

TABLE V *Type IV (Morquio's Syndrome)*

Ref No.	Sex	Age		UA/C ratio	HyalR ratio	Hex/UA %	Hexosamine % GluN	GalN	Screening test
65	M	13y		9·7*	22*	1·075	39·7	60·3	+ weak
		15y		7·6*	14*	1·890	67·2	32·8	neg.
76	F	2y		29	19*	1·120	10·5	89·5	+
		2y	11m	33	26*	0·865	22·2	77·8	+
190	F	42y		6·0*	7*	1·019	48·5	51·5	neg.
195	M	2y	6m	63	14*	1·860	36·9	63·1	+
		3y	2m	38	60	1·820	44·3	55·8	+
208	M	6y	5m	21	23*	0·766	41·3	58·7	+
		6y	9m	37	27*	0·910	38·3	61·7	+ weak
209	M	5y	4m	53	25*	1·014	34·7	65·3	+

* = Normal

above would show a high hexN/hexuronic acid ratio, a high HyalR per cent and gluN as principal hexN (Kaplan did not include a study of this condition in his classification of GAG excretion). A study of the results in Table V clearly shows this not to be the case. Indeed, were it not for a positive screening test and raised UA/C ratio associated with a high index of clinical suspicion, many of these patients would have been regarded as normal GAG excretors. However, in some of these cases a band migrating as KS was found on thin layer chromatography associated with a predominant CS band. When the samples were digested with testicular hyaluronidase, KS remained as the only prominent band. In the adult patient with this disease no such abnormality was found while in two children no abnormality was found on initial examination but an increased amount of KS was found on examination of a further sample at a later date. In one patient (No. 195) KS became the predominant GAG and the gluN per cent rose as well as the HyalR per cent. It would seem therefore that abnormal KS excretion may appear late in the development of the disease and disappear again in adult life. Furthermore, KS excretion must be specifically looked for and, in view of the fact the CPC may be poor precipitant of KS, alternative methods may be required to detect this condition and to study normal KS excretion in childhood as well as to follow its excretion pattern in Morquio's disease.

The final group of patients presenting difficulty to interpretation of results are shown in Table VI. They are a mixed group and require individual discussion to highlight the particular problem encountered.

The first patient (No. 43), although giving a positive screening test, gave a UA/C ratio within the normal range for her age (8 months). She was the child of Portuguese parents who are first cousins. Gestation and delivery were normal but at the time of examination she presented with delayed motor development, odd facies and a large protuberant tongue. There was difficulty in abducting both legs and a marked lumbar lordosis. There was no hepatosplenomegaly and the rest of the physical examination including retinoscopy was normal. Radiological examination showed a normal bone age but the pelvis showed abnormal acetabular angles and lumbar vertebrae showed abnormalities consistent with Hurler's syndrome. The patient subsequently died of bronchopneumonia and post mortem examination was refused. Further analysis of the only urine sample obtained showed an intermediate abnormal HyalR per cent and an atypical hexN ratio. It is possible that this child was a case of Hurler's syndrome or was an atypical mucopolysaccharide disorder, and raises the possibility that the full features of abnormal GAG excretion may not be present in infancy but may develop progressively.

The second patient in this group has clear radiological and clinical features of Engelmann's disease, a progressive diaphyseal dysplasia (Lennon, Schechter and Hornabrook, 1961). Samples from this patient gave positive screening tests, a raised UA/C ratio and raised HyalR per

TABLE VI   *Other Abnormal Samples (with positive screening test)*

| Ref No. | Sex | Age | | UA/C ratio | HyalR % | Hex/UA ratio | Hexosamine % | | Diagnosis |
							GluN	GalN	
43	F		8m	31	56	1·427	54·2	45·8	Type IH (Hurler)
44	F	17y		13·8	56	1·024	45·8	54·2	Engelmann's disease
89	F		6m	38	54	1·171	56·5	43·5	Perinatal anoxia
106	F		8m	152	62	0·742	57·5	42·5	Unknown
		2y	4m	20	36	0·850	35·5	64·5	

cent. The hexN ratio does not differ significantly from normal adults in whom HS excretion represents a higher proportion of GAG than in childhood (Manley *et al.*, 1968). However, electrophoresis and thin layer chromatography showed that a significant band of DS was also present and the possibility that this disease is a mucopolysaccharide disorder requires further study.

No explanation can be offered for the results on the third patient (No. 89) who died of bronchopneumonia and had hypertonia and deteriorating vision thought to be the result of cerebral damage due to perinatal anoxia. Although the urine results are similar to the first patient in this group, this infant had none of the features of Hurler's syndrome.

The fourth patient (No. 106) also gave abnormal results on a sample collected at 8 months of age with a prominent band of HS present on electrophoresis and a tentative diagnosis of Sanfilippo syndrome was made. She presented at 2 months of age with a large protuberant tongue, marked lethargy and bilateral optic atrophy. Although she looked hypothyroid, serum thyroxine was within normal limits. Radiological examination showed periosteal new bone formation in both femora and no other abnormality. Urine examination at this time was normal. The urines examined at 7–8 months gave the results shown in the table and electrophoresis (barbitone buffer) showed a band migrating as hyaluronic acid which represented 30 per cent of the isolated material. The remainder migrated as HS and CS although the latter band was thought to be mainly DS. More recently there has been a progression of her optic atrophy but no new radiological features. The diagnosis remains unknown but a urine sample gave a negative screening test, normal UA/C and almost completely normal GAG pattern with CS predominant (by TLC). There would appear to be no explanation for these bizarre findings except to say that retrospective investigation of drug treatment shows that she was briefly treated with thyroxine at the time of the initial examination in view of the tentative diagnosis, at that time, of hypothyroidism and it may be that the abnormal GAG excretion pattern reflects an effect of thyroxine.

In conclusion, apart from the anomalies detailed above, the simple series of urine analyses described are of value in the detection of mucopolysaccharidoses and the certain diagnosis of Hurler's, Scheie's and Sanfilippo syndrome. The difficulties encountered with Hunter's syndrome and Morquio's disease are common to many other methods and do not necessarily detract from the value of the simpler methods described here. These methods have a distinct advantage in their simplicity and are recommended to clinical laboratories for this reason as a useful first approach to the study of abnormal glycosaminoglycan excretion.

Acknowledgements

I am indebted to Professor N. R. Butler and Drs Beryl D. Corner, J. Apley, D. Burman, P. Dunn, W. Schutt for allowing me to study patients in their care at Bristol Royal Hospital for Sick Children and Southmead Hospital, Bristol, and to Dr G. K. McGowan and Professor N. R. Butler in whose laboratories this work was done. Samples from patients with mucopolysaccharidoses were also sent by the following people to whom I am also grateful: A. D. Griffith (Abergavenny), J. M. Davies (Bath), B. A. Wharton (Birmingham), N. J. Brown and J. Jancar (Bristol), P. Harper (Cardiff), P. Jenkins (Carmarthen), D. G. Vulliamy (Dorchester), J. Keenan (London), A. T. Howarth, T. V. K. Nasir and R. Smith (Newcastle), R. H. Lindenbaum and R. Smith. (Oxford), P. R. Evans, J. N. Montgomery and Janice Went (Plymouth), R. T. T. Harrison (Taunton) and G. Manley (Torquay).

This work was initially supported financially by the Medical Research Committee of the United Bristol Hospitals and is currently supported by the Bristol Good Neighbours Trust to whom I am most grateful. Finally my thanks are also due to the members of the Bristol and South West Bone Dysplasia Registry for advice on some of the problem cases, especially Dr I. R. S. Gordon for his much valued radiological opinion.

REFERENCES

BERRY, H. K. & SPINANGER, J. (1960) *Journal of Laboratory and Clinical Medicine*, **55**, 136.

BITTER, T. & MUIR, H. M. (1962) *Analytical Biochemistry*, **4**, 330.

CANTZ, M., CHRAMBACH, A., BACH, G. & NEUFELD, E. F. (1972) *Journal of Biological Chemistry*, **247**, 5456.

CONSTANTOPOULOS, G. (1968) *Nature*, London, **220**, 583.

DEAN, M. F., MUIR, H. & EWINS, R. J. F. (1971) *Biochemical Journal*, **123**, 883.

DENNY, W. & DUTTON, G. (1962) *British Medical Journal*, **1**, 1555.

DI FERRANTE, N. M. (1967) *Analytical Biochemistry*, **21**, 98.

DI FERRANTE, N. & LIPSCOMB, H. S. (1970) *Clinica chimica acta*, **30**, 69.

DORFMAN, A. (1958) *Pediatrics*, **22**, 576.

HARDINGHAM, T. E. & PHELPS, C. F. (1970) *Biochemical Journal*, **117**, 813.

HUMBEL, R. & CHAMOLES, N. A. (1972) *Clinica chimica acta*, **40**, 290.

KAPLAN, D., McKUSICK, V., TREBACHI, S. & LAZARUS, R. (1968) *Journal of Laboratory and Clinical Medicine*, **71**, 48.

KAPLAN, D. (1969) *American Journal of Medicine*, **47**, 721.

LENNON, E. A., SCHECHTER, M. M. & HORNABROOK, R. W. (1961) *Journal of Bone and Joint Surgery*, **43b**, 273.

LIPIELLO, L. & MANKIN, H. J. (1971) *Analytical Biochemistry*, **39**, 54.

MANLEY, G. & HAWKSWORTH, J. (1966) *Archives of Diseases of Childhood*, **41**, 91.

MANLEY, G., SEVERN, M. & HAWKSWORTH, J. (1968) *Journal of Clinical Pathology*, **21**, 339.

MAROTEAUX, P. & LAMY, M. (1967) *Lancet*, **ii**, 510 (Correspondence).

MAROTEAUX, P. (1970) *Revue European Etudes Clinical Biology*, **15**, 203.

McKUSICK, V. A. (1972) In *Heritable Disorders of Connective Tissue*, Fourth Edition, p. 525. C. V. Mosby. St. Louis.

MURPHY, D., PENNOCK, C. A. & LONGDON, K. (1974) *Clinica Chimica Acta*, **53**, 145

PEDRINI, V., LENNZI, L. & ZAMBOTTI, V. (1962) *Proceedings of the Society for Experimental Biology and Medicine*, **110**, 847.

PENNOCK, C. A. (1969) *Journal of Clinical Pathology*, **22**, 379.

PENNOCK, C. A., MOTT, M. G. & BATSTONE, G. F. (1970) *Clinica chimica acta*, **27**, 93.

PENNOCK, C. A., WHARTON, B. A. & WHITE, F. (1971) *Acta paediatrica Scandinavica,* **60,** 299.

PENNOCK, C. A., WHITE, F. & WHARTON, B. A. (1972) *Acta paediatrica Scandinavica,* **61,** 125.

PENNOCK, C. A., WHITE, F., MURPHY, D., CHARLES, R. G. & KERR, H. (1973) *Acta paediatrica Scandinavica,* in press.

PROCOPSIS, P. G., TURNER, B., BUXTON, J. T. & BROWN, D. A. (1968) *Journal of Mental Deficiency Research,* **12,** 13.

RENUART, A. W. (1966) *New England Journal of Medicine,* **274,** 384.

SCOTT, J. E. (1960) *Methods of Biochemical Analysis,* **8,** 145.

SEGNI, G., ROMANO, C. & TORTOROLO, G. (1964) *Lancet,* **ii,** 420.

TELLER, W. M., BURKE, E. C., ROSEVEAR, J. W. & MCKENZIE, B. F. (1962) *Journal of Laboratory and Clinical Medicine,* **59,** 95.

VALDIVIESO, F., MARTINEZ–VALVERDE, A., MATIES, M. & UGARTE, M. (1973) *Clinica chimica acta,* **44,** 357.

WESSLER, E. (1968) *Analytical Biochemistry,* **26,** 439.

WHITEMAN, P. (1975) In *Inborn Errors of Skin, Hair and Connective Tissue, S.S.I.E.M. Symposium No. 11.* Edited by J. B. Holton and J. T. Ireland. Lancaster: Medical and Technical Publications Co.

DISCUSSION
(of papers by Drs Lewis, Kennedy & Raine, Dr Sabater, Dr Whiteman and Dr Pennock)

Logan (Glasgow). We have adopted the same empirical approach, we think that these methods should be designed for the benefit of the clinician and I have the same antipathy for column chromatography which involves a great deal of work for routine testing. On this basis, from the literature, simple screening tests such as toluidine blue and alcian blue as spot tests based on a fixed amount of creatinine should be the most useful method for routine screening in high risk cases. If these are then positive we do a differential staining with magnesium chloride in increasing amounts and by this means we're able to detect keratan sulphate if present. Then we go to the CPC precipitation with dialysis. We measure the uronic acid content of this material. Electrophoresis is the next step in barium acetate or hydrochloric acid, the one being based on the charge on the molecule and the other the backbone structure. By this procedure we feel that we can differentiate between the different conditions which are present with a fairly high degree of certainty.

We have applied this to prenatal diagnosis as well as investigations of urinary samples and so far our experience is limited to one Sanfilippo case which proved to be positive in various other laboratories. We would be very interested to investigate any other suspect cases. We have shown that for 30 weeks hyaluronic acid is predominant in the amniotic fluid, whereas, after 30 weeks the slower of the two slow moving bands is predominant. It is very important to do as we have done to find the normal range of the uronic acid content at the various stages of gestation. We have done this between 10 and 40 weeks and also the individual components. We have extended it to try and see if the contribution from the urine being secreted into the amniotic fluid was an important factor in varying the amniotic fluid content.

Using these techniques we think that we have a fairly high chance of detecting cases but I should stress that, like previous speakers, one technique is not enough and that enzyme analysis is obligatory to back up.

Blau (London). We have tried the method of Pennock in an automated form for screening. We worked out a special autoanalyser manifold which we can use to monitor the fluid from chromatographic columns. The precipitate is measured by nephelometry and in fact we have had to dilute Pennock's reagent considerably in order to obtain optimum results. This method is very suitable for the analysis of very small samples on columns and also on samples of urine that had to be diluted. It can be run at forty samples per hour. The method can also be used to follow column chromatographic separations for GAG mixtures continuously.

Sabater (Barcelona). According to our experience, if the CPC-citrate turbidity test is the only test to be used in screening, it is necessary to correct the values obtained (as turbidity units) according to the urine specific gravity. Urine with high specific gravity can give false positive results and also, and this is very important, dilute urines with low specific gravity can give negative or 'normal' values for the CPC test despite being from a patient with mucopolysaccharidoses.

Dorfman (Chicago). A number of people have raised the question as to when the urine becomes positive. We have had two cases in which we have examined the urine on the first day of life from a patient with Hurler's syndrome and it was strongly positive, way above normal.

The question of heparan sulphate standards that is troubling a lot of people. The material that we have supplied to people all over the world is high molecular weight material not comparable to urine material and is not meant to be a standard for this purpose, originally it was prepared for chemical studies. I suspect that it might be useful if someone made a standard from one of these patient's urines or tissues. According to the paper from Dr Konecka in 1967 it is much more than likely that it is polydispersed and I don't know the differences between Hunter's, Hurler's and the two Sanfilippo's because we didn't do that in great detail, one of these patients studied was a Hurler or Sanfilippo and both were polydispersed and very low molecular weight in the range 2,000–7,000.

Finally I would like particularly to complete the comment yesterday that I am extremely interested in the laboratories that are using chemical methods for amniotic fluids and I didn't mean by my comments yesterday that I was opposed to this. It could have very great advantages over fibroblast culture in terms of time and I hope that the people who are doing this work make the cases that are positive and negative known in the literature, because the reports here suggest to me that it would be worthwhile. In all the amniocenteses being done around the world, the three methods are being compared—enzymology, the sulphate uptake and the chemistry. It may well be that the chemical method may be the best method. It would be a great advantage in time, cost and early diagnosis.

Index